1987

VALUES IN
HEALTH
CARE

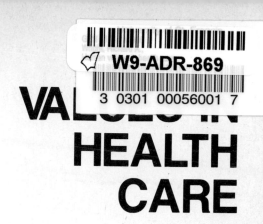

HUMAN VALUES IN HEALTH CARE: THE PRACTICE OF ETHICS

Richard A. Wright, Ph.D.

University of Toledo

McGRAW-HILL BOOK COMPANY

New York   St. Louis   San Francisco   Auckland   Bogotá
Hamburg   Johannesburg   London   Madrid   Mexico   Milan
Montreal   New Delhi   Panama   Paris   São Paulo
Singapore   Sydney   Tokyo   Toronto

For Sandy and Eric

HUMAN VALUES IN HEALTH CARE:
THE PRACTICE OF ETHICS

1 2 3 4 5 6 7 8 9 0   DOCDOC   8 9 2 1 0 9 8 7

ISBN 0-07-072076-2

This book was set in Helvetica by J.M. Post Graphics, Corp. (ECU)
The editor was Stephanie K. Happer; the cover was designed by Carla Bauer;
the production supervisor was Friederich W. Schulte.
Project supervision was done by Chernow Editorial Services, Inc.
R. R. Donnelley & Sons Company was printer and binder.

Library of Congress Cataloging-in-Publication Data

Wright, Richard A.
  Human values in health care.

  Includes bibliographies.
  1. Medical ethics—Philosophy.   2. Medical care—
Decision making—Philosophy.   3. Medical ethics—
Case studies.   4. Medical care—Decision making—
Case studies.   I. Title.   [DNLM: 1. Ethics, Medical.
2. Philosophy, Medical. W 50 W952h]
R724.W73   1987   174'.2   86-18590
ISBN 0-07-072076-2

ABOUT THE AUTHOR

The author is a graduate of Baylor University and the University of Illinois at Urbana-Champaign. He has a Ph.D. in Philosophy with a wide range of teaching and professional experience. He is particularly active in the area of health care ethics, as a teacher, lecturer, workshop presenter, and writer. In addition, he continues a seven-year clinical practice, serving as a consultant to health care professionals, and as a clinical instructor of medical humanities. His experience includes teaching and working closely with all of the health care professions. He is currently an Associate Professor of Philosophy at the University of Toledo, Clinical Professor of Medical Humanities for the Department of Pediatrics at the Medical College of Ohio at Toledo, and Adjunct Professor of Ethics for the School of Nursing at the Medical College of Ohio at Toledo.

CONTENTS

CHAPTER 3   SITUATION ASSESSMENT PROCEDURE: THE PROCESS OF ETHICAL DECISION MAKING   44

CHAPTER 4   PRIVACY AND CONFIDENTIALITY   64

CHAPTER 5   COMMUNICATION IN HEALTH CARE: INFORMATION, DECEPTION, AND INFORMED CONSENT   84

CHAPTER 6 DECISIONS FOR OTHERS: PROXY CONSENT AND PATERNALISM

CHAPTER 7 PERSONS, CARING, AND COMMUNITY: THE ETHICAL BASIS FOR HEALTH CARE

SELECTED READINGS 137

APPENDIX 281

INDEX 297

PREFACE

If I teach you something supposedly "relevant," I am guaranteeing irrelevance. If I teach you how to work, to have good attitudes, to take responsibility for your own ideas, to communicate and to think a problem through, no matter what subject matter I use in order to get those basic skills of mind and intellect across, then I am giving you something you can use for a very long time. These skills will never change.

Jacob Neusner
How to Grade Your Professors

A FRAMEWORK FOR STUDY

This book is an introduction to ethics designed for the people with no philosophy background, who are primarily interested in health care either as a member of the health professions or as a potential user of the health care system. The guiding feature of the text is the attempt to help those with little background in the humanities develop a philosophical perspective on the ethical issues which pervade health care practices. By using case studies as a starting point, the text is designed to help readers achieve a deeper understanding of the philosophical basis for ethical decisions. It is also intended to help them develop an appreciation for the rich philosophical frameworks upon which one may base an understanding of those issues.

Because each individual brings to the study of ethics a set of personal values and because those values are frequently accepted without critical reflection, the emphasis of the philosophical perspective is to develop reflective skills relevant to ethical decision making. The primary text users will not be philosophy majors; thus four assumptions are made: (1) because health care is essentially case-oriented, the best way to introduce the issues is through a case study approach; (2) because most readers are not humanities majors and, in fact, are technically oriented, introductory work in ethics must be in the context of a general introduction to humanistic thinking; (3) because no prerequisite or subsequent philosophy may be assumed, the text must address itself to the *doing* of philosophy, not to a recitation of philosophical viewpoints; and (4) because professional education is aimed at application of skills to specific situations of practice, the study of ethics, to be "relevant," must be similarly aimed.

CASES AS LEARNING TOOLS

Case studies are an integral part of this book. Throughout, cases are used to introduce, explicate, and illustrate the ethical dimension of health care practices. A primary basis for this approach is that health care is *not* a science, but the application of science to the human condition. More important is the fact that ethics is a *part* of health care. Because health care consists of interpersonal relationships, one cannot be involved in health care, either as a practitioner or as a consumer, without at the same time *doing* ethics. It is therefore impossible to study the ethical issues in health care without using case studies.

The use of cases may seem artificial to some readers, and in a way it is artificial, because no written presentation can capture the full dimensions of the actual experience. At the same time, we cannot all go into the health care setting to observe instances of the sort that need discussing; the case study is thus the next best thing to being there. An additional artificiality is the limitation of information available in the written case. This is dictated in part by space limitations but also by the need to focus attention on certain issues and problems. Readers will, at some point, want more information than is given; but then they must ask, "Why? What more is needed? Why is that needed?" It is easy to avoid thinking and decision making by saying "I need more information first." The cases are designed to encourage overcoming that response and learning to work with the information given.

Some people might find it difficult to work with cases which try to put them in the position of a professional. The usual comment is, "I'm not a(n) X (where X is a profession), so how can I think about this case like a(n) X?" Although that is certainly a problem in the technical sense, there is no real difficulty in the philosophical sense. One point of this book is to show that ethical problems are problems of *persons* who just happen to be professionals or *persons* who just happen to be recipients of health care. I may not know how to perform a leg amputation, but I can still understand what it means to have informed consent for that amputation; and I do not have to have had a leg amputation to know whether the person who did have it consented to it. In short, the issues are ethical, not technical. They just happen to occur in a technical context. There is thus no need to worry about technical knowledge. Instead, make an effort to take the place of the person confronted with the problem, and try as much as possible to understand what he or she[1] is facing. If all else fails, change the professional context of a problematic case so that it fits into your experience, and work from there.

One danger of the case study approach is that the ethical issues become trivialized or submerged beneath the empirical data of the cases. In developing the situation assessment procedure used in the book to analyze cases, every effort has been made to avoid that problem. Throughout, the attempt has been to show that the case study, which is concrete and particular, leads logically to the ethical study, which is abstract and general, which, through application of the ethical study to cases, leads back to the practical. Thus the doing of ethics is seen as a recursive activity, a process that is never really complete but always making progress.

Another danger of the case study approach is that the philosophy of ethics is trivialized, and not enough "hard core" ethics is learned. The basic assumption of this book is that an introduction to ethics, at this level, should be generally nontechnical, serving as an overview which may be used as a foundation for later development of more detailed knowledge. While presenting that overview, however, every effort has been made to avoid trivialization and develop a reasonable perspective for study. In particular, the theories have been developed by types, as opposed to "isms," thus making them more readily applicable to situations a person may encounter in life-after-class. The aim throughout is to introduce important questions and encourage a willingness to understand and to deal with those questions from legitimate philosophical bases.

ETHICS AND THE LAW

There is always a temptation to deal with the law when ethical issues are discussed, particularly in the health care context. This book tries to avoid that mistake for several reasons. First, ethics and the law are quite different sorts of undertaking. Second, to lump law and ethics together is to mistakenly suppose that what is legal is ethical and what is ethical is legal, when obviously neither assumption is correct. Third, because law is case precedence oriented and the jurisdictions of precedence are often quite narrow, legal decisions are frequently contradictory to each other, thus not especially helpful. Finally, legal decisions are made by individuals, judges, and juries; as a result, they are really reflections

---

[1]The problem of how to refer to individuals is particularly troublesome. The generic *he* is not acceptable, since not all persons are he's. On the other hand, neither are all persons she's. Extensive use of *he or she* is cumbersome, so in the text I have chosen to simply switch back and forth between *he* and *she*, with no regard to professional stereotype or anything else. I have not counted to be sure the distribution is even, however; so apologies to anyone offended by disproportion—it was not intentional.

of individual value judgments which themselves need to be examined, not just automatically accepted.

There is an added practical reason for avoiding legal discussions in this book, namely, that the law gives the impression that matters decided within its jurisdiction are settled once and for all. Ethical decisions may resolve a case in a specific set of circumstances, but the basic tenet of philosophical reasoning is that everything may be, and should be, reconsidered. Philosophy recognizes the fallibility of the human endeavor, while law tends to immortalize those failings through decisions which serve as precedent and are thus frequently difficult to overturn.

Despite these problems, legal reasoning often offers insights which may be applied to philosophical thinking. We must then take account of that reasoning in the overall effort to understand any given ethical problem. The point to be emphasized, and not forgotten, is that the law is only *one* dimension of that overall effort and must be treated accordingly.

TOPIC COVERAGE AND ORGANIZATION

Unlike most other books on the market, this one does not purport or intend to cover all the traditional topics in biomedical ethics or to present all the classic articles on the topics covered. The basic reason is that the intention here is not to develop encyclopedic knowledge of every imaginable issue. Instead, this book aims to aid the reader's understanding of issues which are fundamental to ethical thinking. Rather than see how many concepts and points can be introduced per page, the focus is on a well-developed, well-understood core of basic concepts. Obviously, this is a trade-off between gathering a lot of information and clearly developing a small amount of information. But doing ethics is not easy, and developing an understanding of ethical issues and concepts takes a good deal of thinking time. I have thus chosen to extend the thinking time by developing each topic in more depth, with the hope that the basic understanding will be deeper and more lasting.

Although the text covers most traditional topics in biomedical ethics, there are several important, unique aspects to the presentation. First, the topics have been arranged to allow development of the philosophical concepts from a basic to a more complex level. The discussion of specific issues is delayed until the basic framework is established in Chapters 1 to 3, so that there is a philosophical basis for understanding the issues in Chapters 4 to 7. The issues presented are "basic" in that they occur in every dimension of health care practice. They are also basic because the concepts involved in understanding the issues presented are prerequisite to understanding the more complex issues, such as abortion, euthanasia, genetic control, allocation of resources, and so on. Second, the issues covered were selected for discussion because of their bearing on clinical practices, and they include things which are likely to be encountered in regular health care situations. In this way, the text has a very practical application. Finally, the aim throughout the text is to show ethical questions not as isolated from each other but as a complex of issues whose basic character is identifiable in the mainstream of issues concerning human values.

The readings and codes in the Appendix which accompany the book are intended to develop depth of understanding by showing detailed analysis of specific issues. When they are used together with the text chapters, the readings foster three basic philosophical skills necessary for doing ethics. The first is to develop an ability for in-depth questioning. A person who cannot ask relevant questions, or understand when they are being asked, does not have a basic ability which any serious thinking requires. The method of presenting lots of cases, with different viewpoints and questions, coupled with readings, is aimed at stimulating such development. The second skill is the ability to understand different points of view. The aim here is to make a reasonable, empathetic effort to understand another person's viewpoint, regardless of whether it agrees with one's own. No one can effectively deal with a view he or she does not understand; certainly, I can say, "Yes, I can recite your stupid argument," but can I say, "Is this your argument, fairly stated?" and have the other person respond yes? The third skill is the ability to engage in dialectic exchange. The basic premise here is that we need to be able to learn from things that we disagree with, as well as from those that we agree with. More than that, however, we must learn to engage in dialogue with others, through reading, writing, or speaking, which can result in *both* parties learning something. The purpose of philosophy is *not* to learn the best way to destroy another person's viewpoint, although it could certainly be used that way. To do philosophy is to engage in a process, of which we are all a part. To do ethics is to engage in that same process.

A FINAL NOTE ON THE CASES

All cases used in this book are fictitious, unless citations are given. At the same time, all the cases are derived from actual experiences of actual persons in actual health care situations. Drawn from published cases, as well as those given to me by my colleagues, students, and friends from around the country, the presented cases are composites. Any resemblance of these cases to actual cases, except where footnoted to public sources, is purely coincidental. The resemblance, however, to cases with which we are all familiar shows that the issues and problems are not singular, but general and pervasive of the system. And it is to that generality that we now turn.

ACKNOWLEDGMENTS

This book is the result of several years' work. Over that time, there have been many people who have assisted in the project and to whom I owe my thanks. First, and foremost, are the hundreds of students at the University of Toledo, the Medical College of Ohio, and the Toledo Hospital School of Nursing, whose use of manuscript versions of this text helped to shape and sharpen the present book. I am particularly grateful to my friend Pierre Vauthy, M.D., for taking me into the world of medicine and helping me to learn its intricacies and understand its complexities. My colleagues Jim Campbell, Steve Knaster, and Lynn Lumbrezer deserve special thanks for teaching from manuscript versions and supplying extensive, helpful comments during the revision process. Finally, I also benefited from the suggestions of many health care professionals and the following reviewers: Robert Davis, M.D., Providence, Rhode Island; Judith Erlen, University of Pittsburgh; Susan Lowndes, Rockland Community College; David Ozar, Loyola University of Chicago; Leslie Mayrand, Angelo State University; and Caroline Spana, Incarnate Word College. Basic work for Chapters 5 and 6 was supported in part by a grant from the de Arcex Memorial Endowment Fund of the University of Toledo. Any remaining errors are, of course, my own.

Public thanks are also due to those who helped in preparing the manuscript and associated materials. Sandy and Pat Wright helped with typing and permissions, while Lynn Lumbrezer helped with the bibliographies. The editors at McGraw-Hill deserve a special vote of thanks for their patience, wisdom, and assistance.

My thanks to you all!

Richard A. Wright

CHAPTER 1

HUMAN VALUES, ETHICS, AND HEALTH CARE DECISION MAKING

Moral values are more basic than all other values, because moral values touch, not just on what we do or experience or have, but on what we are.

Daniel C. McGuire*

MAKING CHOICES

Every person who lives a normal life frequently faces situations in which choices must be made: Which shirt should I wear? Should I buy a new car? Should I get married? Should I turn in a coworker who is stealing from the company? The sales clerk gave me too much change; do I keep it or give it back? I was asked to keep something secret; will I do it, or will I share the information? I accidentally hit a pedestrian with my car; do I stop or drive on, hoping not to be caught? I see someone shoplifting jewelry from a store; do I ignore it or do something to prevent it?

People often make such choices even though they are uncertain what would really be best, and sometimes mistakes are made. Yet choices must still be made, because that is part of living a normal life.

Ethics is about choices—not all choices, only those that have to do with what is morally right and wrong. Which dress a person chooses to wear, or

*The Moral Choice, Doubleday & Co., NY, 1978, p. 3

whether she buys a new car, is not ordinarily a matter of ethics; whether a person steals, keeps a secret, or drives away from an accident—these are a matter of ethics. In health care, whether a person is a professional giving care or a person receiving care, ethical questions are a fact of life, and ethical decisions are made many times a day. Why, then, does anyone need to study ethical problems in health care, if ethical decisions are already being made all the time? There are three reasons. First, the fact that people make ethical decisions all the time does not mean the decisions are properly or adequately made; studying ethics helps improve ethical decision making and thus the quality of health care. Second, with recent advances in health care technology, some health care decisions are literally a matter of life and death. The capability for prolonging life already exists, which makes it possible to decide *not* to prolong life; because of their importance, such decisions need *very* careful attention. Third, ethical issues in health care have been seen historically as primarily the concern of physicians. Now, however, health care roles have changed so that such issues affect all health care professionals as well as each person receiving care. Not all ethical decisions are life-and-death matters. A whole range of questions arise simply because health care is based on human interaction, and ethics is part of human interaction. So it is very important for everyone to become familiar with these issues and learn about resolving[1] the problems that they raise.

But what exactly *is* ethics, and what makes a problem ethical? To answer that question, first notice that the word *ethics* is often used to mean at least two different things—etiquette and morality. Matters of *etiquette* are social rules, sometimes called *manners,* which describe how one person should act in the presence of another person. Florence Nightingale's requirement that nurses stand in the presence of a physician is a good example of a rule of etiquette. *Morality* has to do with right and wrong conduct. In this context, Was that ethical? means Was that action morally correct? Notice that there is no moral value to the requirement that nurses stand in the presence of a physician; it is simply a statement of the etiquette of the time. If a nurse does not stand for a physician, we do not ask if she or he has acted in an immoral way, although we might ask if the nurse was impolite. On the other hand, if a social worker divulges con-fidential information about a client, in order to make interesting cocktail party conversation, we certainly question the moral correctness of that action.

This book is concerned with ethics in the sense of "morality", and we will focus on situations where personal choices, and actions, may in fact be right and wrong, good and bad. This will mean paying attention to both the *type of situation* and the *process* used to figure out what is right and wrong. The basic problem, then, is to learn enough about ethics to identify moral situations and figure out the right and wrong actions when an ethical decision has to be made.

---

[1]The word *resolve* is used instead of *solve* to discuss the outcome of ethical problems in order to avoid the mistaken view that they can be "fixed" once and for all. The resolution to a problem may not solve the basic issues, but it may allow us to get on with other things.

CASE STUDY APPROACH

Learning more about ethics is best done by working with actual situations in a context designed to increase basic knowledge. This requires spending a lot of time examining cases in which ethical problems arise. Without cases it is hard to keep our discussion connected to real life, and the study of ethics can easily become little more than an abstract intellectual exercise. Real-life cases raise the basic questions that need answering and give a "target" for ethical inquiry. The complete analysis of a case, however, requires a systematic way of thinking which will adequately handle those questions. A systematic approach will not accomplish much without basic knowledge to use in that system, so it is also necessary to learn basic ethics. Once the fundamental questions are raised by the cases, then the issues and problems may be analyzed by using the system and a knowledge of ethics. The following cases will help to clarify how this works.

CASE 1.1

Beverly Williams is a pharmacist who has filled a physician's order for a sugar-pill placebo. She gives the bottle of pills to the patron and recites the physician's instructions for taking the pills. When she is finished, the patron asks her, "What are these pills anyhow? Is this really an experimental painkilling drug?" Beverly wonders what to tell the patron.

Beverly must decide whether she should tell the patron the truth about the prescription or go along with the physician's "experimental drug" explanation. In reaching her decision, Beverly will have to consider a number of values: telling the truth seems to be important to society, thus the laws against perjury. Health professionals, however, often say that patients should not be told the truth, for their own good, and expect others to cooperate. Beverly personally believes that it is wrong to withhold information from a person who has asked a specific question; yet she also knows that the patient cannot know about the placebo or its use will not be effective. What is important is that whether to tell the truth is a moral consideration, so her answer will result from an ethical analysis, not her technical skill as a pharmacist.

CASE 1.2

Joan Samuelson is a student nurse caring for a patient who is uncooperative and verbally abusive. It is time for the patient's treatment, but the patient is refusing to allow Joan to carry out the treatment. Joan wonders whether to do the treatment anyhow, ignoring the patient's refusal, or try to trick her into agreeing to the treatment.

Joan's problem is whether to force the patient to do something she does not want to do. As a nurse, Joan believes that the treatment is really quite necessary for the patient's recovery; yet hospital policy allows patients to refuse treatment if they wish. The doctor has told Joan how important the treatment is and has asked Joan to do everything possible to get the patient to accept the treatment. Legally Joan must honor the patient's wishes, since to treat her without consent is assault and battery, for which she could be sued. At the same time, if she could talk the patient into agreeing to the treatment, no lawsuit is likely; but that would also be coercion, which Joan believes is not morally right. What Joan does will result from a weighing of ethical values, not just from her training and skill as a nurse.

CASE 1.3

Lisa Andrews is a public health agency clerk. While processing a venereal disease (VD) report, she recognizes her roommate's boyfriend as the client. What worries Lisa is that the boyfriend has not listed her roommate as a contact and Lisa knows they have been spending weekends together at his apartment. Lisa wonders whether to tell her roommate what she has learned.

Lisa must balance confidence and privacy against the prevention of harm to her roommate. She does not know for sure that her roommate's boyfriend has failed to tell her about his infection, but she does know that they spend weekends at his apartment, which means the roommate could be infected and not know it. Society, by placing Lisa in a position of handling confidential materials, has entrusted her with upholding the social values of privacy and confidence, and office rules certainly prohibit divulging confidential information. Yet she also feels obligated to try to protect her roommate from harm. Should she tell her roommate about the boyfriend's infection? Her professional values might say no, but her personal values might say yes. Her skill as a clerk is of no help in resolving the matter.

CASE 1.4

Ralph Davis is a social worker for the Children's Services Agency. As part of a routine case review, he discovers that one of his clients has been receiving aid payments which are more than her entitlement. He checks her account and discovers that she has been receiving the same amount since her first check. Ralph knows that she needs the extra money, and by signing the case review he would ensure that she would continue to receive the extra money. Ralph wonders whether he should sign the review.

Ralph faces a decision which involves not only himself but also his client, the agency, and society (via the expenditure of public money). Social services are intended to be fairly distributed, with no one receiving more than his or her share. The agency and its employees thus have a social obligation to see that expenditures are proper. Ralph also believes that he should help his clients as much as possible, especially those who have special needs. Since the agency has legal means for accomplishing that goal, he wonders whether the end of supplying his client with needed money will justify the means of getting that money to her. Should he follow the values of the agency, thus society, or sign the review and support his own values? His training and experience as a social worker give him no immediate answer to that question.

These cases involve different persons in different health care professions; yet they are all similar because each person is trying to resolve a conflict of values. Moreover, the decisions to be made go beyond technical expertise, requiring the use of more than just technical information or professional training. Each person is free to decide how his or her own situation is to be resolved, according to an individual decision process, utilizing individual values. This freedom of decision, called *autonomy,* is the cornerstone for doing ethics, as well as for the study of ethics. At the same time, even though each person may decide as he or she wishes, not all decisions are necessarily correct, and not all decisions are equally good. Autonomy is the cornerstone of ethics, thus a precondition of doing ethics; however, autonomy alone does not determine correctness or goodness. Let us look now at some suggestions about how to make that determination.

ETHICS AND PERSONAL FEELINGS

Usually when people talk about ethics, they want to discuss emotions and feelings—How do you feel about this? What are your feelings? Do you feel this is right? Why do you feel that way? In fact, people are often reluctant to consider ethics as anything more than an expression of feelings, not in the least subject to any process of thought. This idea is mistaken though, because doing ethics requires assessment of reasons, which in turn means that doing ethics requires reasoning. Ethics is a rational enterprise, and ethical judgments need to be based on careful processes of thought. But people are human beings, with emotions and feelings; does this mean that to do ethics a person must become cold and calculating, like a computer? Not at all! As Vincent Ruggerio points out.

There is an unfortunate tendency among many to view feeling and thought as mutually exclusive, to force a choice between them. . . . But this is mistaken. Feeling and thought are perfectly complementary. Feeling, being more spontaneous, is an excellent beginning to the development of conclusions. And thought, being more deliberate, provides a way to identify the best and most appropriate feelings. . . . Thinking, however, is less automatic than feeling. To do it well demands a systematic approach guided by practice.[2]

Feelings and emotions must therefore be balanced with thoughtful reasoning; but how and when they should be used remains to be seen.

Some people say that we should decide what is right according to the values our society accepts as important. This idea seems plausible at first, but relying on "social values" to resolve ethical problems is easier said than done. One problem is that there are many different types of social values—political, religious, economic, legal, ethical, etc. Which ones should a person honor, and in what order of preference? For Ralph, in Case 1.4, political, economic, legal, and ethical values are all in conflict; which should he take as most important? In any particular group, someone will probably give reasons for each one; but how does Ralph decide who is right? Another problem is the extreme difficulty in saying precisely what specific value a society supports. For example, polls taken on abortion regularly show different percentages of society to be for or against abortion. Thus there seems to be *no* unified social position regarding abortion. In any society, there are usually different opinions on almost any issue, so how can a person know what to uphold when making a decision? Using Case 1.2 as an example, what could we tell Joan? Is our society in favor of coercing patients into treatments they don't want but which would be good for them? If free, autonomous decisions are most important, then probably not; but if life is at risk, then maybe some coercion is OK. The problem for this position is how to determine a society's value so that it may be used to make a decision. Must we take a poll each time before making a decision and then do what the majority would do? What if (as in most cases) there is no clear majority view?

PROFESSIONAL VALUES AND VALUES CLARIFICATION

An alternative to using social values as the basis for ethical decisions is to use professional values. To begin resolving an ethical problem on this basis, however, those involved must first see what values are important to the profession and how those values influence the correctness of the decision made. One step in this process is called *values clarification,* a process by which individuals come to understand what values they hold and the importance of each of those values relative to others.

There are values which cover all areas of our lives; religious, political, economic, legal, social, and moral values all enter into our decisions in one way or another. Sometimes the values are explicit, clearly identified because they are stated as part of the situation. For example, when a pregnant teenager says, "I won't have an abortion because I think abortion is wrong," she has made the value involved explicit. Other values that she holds, which cause her to say that

---

[2]Vincent Ruggerio, *Beyond Feelings: A Guide to Critical Thinking,* 2d ed., Mayfield Publishing, Palo Alto, CA, 1984.

abortion is wrong, are not stated and thus are implicit, that is, built into the decision but not stated. If we then ask, "Why do you think abortion is wrong?" and she says, "Because it is wrong to take a person's life except in self-defense," she has made an implicit value explicit.

The basic procedure of values clarification is, first, to discover one's implicit values by thinking about how to act in the type of situation under consideration. For example, a person might determine his or her values concerning terminally ill patients by thinking about possible responses to such patients. This may be done with a series of questions, for instance, Do I dread having to take care of someone who is dying? Do I feel good about death? Do I tend to avoid terminally ill people? The second aspect of values clarification is to rank specific values against each other. Suppose, as an example, that someone were to identify his or her occupational values as high pay, job security, status, and enjoyment of the work. Before looking for a job, the applicant would need to list these values in priority order, in order to decide what to do if no job fulfilled each quality. Or, if the same person were employed and faced a conflict, such as choosing between high pay and job security in a strike situation, that person could make a choice which reflected these values and their priority order.

As a matter of fact, we all do something roughly like values clarification on a regular basis; we just do not often recognize the process. Recognizing and intentionally engaging in the process are, however, a precondition to a well-developed ethical process. Individual values *do* enter into the ethical decision process; it is thus important to identify the specific values operating in a given situation. Broadly speaking, values influence our ethical decisions in three ways:

1 *Values frame the problem.* We "see" a problem (or fail to see one) on the basis of the values we apply to the situation.

2 *Values supply alternatives.* The alternatives that we consider as possible resolutions for a problem are determined on the basis of the values we apply to our potential actions.

3 *Values direct judgment.* The judgment (reasoning) on the basis of which a problem is resolved is framed by the values we wish to uphold or promote.

If the role of values in ethical decisions is not recognized as occurring in each of these ways, then important values will be overlooked in reaching a decision.

Before we specifically consider professional values as a source for resolving ethical dilemmas, the following case will help show how values can influence judgment and so must be kept clearly in mind.

CASE 1.5

Mirium Markowicz, 83 years old, was admitted to the hospital for tests to determine the cause of her high blood pressure. From the time of admission she returned her meal tray with the food untouched. At first the nurses thought it was simply because she was not feeling well, and so they encouraged her to eat but made no issue of her not eating. On the second day, when John Robinson, her primary nurse, asked her to eat and she refused, he made the following note in her chart: "Patient uncooperative, refuses to eat or drink." John then contacted her physician, who said she would talk with Mrs. Markowicz the next day. When Dr. Thergan made her rounds, she asked Mrs. Markowicz why she was not eating. Her reply was, "The food and utensils are not kosher."

In that case, no one noticed Mrs. Markowicz's religious values. As a result, not only did she spend 2 days without food, but also she was treated as an "uncooperative" patient. The nursing staff was looking at the situation from the perspective of *medical* values and so labeled her as "uncooperative," a label the physician obviously accepted, since she waited until rounds to deal with the problem. This way of "seeing" the case also meant that the options for solving the problems were quite limited. As a result, the staff did not spend the necessary time with Mrs. Markowicz to uncover the real source of the problem. Finally, because of the values the *staff* was using, the problem was resolved by turning to the doctor, when it could have been easily handled by the nurses before it became an issue, the resolution of which made the nurses look unprofessional.

Are there professional values which may be identified and utilized in resolving ethical dilemmas? To begin looking at that question, consider the following case.

CASE 1.6

Bill Anderson, 37 years old, is brought to the emergency room by ambulance after passing out in a nearby supermarket. Although unconscious when first admitted, Bill regains consciousness and appears to be alert and lucid. After examination it is determined that Bill is suffering from an ulcer which has perforated his stomach wall. The problem is made considerably worse because Bill is also on anticoagulant medicine for a blood-clotting disease. Because of the perforation, the usual treatment of washing the stomach with ice water to slow the bleeding cannot be done; yet the bleeding is so severe that Bill's life is clearly threatened. When told of the need for immediate transfusion to save his life, Bill, a Jehovah's Witness, refuses on the basis of his religious beliefs. He soon slips into semiconsciousness because of the blood loss, and the medical team must decide what to do, because Bill is bleeding to death very rapidly.

The members of the medical team caring for Bill are facing an ethical dilemma: If they give Bill the blood, they will save his life but violate his religious beliefs and his expressed wishes; if they honor his beliefs and his wishes, they will not be able to save his life. In this case, the medical team is *not* trying to decide on the proper treatment for Bill—the members already agree that he needs to have the blood. What they are trying to decide is whether they *ought* to give him the blood in spite of his expressed wish not to have it. Resolving dilemmas such as this one is not just a technical decision then, but a complex value decision.

Each member of the medical team caring for Bill had a view on the case which was formed by making a value judgment. We'll look at those views in a moment, to see what ideas and values each one expresses. But first, stop for a moment and think about this case; what would *you* do if you were on the medical team? You have an opinion, right? What is your opinion? More important, do you know *why* you have that opinion? What values are you using in forming that opinion? Are you prejudiced in one way or another toward Jehovah's Witnesses? Do you think Bill is committing suicide? Are you afraid of death, thus want to try to prevent it? Do you believe that all life should be saved no matter what? What sorts of values are influencing this case? What *do* you believe, and *why* do you believe it? Before you read further, give these questions some thought and write down what you think ought to be done and why you think that is the right thing to do.

Formulating answers to such questions is crucial because the process forces an examination of individual values, and that is the first step in doing ethics. Now look at each team member's views, trying to see how the values affect their decisions and how the expressed values match or differ from your own.

Dr. Ralph James:

As a physician I have no choice but to go ahead and give him the blood. I am obligated by my professional code to save his life; besides, religious beliefs are not a good reason to die needlessly. Let's order the blood and do it; in the end he'll be glad we did.

Nurse Susan Livingston:

I disagree with his reasons and wouldn't do it myself, but the patient made his wishes clearly known, so we must honor them. He was alert and lucid when he made the request, and his wallet identification makes a similar request, so we know it was a genuine request. I think he should have the blood, but we have no right to go against his wishes and give it to him if he doesn't want it.

Dr. Marcia Latimer:

I agree with both of you that he needs the blood, and I agree with Susan, in principle, that his wishes should be honored; but I don't want to risk a lawsuit by the family. Suppose this guy has a wife and eight kids who can't support themselves if he dies; do you want to be responsible for a bunch of starving kids? Besides that, can you imagine the bad press the hospital will get if word of this gets out? I say we should give him the blood, but let's get a court order to do it.

Each participant in this case saw the problem as whether Bill had a right to decide his own fate, and each selected a resolution for that problem on the basis of specific values. The disagreement among team members over the course of action to take is a direct result of differences in their values. For example, Bill holds his religious beliefs, including his belief about transfusion, to be more important than his physical life. (Notice that the transfusion itself has a neutral value; it is the value which Bill attaches to it that causes the problem.) As the team tries to decide what is right, each individual's beliefs about transfusions, attitudes about Bill's beliefs, and professional and social values all come into play. Ralph James obviously believes that the preservation of life must be given priority over religious beliefs; Susan Livingston is concerned with Bill's right to make his own decisions; and Marcia Latimer seems most concerned with protecting herself and the hospital from consequences she thinks are unaccept- able, namely a lawsuit and bad publicity for the hospital. Overlapping each individual's values are the social values of preserving life and honoring diverse religious beliefs, the professional value of preserving life, the institutional value of providing the best possible care for patients, and the emergency-room (ER) value of doing everything possible to save a patient. Noticing these values does not alone resolve the problem of whether to give Bill the blood, however; we need to find out which values ought to be respected in this case, which may be passed over, which are to outweigh the others, and so on.

Although the values operating in this case are now relatively clear, a short- coming of values clarification is also clear, namely, that even with the values clarified, no resolution to the problem is readily seen. This is because clarifying values does no more than *describe* what values a person has; it does not allow the person to know whether those values *ought* to be used, which ones are *most important,* and *why* those values should be upheld. For example, suppose some- one were asked, "What three things do you value in a job?" and she said, "Good pay, short hours, and a nice office." If she were then asked, "Why is good pay more important than good fringe benefits?" or "Why is a nice office more im- portant than a nice boss?" she could have no possible response based just on values clarification. Clearly she is being asked to *justify* her values, not just describe them. How, then, are judgments justified, once the values involved have been clarified?

DECISION BY AUTHORITY

One way to resolve such cases is to ask a question of procedure, namely, Which person's values should be accepted? Or, to put it differently, How do we decide who decides in such cases? As a matter of practicality, there are usually rules (often unwritten) which specify who is in charge. In the hospital, for example, nurses, therapists, technicians, and others usually follow the traditional rule that the physician is the decision maker. But in this case there are *two* doctors, so whose view should be accepted? If we say, "Accept the view of the physician in charge," then we must ask how the accidental factor of being in charge of a case makes one person's moral values better than another's. The attending physician certainly has a *legal* responsibility for the *medical* care of the patient, but does that automatically make the doctor's *ethical*[3] judgment correct? Can we automatically accord the decision to the doctor by claiming that it is a medical decision and doctors should make medical decisions? Perhaps—if it is, in fact, a medical decision. As Norman Fost, a physician, points out, however,

[This sort of judgment] . . . is a value judgment, based on a complicated mixture of fact, ignorance, prejudice, mixed loyalties, feelings and philosophy. [It] is not a medical decision. It does not become medical simply because it is shared by a doctor.[4]

Mila Aroskar, a nurse, has made a similar point:

Certain medical decisions (such as continuing treatments that cause a patient to suffer unnecessarily) cross into the domain of ethics. . . . [In such cases] an incorrect assumption—that a physician's technical/professional expertise transfers to the ethical/moral realm—may be made. No one should accept this. [No one's] obligations . . . include following physician's [or anyone else's] orders unquestioningly.[5]

A physician's moral judgment is thus not automatically better than anyone else's *just because that person is a physician.* Why do people so often believe that the physician's opinion is most important in ethical decisions? Usually it is because they respect the physician's *medical* judgment, but fail to recognize that not all decisions made about patient care are purely medical. If a decision made by a health care professional hinges on the application of values and factors which are *not* a matter of technical expertise, the decision is *not* medical and thus is *not* the prerogative of the professional.

What about Bill's wishes? What about Ralph or Marcia? To assume that any particular person automatically has the unique right to make ethical decisions is to completely misunderstand the nature of such decisions. For whether something is right depends not on who says it, but on the reasons we have for accepting the claim as correct. The position or professional stature of people is not automatically a relevant criterion for the correctness of their judgments; instead we must look at the validity of the *reasons* they give to support their views. We must thus reject the simple fact that someone believes something is correct as proof that the belief is correct, and we must ask instead for reasons why that belief is correct.

---

[3]The word *moral* and the word *ethical* are sometimes used to refer to different realms, with *ethical* used in connection with philosophical theory and *moral* used in connection with individual action. Except when we are talking specifically about theory, in which case we will use *ethical,* the two words are used interchangeably.

[4]Norman Fost, "Putting Hospitals on Notice," *Hastings Center Report,* vol. 12, no. 4, August 1982, p. 5–8.

[5] Mila A. Aroskar, "The Choice: Two Experiences. An Ethicist Comments," *American Journal of Nursing,* vol. 82, no. 11, November 1982, p. 1770.

PROFESSIONAL CODES AND ETHICAL DECISIONS

What sorts of reasons are appropriate, if we cannot rely on social values, personal feelings, professional values, or authority? Some people suggest that the professionals involved should simply apply their professional code of ethics and decide on that basis what to do. A problem with that approach, though, is that professional codes are often not specific enough to handle cases. For example, there is nothing in any known professional code which says whether a Jehovah's Witness should be given a blood transfusion. In fact, if you look through the various codes contained in the Appendix, you will see that they are all very general, covering a wide range of issues. Because they are so general, they are often interpreted very differently. For example, a basic principle for most health profession codes is some form of the requirement to "do no harm." We see in Case 1.6 a group of professionals agreeing that a patient needs a blood transfusion; yet they still disagree as to whether the patient ought to be given the blood. They no doubt believe that they should "do no harm," and yet they disagree about whether giving or not giving the blood would be harmful. The professional code is thus not helpful in this case because it is too general.

However, professional codes do have some elements which are quite specific. Are they, then, useful in cases where they directly apply? Let's look at such a case.

CASE 1.7

As Helen Jones is preparing to leave the hospital, she is talking with Lorraine Williams, her primary care RN, and tells Lorraine that she dreads going home because she knows that her husband has been physically abusing their 14-year-old daughter. She says that she has already decided not to make an issue of the matter, but to accept it, since "parents have a right to do as they wish with their children." She says, "I don't like what he is doing, but he says she needs the discipline. I don't agree, but then we don't see eye to eye on a lot of things." She then says, "Please don't tell anyone about this; I just told you because I needed to talk to someone about it."

What ethical problems is Lorraine facing in this situation? First, there is the problem of confidentiality, since Mrs. Jones has asked Lorraine not to tell anyone about her situation. Second, there is the problem of preventing harm to the child through prevention of child abuse.

Confidentiality is a primary problem in this case because Lorraine cannot do anything to correct the abuse situation without first deciding what to do about Mrs. Jones's request that she say nothing about the abuse. As we saw before, values will determine how a problem is seen, what alternatives are considered to resolve that problem, and what resolution can be adopted to take care of the problem. Suppose Lorraine believed, as many people do, that her professional ethics code would help resolve the problem. If she looked at the nursing code, she would be told that "The nurse safeguards the client's right to privacy by judiciously protecting information of a confidential nature."[6] This certainly seems to be a code item which applies directly to a situation; yet we must ask how well it applies.

To begin, the code statement is vague because we are not sure what things a nurse should do to "judiciously protect" someone's privacy. If the code is to clearly apply, that vagueness must be eliminated. Perhaps more important is the fact that the code is contradictory since in another section it also requires a nurse to obey the law. Because there is a state law requiring that suspected abuse be reported, Lorraine would have to violate the code requirement for confidentiality to maintain the code requirement for obedience to the law; or she would have to violate the code requirement for obedience to the law in order to maintain the code requirement for confidentiality. Importantly, the code cannot help alleviate this dilemma because it says nothing about how to resolve conflicts between code elements. This is a second shortcoming of codes, albeit not unique to the nursing code, since when *any* of the codes in the Appendix are used in this case, a similar dilemma arises. Although there are other problems with codes, on the basis of just these two it is clear they cannot serve as a means for resolving specific ethical dilemmas.

If one cannot rely simply on emotions, authority, professional codes, or social values to justify decisions, what *can* be used?

BASIC PRINCIPLES IN PROBLEM SOLVING

As mentioned earlier, justification of ethical decisions requires the use of values, together with an understanding of ethics and a system of problem assessment. Although it is true that emotions, social values, and professional codes cannot alone justify an ethical decision, they are not totally unconnected to those decisions. Emotions influence our judgments, and personal values reflect an individual interpretation of the general social and professional values. Usually the various values are embodied in rules, or principles, which form the basis for making decisions. For example, a person who strongly values family relationships will follow principles which support family relationships. Such principles have many different sources, including law, religion, and personal viewpoint. The important thing is to know what principles are being used, how they are being used, and why they are being used. To see how this works, let's continue to look at Case 1.7.

---

[6]Item 2, "Code for Nurses," The American Nurses' Association, ANA Publication no. G-56 25M, Kansas City, MO, 1976.

Lorraine is facing an ethical dilemma which she can resolve by making an ethical judgment. To do so, she must first identify the values at issue and then identify the problem she must resolve; once she has done that, she must decide what her options are and make a decision how to act. As an example, suppose she were to think the problem through in the following way:

> To solve this case, either I must violate Mrs. Jones's privacy and tell someone of the abuse, or I must violate the law and not report the abuse. The nursing code says that I must maintain confidence and that I must obey the law. Since I can't do both, I will choose to obey the law, because every citizen has a duty to obey the law above all else. The law will then protect the child from further harm, and that protection is important.

Lorraine has resolved the contradiction of the code by using the basic principle "Obeying the law is more important than maintaining confidentiality." That principle is then the basis for her decision—the primary value she is incorporating into her decision process.

Notice that if Lorraine had used a different set of values or applied a different basic principle, she would have thought through the case in a different way and perhaps have reached a different conclusion. For example, Lorraine might have seen the problem not as one of obeying the law but, instead, as one of protecting the rights of those involved. Using this basis for thinking, she might have worked through the case in this way:

> As a professional, I must protect the rights of other people. The family has a right to privacy, but the child also has a right not to be abused. I cannot honor both rights; because protection of the child is more important than the family's privacy, my duty is to the child. The fact that the mother doesn't seem to see this means that I have to help. I will tell her that I will have to report the matter, because the child's right to protection is more important than anything else here.

The result of this deliberation is essentially the same as before, because Lorraine has decided that action is needed to prevent the abuse of the child, even if that means violating confidentiality. In this version, however, Lorraine's action is based not on her duty to the law but on the child's right to protection from harm. She is using a different basic principle here, namely, "A child's right to protection is more important than a parent's right to privacy."

The application of different principles to the same situation will change the way in which one thinks about that situation; and different thinking may result in a different solution. Suppose, for example, that Lorraine were to still see rights as the most important thing, but instead of focusing on the child's rights she focused on the parents' rights. Her thinking might then go like this:

The mother is correct—parents do have a right to do what they want with their children. I certainly would not allow my children to be treated that way, but who am I to question the values of someone else's family? Beside that, the nursing code tells me to keep the confidence of my clients, so that is another reason for not doing anything. It is a shame that the child has to suffer; but if the mother does not want to do anything about it, I have no business interfering.

Here Lorraine is also using a basic "rights" principle, although she is now counting the parents' rights more than the child's rights. Notice that she also uses a second basic principle, namely, "What people do is up to them, and nurses cannot impose their values on the client if they disagree." Rights are considered at length later, so a look at the second principle is in order here.

VALUE NEUTRALITY AND ETHICAL DECISIONS

The principle "What people do is up to them" is frequently translated into a rule that health care professionals should be "value-neutral" and "nonjudgmental" in their professional roles. According to this rule, no matter what values the professional holds, he or she must remain neutral relative to the values of the care recipient. On this view, there must be

> . . . a commitment to clients whether or not the nurse [or other professional] and the clients hold the same values. The [professional] does not assume that personal values are right and should not judge the client's values as right or wrong depending on their congruence with the [professional's] personal value system.[7]

Although this view is certainly reasonable in some situations, it is not valid in all situations. First, this view incorrectly assumes that there is radical disagreement on ethical matters and that no two people's values will be in agreement. We would, for example, find few people who would say that it is morally right for men to rape schoolgirls, or for mothers to sell their babies into slavery, or for Hitler to do what he did to the Jews in Nazi Germany. And, if we did find such people, we would all agree that something was wrong with them, because such acts are simply not acceptable. Without question, if Hitler were hospitalized, he should be cared for as a person, treated humanely, etc.; at the same time, it makes no sense to say that the care giver should not judge Hitler's values as right or wrong. Hitler's values *are* wrong, and there is no problem in recognizing that or even in saying that to him. The problem arises if his treatment is substandard because of his values.

This raises a second, more serious problem with the value-neutral idea—it is

---

[7]Shirley Steele, *Values Clarification in Nursing*, 2d ed., Appleton-Century-Crofts, Norwalk, CN, 1983, p. 27.

simply not morally permissible to maintain, even though it can be stated, as the following case shows:

> LuAnn Carter, a student nurse, was assigned to care for Milton Gregory, who was recovering from a gunshot wound. Milton had been shot by the jealous ex-boyfriend of his wife, Julie, and although not seriously wounded, Milton was extremely angry. Several times he told LuAnn that he was going to "get even" with the man who had shot him and "then he won't be shooting anybody again." When LuAnn talks to Milton about this, he says his motto is "Don't get mad, get even." LuAnn is concerned that Milton will try to kill the ex-boyfriend. Also, Julie's comment that he has "quite a temper" adds to her concern and convinces her that the ex-boyfriend is in grave danger once Milton is released from the hospital.

If LuAnn believes that Milton will attempt to kill or seriously harm Julie's ex-boyfriend, she cannot remain value-neutral and nonjudgmental; she has a clear obligation to act in an attempt to prevent harm to another person. Although Milton has values that differ from LuAnn's, she must make an effort to prevent him from acting on those values. What action she takes is, at this point, irrelevant. The crucial thing is that she must act. Value neutrality is simply not morally permissible.

Values are so much a part of one's personality that operating without them would leave nothing with which to operate. To put it in a different way, although theoretical discussion separates values from the person holding the values, such separation is not possible in practice. The person and the held values are one and the same; it is then impossible to operate as a human being, in a real situation, without values entering the picture. As John Hoffman has said, health care

> . . . is conducted in a real world where human beings . . . dream and build, curse and kill, laugh and love, suffer and die. To be mentally whole is to be able to cope with such a world. If you and I would be mentally whole, we cannot deny entire dimensions of reality and live as if there were no question of moral values.[8]

As a result, value neutrality is really nothing more than an excuse to not deal with ethical problems and to avoid facing the real problems of the world. Instead of an ethical rule, the call for value neutrality is more reasonably understood as a request for tolerance and recognition that there are acceptable alternatives to *some* of one's own values. That, however, does not lead to the conclusion that the correctness of moral judgments is solely a matter of unquestionable individual preference. What does follow is that we have an obligation to consider the reasons supporting adherence to certain values, consideration which may lead to either acceptance or rejection of those values.

[8]J. C. Hoffman, *Ethical Confrontation in Counseling,* University of Chicago Press, Chicago, 1979, p. 3.

RESPONSIBLE ETHICAL DECISION MAKING

It may seem that there is no way to work with ethical problems so that a satisfactory resolution may be achieved, because fault may be found with any approach one might suggest. Despite the appearance, however, that is not so; what we *have* seen are a number of "popular" approaches which do not work independently of one another, because each is too narrow. Moreover, each is usually seen as a "quick fix," an easy solution, an automatic way to eliminate a problem. On examination each is seen to be superficial, failing primarily because no thought is required and problems are covered up instead of resolved.

Ethical problems arise in many contexts, and the specific problems that one professional faces in a situation may differ from those faced by another professional in a similar situation. Moreover, ethical problems are very complex, have no simplistic answers, and usually cannot be adequately handled without thought and understanding. But what is this thought like, and what is the best way to go about doing it?

First and foremost, doing ethics is not simply the learning of another set of facts which may be recited on command. There are indeed facts to be learned, but they are only tools for later use in making decisions. The facts are not *the* answers to ethical questions or *the* resolutions to ethical problems. Rather, they are facts about ethics, and the ethical decision process, which serve as the basis for a person's ability to handle ethical problems. Development of that ability also requires coming to understand yourself and how you already think. This in turn requires confronting your personal beliefs, examining them, and deciding how they should be utilized. Because different people have different values, and those different values cause problems to be viewed in different ways, it is also important to learn how to understand the views of other people and how different ways of thinking may be used to resolve a problem. All this will then become part of the process used for ethical problems in everyday life. It will form a basis for deciding what *ought* to be done and *justifying* that decision.

The key to resolving ethical problems is decision making. Decision making is a specific type of thinking process which does not apply in every situation, but does apply to problem-solving situations, including those in which ethical problems arise. Unfortunately, it is possible to handle problems without using a decision process, by using dogma, authority, force, and other undesirable means. The main theme of this book is that a morally responsible person will utilize decision making to resolve ethical problems. The decision process in dealing with ethical problems is, then, a primary concern, and our efforts must be directed toward developing the skills necessary to use that process effectively.

The word *process* has been used several times in the past few paragraphs. That is no accident, for another basic theme of this book is that ethics is something we *do,* and the rational doing of ethics is a process. The process is an active, ongoing event in one's life. It is a conscious development of the knowledge and sensitivity which is crucial to having moral integrity. Moral integrity, that aspect of character according to which a person tries to act in a morally correct way, also involves an expanding, developing capacity to used the ethical process. In this way, doing ethics is not a peripheral extra in a person's life, but is at the core of living. Since one's professional activity is part of one's overall life, ethics is at the core of professional activity. The process, guided by moral integrity, is part and parcel of being a person.

Moral integrity must guide the process in order to maintain the role of emotions and feelings in the ethical decision process. What is moral integrity?

> At the simplest level, an individual with integrity is expected to be truthful, impartial, consistent, and whole within oneself. In relation to others, the indvidual with integrity is expected to act honestly and fairly, to behave with consistency through time, and to fulfill an essential function in interdependent interaction with parts of the whole.[9]

While the remainder of the book will help develop and clarify this idea of integrity, a few comments are in order here. First, integrity requires the individual to recognize the values which affect relations with others. All of us must know what we believe and why, if there is to be any hope of consistency. This will require a good deal of self-examination, since many of our beliefs are deep-seated and automatic.

Second, we must hold ourselves accountable for our beliefs and the moral reasoning which we base upon them. Without such accountability, we have no assurance that our actions are not based simply on prejudice, irrelevant emotions, irrationality, or other nonsense. Third, the truth element of integrity is truth to oneself. Moral persons must be honest about their beliefs, both to themselves and to others.

Finally, we must recognize that autonomy, the freedom to choose, is a fundamental element of moral integrity. Without freedom, there can be no morality, and integrity only means acting as a machine. This idea of autonomy poses a problem though—there will be disagreement about what ought to be done. In the spirit of integrity we must, in general, accept other people's beliefs, and sometimes compromise is required to resolve an ethical problem. At the same time, integrity means that we do not have to accept as correct whatever belief anyone else might have. Because, as we saw above, it is impossible to be value-neutral and nonjudgmental, there will be many occasions for thinking someone else is wrong. The perspective of moral integrity requires the ability to identify those situations in which a personal value cannot be compromised and to make reasoned objections, even to the point of refusing to act. Again, however, note the need for a decision process.

Health care is a process through which human beings try to do the best they

---

[9]C. Mitchell, "Integrity in Interprofessional Relationships," paper presented to the 11th Trans-disciplinary Symposium on Philosophy and Medicine, 1981.

can to promote the well-being and preserve the rights of a person receiving care. As such, it is essentially an ethical activity. Health care is *not* a science; it is the *application* of science to human beings. The process of ethics, framed by moral integrity, is therefore inseparable from health care. As a means for learning this process and developing a perspective on moral integrity, the remainder of the book focuses on three things: (1) developing a better understanding of the role of values in ethical decision making, (2) understanding the basic ethical frameworks for decisions, and (3) developing a systematic approach to ethical judgments in practice. As an introduction to that work, consider this passage from T. H. White's *Book of Merlin:*

> All thought, in its early stages, begins as action. The actions which [we] have been wading through have been ideas, clumsy ones of course, but they had to be established as a foundation before we could begin to think in earnest. [We] have been . . . think[ing] in action. Now it is time to think in our heads.[10]

STUDY GUIDE

The study guide for each chapter is intended as a follow-up to the work of that chapter. Each study guide will have three parts: a list of relevant readings from the second part of the book; a series of questions for reflection, to help guide further thinking; and a series of case studies to analyze by using the chapter materials, readings, and prior discussion. Following the study guide will be a bibliography of additional readings on the topics in the chapter.

READINGS

D. Callahan, "Competency in Medical Care," p. 137.

QUESTIONS FOR REFLECTION

1 Using your own experiences, describe two situations in which you believe that what someone else thinks is right is, in fact, wrong.
2 For the two instances in question 1, make a list of the values that you hold important and the values the other person holds important; then compare the two lists.
3 Carefully describe two social values which you believe give direct guidance to health care professionals making ethical decisions.
4 For Cases 1.1 to 1.4, how many different ways can you discover to analyze the case? (Use the discussion of Case 1.6 as an example.)

---

[10]T. H. White, *The Book of Merlin,* University of Texas Press, Austin, TX, 1977.

CASE STUDY FOR ANALYSIS

As a social worker for Children's Protective Services, you were sent to visit the Sailor family to determine whether they should have an increase in payments. Mr. Sailor had requested the increase, under a new section of the child support law, in order to help pay the medical bills for care of a child suffering from multiple birth defects and mental retardation. When he requested the increase, Mr. Sailor, a steelworker who has been unemployed for three years, said that he simply did not have enough money to pay all the child's bills.

When you made your home visit, you discovered, first, that the Sailors allow several nonfamily adults to live with them, which is a violation of the agreement for service from your agency. You also found beer and wine in the kitchen but no milk available for the children. In the process of your investigation, you also discovered that the family was still receiving money for a child who died several months ago. You asked Mr. Sailor about this, and he said that this was the only way he could get enough money to even partially keep up with his bills. Later, when you calculated his monthly bills, including food, rent, transportation, and medical expenses, you saw that his basic needs consistently used up all his income.

As the caseworker, you must make a determination of need. What will your determination be? What will you report? Why?

Analysis Questions   As you work on this case, think about the discussion of values in Chapter 1. How do *your* values influence the way you see this case? Make a list of the values involved here. Are there any conflicts? After you have decided what to do, try to identify any *assumptions* you are making. Are there missing data that you supplied, but based on your own experiences, not Mr. Sailor's? Are you biased in your decision? Why? Why not?

BIBLIOGRAPHY

Coletta, S.: "Values Clarification in Nursing," *American Journal of Nursing*, vol. 78, 1978, p. 2057.

Englehardt, H. Tristram: "Explanatory Models in Medicine: Facts, Theories, and Values," *Humanities and Medicine*, vol. 32, 1974, p. 255.

Englehardt, H. Tristram, and Daniel Callahan (eds.): *Knowing and Valuing: The Search for Common Roots*, The Hastings Center, New York, 1980.

Francoeur, Robert T.: *Biomedical Ethics: A Guide to Decision Making*, Wiley, New York, 1983.

Gorlin, Rena A. (ed): *Codes of Professional Responsibility*, Bureau of National Affairs, Washington, 1986.

Greenwald, Harold: *Decision Therapy*, Peter H. Wyden, New York, 1973.

Hall, B. P.: *Value Clarification as Learning Process*, Paulist Press, New York, 1973.

Pence, Gregory: *Ethical Options in Medicine*, Medical Economics Co., Oradell, NJ, 1980.

Rokeach, M.: *Beliefs, Attitudes, and Values,* Josey-Bass, San Francisco, 1969.

Steele, Shirley M., and Vera M. Harmon: *Values Clarification in Nursing,* 2d ed., Appleton-Century-Crofts, Norwalk, CN, 1983.

Stein, Jane J.: *Making Medical Choices: Who Is Responsible?* Houghton Mifflin, Boston, 1978.

Thomasma, David C., and Janet I. Pisaneschi: "Applied Health Professionals and Ethical Issues," *Journal of Allied Health,* vol. 6, no.3, 1977, pp. 15–20.

Tiselius, A., and S. Milsson (eds.): *The Place of Value in a World of Facts,* Wiley, New York, 1970.

CHAPTER 2

AN OVERVIEW OF ETHICAL THEORY

. . . Beware the attraction of the pure *sciences. They are pure only in the way an ancient [person] is—bloodless, without passion. No, no. Stick to the humanistic studies where, though the truth is more difficult to establish and the proofs are more fragile, yet there is the breath of living man in them.*

Trevanian*

WHY ETHICAL THEORY?

Each person operating within the health care environment has a different set of personal values which developed out of individual life experiences, including education and professional training. There are also shared values which give each set of personal values a more general basis of support. For example, health care professionals generally share three principles of practice:

1 Save or preserve life.
2 Relieve or minimize suffering.
3 Avoid harm.

Although different professional codes, and different professionals, may apply these principles in different ways, the principles stay the same.

*The Summer of Katya, Ballantine Books, NY, 1984, p. 284

How does it make sense to talk of both personal values and general principles such as these? The answer is that personal values are examples, or applications, of general principles. For instance, there are many different ways to save or preserve life, and some people may want to use one way while others may choose another. There may also be different ideas about when to preserve life and when to forgo treatment. The important thing is that in each case the basic rule is to save or preserve life; what is at issue is how and when to apply the rule. The rule is the general principle, and the how and the when are the personal values.

Saying that individuals determine for themselves the interpretation of professional and ethical principles does not mean that it is solely up to individuals to determine whether their actions were correct. Rather, it is up to each individual to decide how to act, after which the action may be examined for its correctness. In acting, professionals try to maintain the basic principles outlined above, and the actions taken usually fit the principles clearly enough that the correctness of the action is not questioned. Problems arise, however, either when the principles seem to be in conflict or when someone interprets an action as inappropriate because it is not seen as upholding one or more of the principles. At that point, an explicit analysis of the action becomes necessary to resolve the resulting conflict. The question, of course, is how that analysis is to take place.

The analysis of actions within the perspective of ethics ultimately requires assessing the reasons a person has for the action being questioned. Although the system for that assessment is not complicated, it is important to first have an understanding of the framework upon which the assessment rests, i.e., ethical theory.

An *ethical theory* is a system of related principles which serves as a model for thinking about ethical issues and problems. Ethical theory does not immediately give specific answers to ethical problems; rather, it gives a framework within which the problems may be understood and a means by which they may be resolved. In this way, different theories will apply to the same basic problems, but how each applies and where each leads will vary.

Four types of theory are generally used to do ethics. However, each type of theory is linked to the others in two different ways. First, each is concerned with the actions of human beings in interpersonal relationships. Second, each presumes that, in some case, competent individuals have self-determination; i.e., they are free to make life-directing decisions. What distinguishes the four types of theory is the *way* in which each is concerned with human actions, the *means* to be used in assessing those actions for their moral value, and the *role* of self-determination in moral actions.

Because self-determination is in some way a feature of each type of moral theory to be discussed, we give it general consideration first. The remainder of this chapter is concerned with helping to develop a basic understanding of ethical theory.

AUTONOMY: THE FOUNDATION OF ETHICS

The claim that each person is free to make life-directing decisions is often known as the *autonomy principle*. The concept of autonomy, understood in this sense, is crucial to ethics, because without some sense of autonomy there is no sense of responsibility, and without responsibility we cannot have ethics. Thinking about ethical problems, in order to develop a better perspective from which to do ethics, thus requires understanding autonomy: What do we mean by the word *autonomy?* How does autonomy influence and alter ethical decisions? And how does autonomy fit with other important concepts when we are doing ethics? Autonomy is an extremely complex matter, which will take time to fully develop. This section will help develop familiarity with the basic elements of autonomy and establish an understanding which is expanded and utilized in later chapters.

Although there is some disagreement as to precisely what it means to be autonomous, the following is a good working description:

> Persons are autonomous in the sense in which they are capable of formulating and acting on conceptions of how their lives should be lived. Autonomous agents can conceive of future alternatives; they understand that they can pursue different ends and employ different means. They have conceptions of value which can be used in deciding what ends to pursue and what means are appropriate. They can recognize conflicts between different ends and control their behavior in order to pursue those ends considered most valuable.[1]

Philosophically, the concept of autonomy has featured prominently in ethics and political philosophy since the time of ancient Greece.[2] Moreover, legal thinking and philosophical thinking agree that people usually have a right to make life-directing decisions for themselves roughly along these lines. For the health care setting, it is legally well established that a professional may usually not act against the wishes of a "human being of adult years and sound mind," even if the professional does not agree with the patient's decision.

If people are not able or not allowed to decide how to act, then their actions are not freely chosen; similarly, if people are forced to act in a certain way or restrained from acting, their actions are not freely chosen. The word *autonomy* thus applies *both* to decisions and to actions. Autonomy of judgment (decisions) requires both the freedom and the capacity to utilize reason in making choices; autonomy of action requires both the freedom and the capacity to act on those choices. An autonomous decision (1) is based on the individual's values, (2) utilizes adequate information and understanding, (3) is free from coercion or restraint, and (4) is based on reason and deliberation. An autonomous action is one which results from an autonomous decision.

If either autonomy of judgment or autonomy of action is absent or blocked,

---

[1]Lansing Pollock, *The Freedom Principle*, Prometheus Books, Buffalo, NY, 1981, pp. 111–112.

[2]For a good discussion of the legal and philosophical history of autonomy, see T. Beauchamp and L. McCullough, *Medical Ethics: The Moral Responsibilities of Physicians*, Prentice Hall, Englewood Cliffs, NJ, 1984, pp. 42–50.

then autonomy is limited; and if autonomy is limited, then choice is not free. Since individual choice is an important value, autonomy is a basic element of ethical theory, an element which is always present *unless proved otherwise*. It follows, then, that both ethical theory and practice will need to respect autonomy, unless it can be proved in the given case that such respect is not warranted, e.g., if the person is incompetent. (*Note:* That autonomy is unwarranted does not mean that dignity and rights need not be upheld.)

At this point note that autonomy must be considered at both the abstract and the concrete level. On the abstract level, autonomy is absolute, always present as an element of consideration. On the concrete level, however, degrees of autonomy (both judgment and action) are often possible, so that autonomy may in fact be seen as limited. For example, it makes perfectly good sense to say that a child is less autonomous than a competent adult or that a student is less autonomous relative to class content than the professor. The task of ethical theory is to explain how, if at all, a person's autonomy may be limited, and when, if ever, we may be justified in interfering with a person's choice.

BASIC ELEMENTS OF ETHICAL THEORIES

A theory of ethics is a system of related principles which serve as a model, or framework, for thinking about ethical issues and problems. Though an abstraction, an ethical theory presents a framework for thinking, because it presents a way of understanding; a theory, however, does *not* give a specific set of answers to a specific set of questions. Each of us uses such a framework, and the set of principles which it embodies, because that makes it easier to understand and deal with the complexities of ethical decisions in actual situations. Since it is not possible to present every known ethical theory in this book (there are so many that just presenting the theories would take the whole book), our focus is on four major *types* of theories. By taking this approach, the reader can develop a sense for each type, so that its framework and use may be understood. In this way it is possible to learn about both our own theory and those used by others.

Any ethical theory must address this basic question: What action(s), all things considered, should a person judge to be morally correct? Historically, the answers have come in many different forms, although, in general, each rests on an analysis of three related questions:

1 How do the *consequences* of an act affect its moral worth?

2 What are a person's moral *duties* (obligations), and how do they affect the moral worth of an action?

3 What are a person's moral *rights,* and how do they affect the moral worth of an action?

The difference between any two theories usually depends on what is taken to be most important (consequences, duties, or rights) and how decisions are to be made (with or without a standard for all people everywhere). Depending on which theoretical perspective is taken, consequences, duties, or rights will be the primary consideration in determining the moral worth of an action. This does not mean that a rights-based theory, one which focuses on rights as the basis for moral value, will not take consequences or duties into account; nor does it mean that a consequence-based theory will not have any concern with rights or duties. Instead, the theory will emphasize one particular element as the *primary* determinant of moral value and give the others a value relative to the primary element. The theory type will then depend on which of the three is the base, or primary element, of the theory. A rights-based theory, for example, would use rights as its primary element. It would still incorporate moral duties; however, the duties would originate from the rights. Thus, if someone has a duty to do something for you, it is because you have a right to have that done; without a right, there may be no duty, since the duties are derived from the rights. Similarly, in a duty-based theory we have rights, but the rights derive from the duties.

As we turn now to discussion of the basic types of theory, remember that this is a brief and somewhat superficial introduction. For more depth and detail, see the bibliography at the end of the chapter.

USING CONSEQUENCES TO DETERMINE MORAL WORTH

There is no doubt that all actions have some sort of consequence. There is also no doubt that, under ordinary circumstances, competent people are responsible for the consequences of their actions. Certainly we cannot foresee or be held responsible for accidents and matters otherwise beyond our control; yet there is still a great deal for which we *are* responsible. The important issue, then, is how the consequences of an action should count in determining the moral worth of that action. If the consequences of an action are not good, does that mean the action was bad or wrong? Is an action good only if it produces good consequences? Or, perhaps more important, should we decide what to do on the basis of what we think the consequences will be?

Historically, one major type of ethical theory has assumed that consequences are of primary importance in determining the moral worth of action. Although there are many consequence-based theories, they all require assessing consequences for deciding both what to do and the value of what was done. The primary difference between the various consequence-based theories lies in how the consequences are evaluated. Some people argue, for example, that each consequence must be given a numerical rating, with a plus for good and a minus for bad, and we should do whatever produces the highest positive number. Others, for example, egoistic theories, say that the consequences which count most are those which affect the individual making the decision, so that the right thing to do is the thing that *I* think will do *me* the most good. For still others, such as hedonistic theories, the consequences which count most are those which produce pleasure. And so on.

There are two additional important features of all consequence-based theories. First, each incorporates the autonomy principle, but the extent to which a person may exercise autonomy depends on an analysis of the consequences. Second, each determines a person's rights and obligations *after* consequences are considered.

A Specific Example of a Consequence-Based Theory

Utilitarianism is probably the best known and most widely adopted of the consequence-based ethical theories. Although various elements of the utilitarian theory have been around at least since the time of Epicurus (around 250 B.C.), its best-known modern formulation was given by John Stewart Mill, in his book *Utilitarianism*. In Mill's classic formulation, morally correct action is determined by what he calls the *greatest happiness principle:* ". . . actions are right in proportion as they tend to promote happiness; wrong as they tend to produce the reverse of happiness."[3] Today, this principle is more frequently stated as "Do the greatest good for the greatest number of people." Although that is not Mill's formulation, it captures the basic idea of utilitarianism as a consequence-based ethical theory. The important thing is that, in using this theory, a person must always be guided by the rule "Produce the best possible set of consequences," for only then can an action be considered to have moral worth.

From the utilitarian viewpoint, morally correct activities must incorporate an effort to balance things, doing only good whenever possible, but when it is not possible to do good, doing as much good (or as little harm) as possible. The moral responsibility of each person, then, is to take that action which will result in the best possible set of consequences. Note, however, that right conduct is a matter of how things add up, with each person's "good" counting the same as every other person's "good." Moreover, the good which serves as the basis for decision must not be merely that of the decision maker. As Mill says,

> . . . the happiness which forms the utilitarian standard of what is right in conduct is not the agent's own happiness but that of all concerned. As between his own happiness and that of others, utilitarianism requires him to be as strictly impartial as a disinterested and benevolent spectator.[4]

Since the principle underlying utilitarianism relies on such terms as *good* and *happiness,* and since people define those terms differently, people in the same situation may want to do different things, because each gives different weights and values to the projected consequences. The key point, however, is that each person using a consequence-based theory will decide what to do by weighing the projected consequences of an action and then figuring out which action will produce the best possible set of consequences.

[3]J. S. Mill, *Utilitarianism,* Hackett Publishing Co., Indianapolis, IN, 1979, p. 7.
[4]Ibid., p. 16.

Act and Rule Utilitarianism

There have been two different versions of utilitarianism which have been widely discussed and applied since Mill first formulated the basic theory. These versions, called *act utilitarianism* and *rule utilitarianism,* differ primarily in whether the frame of reference for a decision is a specific action or a general rule which applies to all actions of that type. Act utilitarianism uses only consideration of consequences relevant to a specific set of circumstances. For this version of utilitarianism, there are no general rules which carry over from one situation to another, because each situation is seen as unique.

Rule utilitarianism, however, attempts to develop a set of general rules which may be applied to a wide range of situations. For whatever rule we may want to make, we determine whether it is a good rule by asking, Does applying this rule produce the best possible set of consequences? If the answer is yes, the rule is morally acceptable; if the answer is no, then it is not. Once the rules have been determined in this way, a person only has to follow the rules. If a situation should arise for which there is no rule, then a rule may be formed by using the principle of utility.

Rights and Duties

As mentioned earlier, consequence-based theories always acknowledge the general ethical principles of obligation, rights, and autonomy. However, the interpretation and application of these principles depend on an analysis of the consequences. Thus, if someone has a duty to do something, it is because the analysis of consequences shows that doing it will produce the best possible results. Or, if a person has a right to something, it is because the best possible consequences will be produced by allowing that right. To put it differently, in all cases, the rights and obligations that a person has are a direct result of an analysis of consequences or rules. Similarly, a change in rights and duties will result from the same sort of analysis.

Consequence-based theories are frequently encountered in health care, primarily because one principle of practice is to "do no harm." From this principle arises our concern to weigh the risks and benefits of care. *Whenever* there is a weighing of risks and benefits, we are considering consequences. Similarly, we are *always* considering consequences when making a quality-of-life argument. The only question which remains in either case is whether the consequences are being considered as the sole criterion for treatment, or whether they are a function of upholding patient's rights or professional duties.

The question of rights and duties also comes in here, as we ask, for example, Do I have a right to have good done? Do you have a duty to do good, or simply a duty to refrain from doing harm? If the duty is to do good, is it based on my values or yours? What if we conflict in views of what is good? This also brings in the problem of determining a person's "best interests"—what are they and who decides? These questions, and others, will become key issues as we move on to specific problems later in the book.

Difficulties in Using Consequence-Based Theories

Although it seems intuitively obvious that consequences need to be considered in determining moral worth, and even though it seems easy to say, "This is better than that," analysis of consequences is more difficult than it looks. First, consequences are always *predictions,* never certainties. Thus, in selecting the consequences to assess, one must make predictions about the consequences most likely to occur. Second, the predicted consequences must be analyzed to assess their possible effects and whether those effects are potentially good or bad. And therein lies another difficult dimension of the decision: Whose values should be used to determine whether something is good or bad? Finally, once the relative good and bad aspects of a set of consequences have been established and it has been established whose values will be used, the good and bad aspects must be weighed to see whether the overall result is good or bad. But how is this weighing to be done? What values (whose values) are to be reflected in this balancing? And what do we do when there are conflicting opinions on the analysis?

A potentially serious problem with the consequence-based theories is that it is possible for the good of some to be gained at the expense of others, provided only that the good outweighs the bad. This is what is known as the *problem of justice,* namely, it is possible to have a morally correct action (in terms of consequence analysis) which is nonetheless unjust, thus violating a basic principle of ethics. Although utilitarians have discussed this problem at great length and tried many different ways to solve it, the issue is still very troublesome.

Finally, there is the general problem of trying to determine what constitutes the good and whether there is a single good for everyone or whether each person determines his or her own good. If the last is true, then we are really reduced to relativism (to be discussed later in this chapter); otherwise, we must be able to come to some consensus about what is good for everyone, and that would seem to be a difficult task.

So how, then, are we to even make the analysis of consequences which such a theory requires? Certainly it will not be without some difficulty, *if* we are to do a good job. Many people believe, however, that the problems with consequential analysis cannot be overcome and that the basis for ethical decisions should be something other than consequences, for example, obligations or rights.

USING DUTIES TO DETERMINE MORAL WORTH

The idea of obligations is not unique to ethics. Each person has business obligations, family obligations, social obligations, etc., and a good portion of every day is spent fulfilling these obligations. The difference is that ethical obligations are quite general, not limited to certain people by agreement, kinship, or law.

Instead, ethical obligations apply to any person, provided only that the proper circumstances exist.

Understood in this way, humans have ethical obligations to each other, simply because they are human beings. And, of course, since each person is a human being, there will also be obligations to oneself. Certainly people will sometimes disagree about what these obligations are and how they may best be fulfilled; but people generally do not disagree about the existence of some such obligations.

A second major type of ethical theory is based on people's obligations. The obligations, often referred to as *duties,* are usually expressed in terms of rules of conduct. Duty-based theories are thus a bit like rule utilitarianism because moral worth is based on a set of rules, or guiding principles. Unlike rule utilitarianism, however, the principles of duty-based theories do not come from an analysis of the consequences, but come instead from a recognition of obligation, or duty. Thus you must help someone in need because you have a duty to help, not because helping will produce good consequences. In fact, if your duty is to help, you must help even if it will create some bad consequences. For example, suppose you are on your way to the airport to catch a flight for your European vacation, and you come upon a bad automobile accident. There is no one else around to help the injured people. But if you stop to help, you will miss your flight, your vacation will be delayed, and you will have to pay the tour company a $200 penalty. Should you stop? According to a duty-based theory, if you have a duty to help, you must stop, regardless of the bad consequences you will suffer.

Although it might not seem as if duty-based decisions are very common, in practical situations they may be quite numerous, especially if we think about all the policies, procedures, rules, and laws we must deal with every day. In addition, some fairly important duty bases (sets of duties or rules), from different sources, are used in making decisions. Because the effect and analysis of duties are different, depending on the source of the duties, it is worth taking a moment to look at three major sources and their effect on decisions.

Duties Based on Religion

One source of duties is religion, where one well-known duty base is the Ten Commandments of the Judeo-Christian tradition. But religion-derived duties are much wider, having their roots in church law (e.g., the canon law of the Roman Catholic Church) or tradition (e.g., the Talmud of Judaism) or sacred scriptures (e.g., the Koran of Islam). Religiously imposed duties are traditionally expressed through either revealed or derived rules. *Revealed rules* are those, such as the Ten Commandments, which are believed to have the supreme being as their source and to have been transmitted to the faithful through someone of the faith. The Ten Commandments, for example, are believed to have been revealed to Moses, through their mysterious inscription on two tablets of stone. *Derived rules* are those which come from interpretation of revealed rules and their implications, especially in their application to specific situations. Importantly, derived rules are specifically formulated to uphold the basic belief system of the religion and to reinforce or apply the revealed rules to everyday life. The Talmud of Judaism and canon law of the Roman Catholic Church are two examples of derived rules.

The duties imposed by religious rules are a part of the practice of religion, and people follow the rules either because it is part of their faith, it is the tradition of their religion, the authority of their religion tells them they must follow the rules, or they believe this to be God's will. Regardless of why people honor religiously determined duties, those duties affect their lives. Thus, people may do their duty because they believe that not doing so means they cannot go to heaven after they die, or because the scriptures say to do it, or because they must do God's will. Because of this diversity, the enforcement of religious law is generally a matter of conscience; that is, individuals are responsible for policing their own actions and applying the rules through their own interpretation of the religious beliefs.

Duties Based on Social Rules

A second source of duties is the rules imposed on people by themselves, usually through legislative and institutional systems, for reasons which are understood to be nonreligious. In the health care setting, one source of duties is the hospital, which establishes duties through its policies and procedures; another source of duties is the professional code, which establishes duties for practice. Still another source of secular duties is the law which results from legislative or judicial action. The rules which result from legally or institutionally imposed duties differ from religious rules in their origin, in their scope, and in the way they are enforced. Secular rules generally originate from an actual or perceived potential problem, usually in response to the specific request of an individual or small group.

Although some examples of secular law, such as constitutions, tend to be very general, secular duties on the whole are quite particular, aimed a specific acts and events. In fact, secular law is often so specific that the major problem in its application is determining whether the act in question is "covered" by the law. This problem arises because law is invariably formulated to address an existing problem, and problems tend to be quite specific. Unlike religious duties, secular duties are enforced by the agents of the law, e.g., the police, and are not left to the conscience of individuals. The determination of duty is, then, by authority, with application of the rules similarly determined.

Although violation of religious duties may affect one's spiritual being, violation of secular legal duties may affect one's physical being, through fine, jail sentences, and even death.

A potential problem with duties imposed through religion is that the rules may not be seen as binding by those who do not subscribe to that religion. Throughout history, and even today, for example in the Middle East, different religious groups wage war against one another or against secular states, in the name of their religion, in order to destroy "evil." What has been overlooked is that the conflict of duties and rules may, in fact, be *ethical,* not religious or legal. For example, all religions hold to a general rule equivalent to the commandment "Thou shalt not kill," as does any civilized code of secular law. But the *religious* reason for the rule may be very different from the *secular* reason for the rule. Thus, if people see themselves as nonreligious, they may adhere to a rule not because a religion requires it but because the secular law requires it. However, people who are religious may violate state law because it is seen as violating religious law. This conflict of duties is often the motive for civil disobedience, as exemplified by Mahatma Gandhi and Martin Luther King, in this century, and many religious martyrs through history, such as Joan of Arc and Thomas More.

The third source of duties, philosophical reasoning, attempts to develop a system of duties which can be applied no matter what religion people might adhere to or how they might see their relation to the state or other institutions.

Duties Derived from Reason

The philosophical approach is to rely on reason, logic, and philosophical analysis as the source of duties. The aim, of course, is to arrive at a formulation of duties that will establish moral rules which (ideally) apply to all people, regardless of their religious beliefs or state affiliations. To achieve this end, duty-based theories tend to be formal, that is, based on valid rules of logic and able to be applied via a formula, instead of based on specific instances. Perhaps the most famous philosophical work of this sort is that done by Immanuel Kant, in *Critique of Practical Reason, Groundwork of the Metaphysics of Morals,* and *Letters on Ethics*. In these writings Kant sets out what he calls the *categorical imperative,* a formula for determining whether a proposed rule does, in fact, reflect a moral duty.

Understanding the details of Kant's description of the categorical imperative is difficult and controversial. The main points, however, are quite clear. Kant assumes that the basis for ethics is human reason and that people may make decisions to act in morally correct ways through autonomous decisions utilizing reason. The basis for the decision process, he argues, must be the application of the categorical imperative, which is a formula for determining whether a specific rule is morally correct in all cases. The formula, simply put, asks whether the proposed rule may be equally applied to everyone, without exception, and whether the proposed rule treats persons as ends in themselves and not only as means to some end which is not their own. That is, we must ask whether the proposed rule uses people, thus treats them as objects instead of as persons, and whether the rule applies to everyone, thus does not discriminate or place burdens on some for the benefit of others. Using this notion of duty, Kant would require

both religious and secular laws to apply the categori
whether their proposed rules impose or violate a mc

For Kant, an act has moral worth when it is
recognizes a duty (by applying the categorical imp
simply because it *is* a duty. No further impetus, s
avoidance of jail or any other consequence, is a le
the decision to act out of duty is one which is free
person whose intention is to meet morally imposed obligations.

Difficulties with Duty-Based Theories

Although it seems easy to say, "I ought to do my duty," determining what is a
duty is often difficult. In addition, there frequently are conflicting duties, for
example, duties to yourself and duties to others. To whom does a person owe
allegiance? Is one duty more important than another? In fact, a problem arises
for any duty-based theory when there is a conflict of duties. The difficulty, of
course, is how to decide which duty takes priority. Suppose, for example, that
a person has a duty to tell the truth and a duty to maintain confidentiality. In a
case where both duties cannot be honored, what should be done? Which duty
takes priority over the other? Kant did not recognize and deal with this problem,
but a more contemporary philosopher, W. D. Ross, tries to handle this by arguing
that some duties may be classified as primary while others may be placed in a
secondary role. Others have used different ideas about "levels" of rules which
tell how to resolve differences, for example, by analyzing consequences or
looking for a priority of rights. No matter how it is done, though, any worthwhile
duty-based theory must deal with the issue of conflicting duties.

Another difficulty with duty-based theories is their tendency to consider consequences morally irrelevant. Intuitively, there seems to be something wrong
with causing harm to others. Yet what if that is the result of doing one's duty?
Part of the answer lies in seeing how the harm arises. For example, being put
in jail is harmful to the jailed person; yet there seems nothing wrong with causing
that harm if the jailed person has robbed or raped or murdered someone. The
phrase *causing harm* then needs to be understood to mean "causing harm to
innocent people." Even with that modification, however, a duty-based theory
must still explain and account for the harm caused by obedience to one's duty.

Still another difficulty of duty-based theories is that the rules they impose
often seem too rigid, unable to meet special needs of particular circumstances.
Or these theories are so general as to be essentially meaningless. The saying
"Rules are made to be broken" probably originated in relation to duty-based
theories, as a means for accommodating such particular circumstances. In a
similar vein, such theories seem to downplay initiative and creativity of mind
in dealing with ethical problems. Too often they seem rigidly tied to the rules
and nothing but the rules. As a result, people simply look for a list of rules to

ize so they always "know" what to do and how to stay out of trouble. A based theory, to be adequate, must deal with this difficulty and develop e flexibility needed to work in a changing world.

The final difficulty raised by duty-based theories is that they may not adequately allow for intentions other than the intention to do one's duty. If I am trying to follow a rule, but something goes wrong and I do not, should my trying not count for something? In the most rigid interpretation of duties, what you are trying to do counts only in the doing, not in the failure. An adequate duty-based theory must deal with this difficulty as well as with the other problems.

Duties and Rights

A question which often arises is whether duties lead to rights or rights lead to duties. Is there a direct connection between the two, so that having a duty automatically gives someone a right or so that having a right automatically gives someone a duty? Do duties have rights as their source? Part of the answer depends on whether duties or rights are taken as the most important thing for a theory. On one hand, if rights are somehow independent entities, not derived from anything else, then rights could lead to duties, but duties could not lead to rights. On the other hand, if rights are derived from something, then it is possible that they are derived from duties. Understanding the relation between rights and duties clearly requires a better understanding of rights, so we turn to that now.

RIGHTS—UNDERSTANDING THE BASICS

That human beings have rights is a readily accepted fact. The difficulty lies in determining exactly what those rights are, where they originate, and what their status is in moral considerations. Before we discuss specific rights, however, it is important to recognize that there are different categories of rights, depending on the origin of the right and the exercise of that right.

Origin of Rights

Rights originate in two primary ways; they are either *natural* (inherent, or inborn in some sense) or *bestowed* (given by persons to each other). Natural rights are those which people have simply because they are human beings. We may choose not to recognize, honor, or protect those rights, but they are always present and cannot be taken away. The right to freedom and the right to life are often cited as examples of natural rights. Bestowed rights are those which someone has *only* if other persons specifically give them, and bestowed rights may be taken away in a similar manner. Bestowed rights frequently have specific conditions attached to them or must be "earned" in some way, while natural rights do not. For example, employees of XYZ Company have a right to their paychecks;

however they must first earn the pay by fulfilling the job requirements. Another example of a bestowed right would be the right to drive a car, which depends on being the correct age, not being blind, being able to pass the required tests, etc.

Rights which are bestowed may also be lost: employees may be fired or laid off, thus losing their right to a paycheck; and drivers may lose their licenses by violating the law or becoming disabled. Notice, too, that in each case other rights may be involved. For instance, the law bestows rights on employees via labor relations regulations and on drivers via due-process rules, so that the loss of one right is monitored in the context of another.

Application of Rights

Regardless of their origin, rights are generally either automatic rights or claim rights. *Automatic rights* are those which people have regardless of whether they request them or even know they have them. *Claim rights,* however, require people to specifically request whatever they have a right to, in order for it to be received. The right to drive a car is a claim right, because unless a person applies for a license, passes the test, and pays the fees, no license is received and the person has no right to drive. However, the right not to be murdered need not be claimed to be in force; otherwise, people could legitimately murder anyone who did not specifically request not to be murdered. If a right is automatic, a person need do nothing to receive the benefit of the right; but if it is a claim right, then the benefit must be specifically requested. Notice that this distinction is important for practical as well as theoretical reasons. For example, even if everyone agreed that health care is the right of all people, the design and function of the health care systems would be very different for a claim right than for an automatic right.

Another way to determine how rights apply is to ask whether the right is absolute or conditional. *Conditional rights* depend on certain conditions being met before the right will apply and usually have provisions allowing interference with the exercise of the right. Again, to use driving as an example, the right to drive depends on conditions set up in the law; if those conditions are not met, then the person has no right to drive. But an *absolute right* applies in some general or universal sense with few, if any, exceptions. Unlike a conditional right, an absolute right usually does not permit outside interference, allowing people the freedom to exercise their right as they see fit. Absolute rights also tend to be stated in very general terms, e.g., "Everyone has a right to be treated as a person, not an object" or "Each person has a right to be treated with dignity." Conditional rights, in contrast, tend to be very specific, e.g., "Any person on welfare, with an income of less than $7000 per year, is entitled to Medicare." The *Roe v. Wade* abortion decision by the U.S. Supreme Court presents an interesting combination of absolute and conditional rights. In *Roe v. Wade* the court argued that a woman has an unconditional right to an abortion during the first three months of pregnancy—no one may interfere with or attempt to control the woman's decision or action. After that time the right becomes increasingly conditional; states may regulate abortions during the middle trimester to protect the safety of the mother, and during the last trimester the right is withdrawn except in a very limited number of cases. Although identification of absolute rights may be difficult, this distinction of absolute and conditional rights can help clarify problem situations.

The Force of a Right

The final way in which rights may be distinguished is to determine whether the right is positive or negative. *Positive rights* are usually understood as "a right to" something, while a negative right is "a right from" something. In this way, a positive right results in someone receiving something, while a negative right protects the person from interference. *Roe v. Wade,* for example, articulates a negative right because it prevents states from interfering in an abortion decision; it does *not* give a positive right where, for example, any woman wanting an abortion is entitled to receive one whether or not she can pay for it. Positive rights are frequently referred to as *entitlement*—things to which people are entitled and which they may claim whenever they wish or which they are given automatically. A child's right to an education, in our society, is a positive right, an entitlement which may be claimed for the child and which the child may receive without hindrance. In fact, education is automatic, forced on the child, like it or not, until age 16. Child abuse laws, however, provide a negative right, that is, a right to protection from abuse. Under abuse laws, parents are not required to do anything specific, although they are prevented from doing certain things, and that is the essence of a negative right.

Although it may seem unnecessary to make so many distinctions about rights, it really is not. Our response to a rights claim will be different depending on what sort of right is claimed. And it really is important, in trying to understand a problem of rights, to know what sort of right is at issue. Moreover, since ethical theory is the basis for describing and evaluating rights, to understand a theory it is important to understand what kinds of rights are being described and how they are seen as functioning.

USING RIGHTS TO DETERMINE MORAL WORTH

A theory which is based on rights begins from the position that human rights are the foundation for determining moral worth. Using a rights-based theory, then, means that we must first determine what rights are at issue before we may analyze a situation for moral value. For most instances of such theories, a set of basic human rights is usually taken as primary, while others are secondary to them. In general, these basic rights are usually thought to be natural rights, both positive and negative, although more often automatic rather than claim rights. The most important thing about a rights-based system, however, is that it puts the person at the center of the ethical decision. Consequences and duties may affect a person, but rights help to form the person; however, like duties, rights are something that persons *have,* while consequences are done *to* persons. Also, unlike either consequences or duties, rights are relatively neutral toward secondary values, such as religious or social mores.

Although there have been major rights-based theories throughout history, the understanding of rights as a basis for ethical decisions has been heavily developed only in the latter part of this century. Reflecting Kant's notion that persons must be treated as ends only, not as means to some end, rights-based theories start from the presumption that human beings are inherently valuable *as persons,* regardless of anything else.

In health care areas, the focus on rights has been primarily initiated through the courts; as people sue doctors and hospitals, their rights (e.g., to informed consent, refusal of treatment, and competent practice) have been consistently upheld. Traditionally, however, the focus on rights has its primary basis in natural law theology. This view, developed in medieval times by scholars in the Roman Catholic tradition but now widely held, argues that persons by nature (i.e., by the very fact that they are human beings) have certain rights. Of particular importance is the notion of equality; human beings are essentially equal, and thus a just (moral) system must treat them as such. Importantly, the theological view of rights argues that the rights in question derive directly from people's relationship to the supreme being. On this view of rights, a right which is given by God cannot be taken away by people. The rights are natural and absolute; to deny a person's right is to interfere with the will of God.

There are also nontheological theories of rights which arrive at the same conclusion—that basic human rights cannot be denied a person—but from a different perspective. The primary nontheological approach to rights is through the notion of autonomy. In these theories, the fundamental nature of autonomy, not the will of God, serves as the foundation of the theory. From that foundation the primary line of argument is that since people have a right of self-determination, one cannot interfere with autonomous choices. Obviously people cannot be allowed to do *anything* they want, but then neither can a person be interfered with at will. Unlike the theological perspecitve of rights, the nontheological rights-based theories must rely heavily on secular law for support, and many of the basic rights are seen as needing legislative approval. The important thing which both types of theory have in common, however, is that individuals have basic rights which cannot be interfered with. Moreover, both theories agree that people's duties are derived from the rights of themselves and others, and both theories agree that whether a person has rights is not a matter of what consequences may be produced by exercising the rights.

Difficulties with Rights-Based Theories

Like other ethical theories, rights-based theories have problems. First, and most important, is the problem of clearly specifying a set of rights which is to form the basis for decision. From the religious perspective, these rights are usually determined through revelation or derivation; from the nonreligious view they are determined through reasoning or the law. Second, like the duty-based theories, rights-based theories must be able to settle a conflict of rights. Usually this is done through recognition of primary and secondary rights, with conflicts resolved in priority order or left to the autonomy principle (i.e., what a person chooses as the priority holds for that instance).

Because there are problems with all three theory types discussed so far, some people try to argue that we should give up on these theories and instead focus on autonomy, with action decisions based on individual decisions. This approach creates the fourth type of theory that we will explore—relativism.

USING RELATIVISM TO DETERMINE MORAL WORTH

We have looked at types of theories distinguished by whether consequences, duties, or rights are seen as most important. There is, however, another way to classify theories according to how the most important factor is determined. Historically there are two basic approaches:

1 Each person (or society) is ultimately responsible for determining the moral value of an act, on the basis of factors (usually rules or principles) which apply equally to all persons everywhere.

2 Each person (or society) is ultimately responsible for determining the moral value of any act, on the basis of whatever factors the person (or society) thinks appropriate.

The three types of theory considered up to this point take the first to be most important, while the fourth (and last) type we consider takes the second to be most important.

The ethical theory known as *relativism* is first encountered in the writings of Protagoras, a philosopher who lived in ancient Greece (ca. 480–411 B.C.). Protagoras's famous dictum

> Man is the measure of all things; of things that are, that they are, of things that are not, that they are not.[5]

states the essence of relativism—each person determines right and wrong solely on the basis of his or her own life experiences. Accordingly, one person may not criticize another, because what one thinks is right is based on perceptions

---

[5]P. Wheelright (ed.), *The Presocratics,* Odyssey Press, New York, 1966, p. 239.

or experiences which the other cannot have. This view has come to be known as *individual relativism* and has its expression in the often heard phrase "Well I could never do it, but if it's right for you, you go ahead" or in the question "Who are you to question my values?" or in the claim "What is right or wrong is just a matter of opinion, and one opinion is just as good as another."

Another version of relativism has grown out of sociology and anthropology—*cultural,* or *social, relativism.* The basic principle of cultural relativism is that there are no principles of morality which apply generally to every society; rather, right and wrong are uniquely determined by each society for its own members. This version of relativism grows from the obvious truth, discovered through anthropological comparative studies, that different societies emphasize and reinforce different values. From this fact it is then argued that there can be no standard values that apply to everyone; instead, each society must determine for itself what it will value and how those values will be enforced. Typical examples of this view are expressions such as "When in Rome, do as the Romans do" or "We cannot criticize country A for its record on human rights, since every society is different" or "It is wrong to impose our form of government on another country, since their culture is different from ours."

The most important thing in both versions of relativism is the fundamental claim that right and wrong are to be determined by the individuals involved *and* in whatever way they see fit. At either the individual or the societal level, no one has the moral authority to intervene in the actions of another. A fundamental violation of this theory would be to impose beliefs on someone by force or coercion. On the societal level this occurs most frequently in diplomatic situations, and war is a common end result. At the individual level, this occurs most frequently in a negative way, that is, person A preventing person B from doing something that person B believes is correct and person A believes is incorrect. Suicide prevention is a prime example of such cases.

The second important thing for both versions of relativism is that the basis for moral decisions is up to the decision maker. It is not important whether consequences, duties, or rights are used. For example, a society might decide, by voting in a new constitution, that all citizens must give ultimate allegiance to the state and protect the state above all else. In that society, then, right and wrong will be determined according to whether a particular act supports or undermines the state. Notice, however, that the society could decide to change its values, as happens, for example, when a revolution occurs. When the social values are changed, the basis for determining right and wrong is changed.

Individual relativism follows suit, although within that theory the individual alone decides what is important and how right and wrong will be determined. For example, you may decide that your moral judgments will be directed by the principle "Life is short, so have as much fun as possible while you can." After living by this principle for a while, you may decide that having friends is more important than having fun. So you decide to change your view and determine right and wrong according to the new rule "Life is short, so make as many friends as possible." The important point is that any rules you use are ones *you* consider proper, regardless of what anyone else might say or do. Moreover, those rules will be determined on whatever basis *you* choose.

The theory of relativism, as described above, may initially sound quite reasonable. There are, however, several important problems. First, there is a basic logical inconsistency: The theory requires that there be no rules which apply equally to everyone, yet relativism is itself such a rule. Second, the theory assumes that the existence of variation in viewpoint proves that variation is correct; yet this is a claim that needs proof. The fact that something *is* the case does not prove that it *ought* to be the case. Simply describing different views that people hold does not automatically show that it is correct to hold different views. In fact, after we examine the rules of some societies (such as those in Nazi Germany which caused the execution of 6 million Jews), our intuition tells us that there are at least some exceptions to the claim.

This last point brings us to the third, and most important, criticism of relativism: Following the theory requires that we permit actions which we may find unacceptable, simply because they are acceptable to the person, or society, doing them. The relativist would argue that the individual or society needs to be committed to its views—*sincere* is a common word used here—but think of where that leads. We have Hitler, of whom no one could deny a commitment to his ideas. Yet how can we say his acts were morally correct, even though *he* thought they were?

The basic problem with individual relativism as a theory is that it confuses the *use* of reason with the *certification* of that use. Put differently, relativism confuses *reasoning* with *reasons*. The fact that someone has thought about something does not mean that this person has good reasons for the conclusion reached. It follows even less that a viewpoint without reasons is acceptable simply because a person believes it is right. We might be more comfortable (psychologically speaking) because relativism will prevent criticism of our beliefs, and it allows us the freedom to decide whatever we would like to decide. The price of that particular freedom is very high, however, since we must then accept *anything* as correct, regardless of the consequences.

Cultural relativism, while an improvement because of the checks and balances imposed by society, nonetheless involves two problems. First, there is a failure to distinguish between things properly decided by society (e.g., drinking and driving ages) and things which, even if decided by a society, would be morally improper (e.g., allowing murder or theft of property) and so are not proper social decisions. Second, cultural relativism makes moral decision making a matter of vote or custom. What this does is confuse the *basis* for a decision with the *acceptance* of a decision. That some group accepts something does not prove that it *ought* to be accepted; the fact that some group accepts something as right does not make it right.

At this point someone might point out an obvious fact: Every moral judgment is necessarily personal, as is any thought process. Others may influence our judgments, but in the final analysis the judgment is individual.[6] The question, then, is how to avoid relativism and still be able to make individual moral decisions. This is accomplished in part by learning about other theories and viewpoints, because they broaden our horizons of understanding and help foster a more complete decision process. To that end we have described other views in this chapter, and we continue to work with them throughout the book.

Avoiding relativism also requires understanding and engaging in the moral reasoning process. We are developing that process in this book, especially through the system described in Chapter 3. Through its use you will be better able to develop alternatives and efficiently use that system of analysis as an aid to avoiding relativism.

CONCLUDING THOUGHTS

We have covered a lot in this chapter, much of which may be new and confusing. The purpose, however, has been to help develop familiarity with the basic ethical theories which will surface in any given situation. To understand the situation in which an ethical problem arises, it is necessary to understand the theoretical perspectives of the persons involved in that problem, including yourself. Identifying the base for a theory requires asking what, for that theory, is the most important thing to look at in determining whether an action is morally correct. Put in another way, when you try to determine the moral value of an action, what must be considered as primary? Learning what each theory involves should enable you, first, to come to a better understanding of which theory you are actually using and, second, to understand the views of others who subscribe to a different theory.

A typical reaction of people who read about ethical theory for the first time is, "Why bother? Every theory has problems, so why use any of them? And besides, who's to say what is right?" It is important to recognize that an ethical theory is a constantly evolving *framework,* an ideal we can use as a guide for thinking through problems. We should always strive for that ideal, recognizing the difficulties in fully achieving it and recognizing that it is not irrational to strive. We must be flexible enough to modify the theory when modification is necessary; but it is simply stupid to throw out the theories altogether. In science, for example, no phenomenon is an exact representation of the theory; neither is it in ethics. And just as we would not be willing to throw out science because there are problems with scientific theories or some phenomena don't fit a theory,

---

[6]Coercion seems to be an exception to this claim but is not, since coerced persons either recognize and decide to go along with the coercion or do not recognize it and go along thinking they have made a judgment.

so, too, we should not avoid doing ethics just because there are problems with ethical theory or because our actions (the phenomena) do not seem to exemplify the ideal (the theory). Instead, we must try to address the problems with the theory. Armed with knowledge gained from new experiences, understanding gained from careful thinking, and a willingness to adjust our viewpoint to accommodate new information, we can reformulate the theory to better account for our moral experiences. This in turn will help us approach new situations, from which we may learn and modify our theory, to be applied to new situations.

There is a great deal more to be learned both about ethical theory in general and about specific theories. But in this book we do not present that depth of theory; rather, we present an overview which will be helpful with the practical work of assessing ethical problems. Actually, whole books could be devoted solely to theory, never touching any specific problems or issues. Ethics must also be based on reality, though, so theory must be given a base in reality. Our present goal is to help develop a better sense of the overall perspective, of which theory is one piece. Theory cannot be realistically isolated from experience, however, any more than experience can be devoid of theory. An ethical decision is an empty theoretical gesture if it is not based in a context and tied in to actions which have an effect. Similarly, an ethical decision is also incomplete if it is devoid of concern for the feelings and views of everyone involved. So it is important to learn how all these things fit together in a situation of ethical concern, which is the task of the remainder of this book.

STUDY GUIDE

READINGS

K. D. Clouser, "What Is Medical Ethics?" p. 273.
Select your own from the bibliography.

QUESTIONS FOR REFLECTION

1 Think about your reaction to the cases of Chapter 1. Which type of theory, e.g., consequences, duties, rights, or relativism, are you using to resolve ethical problems?
2 For each case in Chapter 1, determine whether and, if so, how the problem identified might be different for each type of theory. Then determine how the resolution of that problem might be different from within the framework of each theory.
3 Find examples of situations, e.g., in newspapers, magazines, or other media, which show how someone has used a particular type of theory to resolve a problem.
4 Consider your resolution of the case study at the end of Chapter 1. Which type of theory did you use in resolving the problem?
5 As a continuation of question 4, make a list of the consequences you considered, the duties you noted (or followed), and the rights you honored in resolving the problem.

BIBLIOGRAPHY

Bayles, Michael D.: *Professional Ethics,* Wadsworth, Belmont, CA, 1981.

Beauchamp, Tom L., and James F. Childress: *Principles of Biomedical Ethics,* 2d ed., Oxford University Press, New York, 1983.

Beauchamp, Tom L., and Laurence B. McCullough: *Medical Ethics: The Moral Responsibilities of Physicians,* Prentice-Hall, Englewood Cliffs, NJ, 1984.

Benjamin, Martin, and Joy Curtis: *Ethics in Nursing,* 2d. ed., Oxford University Press, New York, 1986.

Engelhardt, H. Tristram, Jr.: *The Foundations of Bioethics,* Oxford University Press, New York, 1986.

Goldman, Alan H.: *The Moral Foundations of Professional Ethics,* Rowman and Littlefield, Totowa, NJ, 1980.

Jones, W. T., Frederick Sontag, Morton Beckner, and Robert J. Fogelin: *Approaches to Ethics: Representative Selections from Classical Times to the Present,* 3d. ed., McGraw-Hill, New York, 1977.

Pellegrino, Edmund, and David C. Thomasma: *A Philosophical Basis of Medical Practice: Toward a Philosophy of the Healing Professions,* Oxford University Press, New York, 1981.

Pollock, Lansing: *The Freedom Principle,* Prometheus Books, Buffalo, NY, 1981.

Veatch, Robert M.: *A Theory of Medical Ethics,* Basic Books, New York, 1981.

CHAPTER 3

SITUATION ASSESSMENT PROCEDURE: THE PROCESS OF ETHICAL DECISION MAKING

By opposing one another, medicine and philosophy can each balance the other's pretension to universality. By converging, they illuminate some of the most important questions of human existence.

Pellegrino and Thomasma*

FRAMEWORK FOR DECISION MAKING

Ethical problems arise in many contexts, and the specific problem that one professional faces in one situation may be different from that faced by a different professional in a similar situation. More important, even though the details of situations are different, there are common types of problems which occur over and over. Not only are the basic problems common, but also the general framework of situation assessment is common because it is a process, not a specific set of facts. Thus, no matter who you are, the *situation assessment procedure* involves the same four steps:

1 Identify the ethical issues and problems.
2 Identify and analyze available alternatives for action.
3 Select one alternative.
4 Justify your selection.

*A Philosophical Basis of Medical Practice, Oxford University Press, NY, 1980, p. 38

These four steps form the basis for ethical decisions no matter who you are or what your profession might be.

DECISION INFORMATION

No matter who is making a decision, information is the first thing that is needed. It is simply impossible to make a decision on the basis of no information, since there is nothing for the decision process to operate upon. When an ethical decision is made, five categories of information are necessary. The categories of information shown in Figure 3.1 are related to each other and to the resolution of the ethical problem.[1]

In Figure 3.1, *all* the major elements are shown by the arrows as having an effect on the decision. Notice also that each element has an effect on some of or all the other elements. Thus, for instance, people's value systems clearly affect how they decide, but their value systems also determine action constraints and how they interpret the data base. As an example, if your value system incorporates a high regard for life preservation, then you will have action constraints preventing the taking of life and you will assess the data base for elements supporting the preservation of life.

In this chapter we first examine these categories of decision information before we commence a detailed discussion of the situation assessment procedure.

---

[1]For a related, though less detailed, analysis, see Mila Aroskar, "Anatomy of an Ethical Dilemma," *American Journal of Nursing,* April 1980, pp. 658–660.

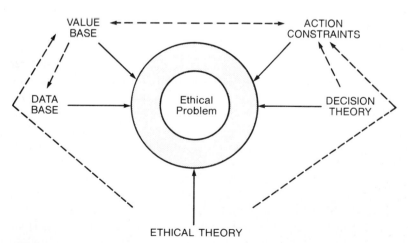

FIGURE 3.1
Categories of decision information.

Data Base

Ethical decisions are not factual decisions; yet ethical decisions cannot be adequately made without a solid basis in fact. When a decision situation arises, all the available information must be considered to determine what applies to the ethical question and what does not. Care must be taken to look not only at the medical data (diagnosis, prognosis, etc.) but also at the human data (age, social and economic situation, family situation, personal values, etc.). The data base of an ethical situation consists of all that information plus the result of identifying and clarifying key concepts.

Clarification of key concepts is a very important aspect of establishing a situation data base. To *clarify* a concept means to determine what that concept means and how it is being used in the situation. For example, in the following case, the concept of quality of life is the key concept. Can you see why it needs clarification?

CASE 3.1

Ruth Miller and Susan Williams are discussing the case of baby Regina Pollard. Regina was born prematurely and suffers from several birth defects, including cleft palate, brain damage (which can cause mental retardation), and duodenal atresia (food cannot pass from the stomach to the intestine). Although the atresia is easily corrected by surgery and the brain damage may not be extensive, Ruth says the baby ought not be treated:

Susan: You are quite wrong! She should be treated because her quality of life is more than adequate. Even if she is retarded, there are sheltered workshops and special schools. She can be a productive member of society.

Ruth: It is quite clear that her quality of life will be minimal. How can she be a productive member of society if she is retarded?

Obviously, Ruth and Susan each mean something different by the term *quality of life;* thus their assessments of Regina's condition differ. They also appear to have different views about what constitutes being a "productive member" of society. Since both are key concepts in their arguments, their usage must be clear before the problem can be assessed. For example, Ruth probably uses *productive member of society* to mean "able to live on her own, earn her own living, and conduct a normal life." Notice that even this does not fully clarify things, since we also need to know how Ruth is using the term *normal life*, before the argument can be understood. Now try to come up with an explanation of the key terms as Susan uses them.

Value Base

The values operating in a situation and the way they are affecting the situation form part of the data for a case. Value data are so detailed and complex, however, that they need to be identified and examined separately from the other data. As noted in Chapter 1, the identification of explicit and implicit values (both your own and other people's) is crucial, since values have such a significant impact on ethical decisions. How do values affect decisions? As you will recall, values affect ethical decisions in three ways:

1 *Values frame the problem.* We "see" a problem (or fail to see it) on the basis of the values we apply to the situation.

2 *Values supply alternatives.* The alternatives that we consider as possible resolutions for a problem are determined on the basis of the values we apply to our potential actions.

3 *Values direct judgment.* The judgment (reasoning) on the basis of which a problem is resolved is framed by the values we wish to uphold or promote.

It is also important to recognize that individual values are not the only ones that affect a situation; there are also group values. Because of this, we can see

MACROVALUES	MICROVALUES	INDIVIDUAL VALUES
Society Always tell the truth	**Family** Never lie to Mom and Dad	**Self** Lie only for self protection
Hospital policy All patients must be coded	**Oncology unit** Never prolong suffering	**Oncology nurse** Never prevent death when the patient is suffering
Society Everyone has a right to good health care	**Hospital policy** All patients must prove they are able to pay before care is given	**Staff physician** I have a duty to care for any person who needs care
Professional code All members must keep their knowledge and skills up to date	**Hospital policy** All staff members must complete 20 CEU's every year	**Therapist** It is wrong for me to neglect my family just for a class
Religion Extraordinary means of life support are not morally required	**Patient's family** We want you to do all you can to keep him alive	**Patient** I refuse to consent to surgery and request that a No-Code order be written

FIGURE 3.2
Comparison of values at different levels.

values operating at various levels, frequently at the *same* time. Depending on the size of the group, values occur on a macro level and a micro level, in addition to the individual level.[2] The macro values are those held by the largest group under consideration, the micro values are those held by the smallest group, and the individual values are those held by a single person. The chart in Figure 3.2 demonstrates these levels through comparative examples. Notice in the chart that the groups at the micro and macro levels vary considerably.

In many instances, the values operating in a situation will coincide at all three levels; at other times, there may be differences both within levels and between levels. Thus the values of two institutions may be at odds, just as the values of two individuals may not agree. There will usually be an ethical problem in those cases where the values do *not* coincide at all levels. The issue of truth telling in health care is a good example of how these levels of values may conflict. In society as a whole (the macro level), telling the truth (being honest) is taken to be very important. There are laws against perjury, and people are thought dishonest if they do not tell the truth. In the health care professions (the micro level), however, the generally accepted principle is that the truth may not be told if the professional believes it will cause harm. If a health care professional believed that the truth must always be told, that person's values would conflict with the micro value but correspond with the macro value.

There are, then, two ways that values must be recognized in situation assessment. First, we must determine what values are operating in the situation. Second, we must determine where there are conflicts, which requires identifying the level at which the values are occurring.

Action Constraints

An inevitable fact of life is that we cannot always do what we would like to do. Nowhere is this more evident than in the practice of a health care profession. Because many practitioners are in the employ of someone else, be it an institution or the person for whom the practitioner is caring, they must operate, at least to some degree, according to the wishes of the employer. Although this is usually not a problem, in those situations where values conflict there may be serious problems. When an ethical decision has to be made, the constraints imposed by the employer may be significant, even to the point where the practitioners may stop work rather than compromise their values. However, the practitioners may compromise their values in order to keep their jobs, thereby operating under the constraints imposed by the employer.

Not all constraints are imposed by employers, however. Society, through its laws and traditional standards, may also place constraints on how a person may

---

[2]This approach was suggested by Raymond Duff, in conversations of October 1983.

act. For example, there are laws against actions which are contrary to social values, such as robbery and murder. These laws, like any others, place constraints on the actions of individuals, by enforcing penalties which are intended, by their severity, to make the doing of the act not worthwhile.

Individuals may also have personal constraints, values which they hold so important as to be inviolable—personal laws, if you wish, that impose sanctions of guilt, remorse, and ill feeling when they are violated. Certainly not all personal values are this strong. The idea is that personal values represent things of importance to us, so by committing ourselves to a value, we commit ourselves to upholding that value. When our values are at odds with those of another, depending on the importance of the value and the severity of its violation, we may see ourselves as obliged to take a particular action. The action we take may be positive, as LuAnn Carter might do if she reported Milton (Case 2.3); or it may be negative, in that we refuse to act because acting would violate the value in question.

In addition to value constraints, several others must be considered in the full assessment of any situation. One important constraint is the capability of the person(s) who must act. If you are incapable of performing an action, then that action is not an option for you, although you may try to find someone to do it for you. For example, if an emergency situation requires surgery and you do not know how to do it, then performing surgery is not an option for you. But knowledge is not the only constraint here; you may know the procedure for surgery, but still be unable to do it, for instance, if you are ill or injured yourself.

Another important constraint is time. Do you have enough time to do what you think is necessary? For example, if someone who has a cardiac arrest has not indicated somehow that she does not wish to be coded,[3] there is no time to make phone calls or search the record to determine the person's wishes. Treatment must be started immediately or not at all, so time is a crucial factor constraining one's action in such situations.

With some thought, you ought to be able to determine other areas where a person's actions may be constrained, for various reasons. It is important for you to think about such constraints, because, like values, constraints may be an important factor in how an ethical problem may be resolved.

Ethical theory

The ethical theories discussed in Chapter 2 are very important to the process of doing ethics, because we cannot understand an ethical problem unless we understand the theories it rests upon. Very often the root of a disagreement lies in the problem being seen in the context of different theories. Someone who is looking at a problem from the consequences-based theory may well disagree

---

[3]Treated with all available medicines and means of resuscitation to try and restore them to life.

with someone looking at that problem from a rights-based theory. If that difference is never identified, the situation will never be fully understood. Moreover, because a theory provides a method for making decisions, understanding the theory a person is using will help in understanding the decision reached.

At the same time, the practical dimension of ethical decision making cannot be ignored. An ethical decision based solely on abstract theories and constructs is only an empty gesture which will not resolve a problem. Certainly one cannot do ethics without consideration of the theories, but theories are not all there is to ethics. At best, a theory is a model, a framework for consideration and a method for decisions. No theory will itself resolve an ethical problem; however, if the theory is coupled with thinking about all the decision factors *as they relate to the situation,* then problems may be resolved. In some ways, the theory can serve as an ideal, something toward which we must strive. But to focus exclusively on the ideal is to play short the entirety of the ethical process.

SITUATION ASSESSMENT PROCEDURE

We have been discussing key elements of a problem situation, but now we turn to the *process* of ethical decision making. Perhaps the best way to see the relation between what has been discussed up to now and the situations upon which that material will focus is to notice that the decision factors just label types of information and ways of thinking. It is the situation which supplies the information to be labeled and thought about. The difficulty is how to work the data and framework into a unified understanding of the situation which can be used in a broader process to resolve the problem.

The process we use is called the *situation assessment procedure.*[4] Designed to formalize the ethical decision process, the situation assessment procedure helps ensure the gathering and utilizing of appropriate information. If you learn this procedure, you will not have to work randomly through the decision factors and will be able to incorporate them into a systematic decision process. The procedure consists of four steps:

Situation Assessment Procedure

1 Identify the ethical issues and problems.
2 Identify and analyze available alternatives for action.
3 Select one alternative.
4 Justify your selection.

In the rest of this chapter we work through each step of the procedure, in an attempt to help you get started using it. We will then continue to use the procedure for case assessment throughout the book.

[4]This procedure was suggested by work of E. Pellegrino and D. Thomasma.

Identifying Ethical Issues and Problems

The primary activity at this stage of situation assessment is the creation of the data base. We went over that in some detail earlier, so we do not repeat it here. Suffice it to say that you must find out the facts, including both the technical and human elements, identify the values operating in the situation, and determine how differences of value affect the situation.

The ultimate aim of your data-gathering activities is the identification of ethical problems and options for resolving those problems. Since correct problem identification is crucial for adequate problem resolution, the data base must be carefully established. Unfortunately, our personal biases often cause us to overlook or discount some information, with the result that our thinking is misdirected. For this reason, it is easy for different people to identify different problems in the same situation.

To avoid this pitfall, you need to recognize that ethical *issues,* which lead to ethical problems, are the same for everyone. An *issue* identifies an area of concern, regardless of whether there is a problem present. Ethical issues are present in every case, but ethical problems are not; at the same time, you cannot have a problem without an issue first being present. Since identification of a problem can only follow the identification of an issue, you must learn to recognize ethical issues, so that you will be able to adequately recognize problems.

As an example of this relation between issues and problems, consider the matter of confidentiality. Clearly, confidentiality is an issue in *every* health care situation, given an individual's right to privacy and the fact that someone other than the patient has knowledge of private, personal information. At the same time, the fact that confidentiality is an issue in each case does not mean that there is an ethical problem of confidentiality in each case. If the situation does not put the private matter at risk of disclosure, then there is no ethical *problem* of confidentiality. Consider the following case to see this difference.

CASE 3.2

Malinda Reeves is a medical records specialist who works for the Public Health Service. One aspect of her job is to review all communicable disease reports for her district. In the process of one such review, she discovers that both the patient and the contact for a venereal disease case are her husband's co-workers.

Confidentiality is always an ethical issue for any records specialist. Only in a situation where that confidentiality may be violated will an ethical problem arise, because without likelihood of disclosure there is no problem. The information above gives no indication of an ethical problem. Suppose, however, that the case were to continue as follows:

Malinda knows from conversation with her husband that the patient regularly dates other members of the office staff. Moreover, right now the patient is dating Malinda's brother Henry. Malinda would like to protect Henry from harm (contracting VD), so she begins to think of ways that her brother can find out about his girlfriend's problem.

Now there is clearly an ethical problem, for Malinda's disclosure would violate confidence, even if she were only to tell her boss so that the patient could be contacted for further information. If Malinda had simply noted the information, with no thought of disclosing her additional knowledge, then there would be no problem of confidentiality (although there might be other problems). Notice, however, that we are identifying a problem, not passing judgment on her actions—that will come later. For now, suffice it to say that an argument may be made both for and against disclosure.

As a means of recognizing ethical problems, it is often helpful to recognize the occurrence of an ethical dilemma. An *ethical dilemma* is a situation in which no matter what a person does, the result will be something which is not desirable. In Case 3.2, for example, Malinda is faced with a choice: either she maintains confidence and risks her brother's health, or she violates the confidence but does not risk her brother's health. She is in a no-win situation; no matter what she does, she cannot both maintain privacy and protect her brother. This either-or situation, from which no clearly correct response arises, is an ethical dilemma, and any ethical dilemma presents an ethical problem.

One caution: When you are identifying a problem, be sure to do so in general terms, not in terms specific to one particular resolution of the problem. An example of an *incorrect* statement of the problem in Case 3.2 is the following: "The problem in this case is whether Malinda should tell her brother about his girlfriend's infection or whether she should tell her boss and have the boss contact her brother." The mistake is that the two things stated are really alternative solutions for the problem. More important, they are alternatives which result from assuming that the dilemma (to maintain confidence or protect her brother) should be resolved in favor of the protection. It is as if Malinda said, "OK, I have to protect my brother, so how am I going to do it?" Granted, how to protect him is a problem, but *only* if it has already been decided that he should be protected.

This brings up another point in regard to identifying problems, namely, that every effort must be made to identify the *primary* problem, not just the *secondary* problem(s) of the case. The primary problem is always the one which presents the broad issues, often in the context of a dilemma. The secondary problem(s) either result from a specific resolution of the primary problem(s) or are additional, though less important, problems in the situation. How Malinda's brother is to be protected is secondary to the problem of whether he ought to be protected *and* is dependent on a specific resolution to that problem. Whenever an ethical problem situation is being considered, we must be certain that the *primary* problem is clear and that it is distinct from any secondary problem(s).

Remember, too, that there is always a need to be careful about clarifying key concepts. *Key concepts* are those upon which the resolution of a problem will depend. In Case 3.2, we need to be clear about the meaning of the term *confidentiality,* since that is the concept on which the problems in this case center. For example, Malinda could notify her boss of the problem, reasoning that this does not break confidence because her boss, as part of the team, has legitimate access to the information. This approach defines *breaking confidence* to mean "giving information outside the team," which is certainly not the standard definition, although it is frequently used in health care practice. A different definition of the concept might be "giving no information to anyone." Clearly the problem will change radically depending on which definition is used. You should keep this need for clarity in mind when presenting your own work, since lack of clarity is a problem no matter where it occurs. *Never* assume that the person to whom you are speaking is using a key concept in the same way as you are; key concepts should *always* be made explicit.

To return to the original matter of identifying issues, be aware that there are several additional issues which occur on a regular basis and thus indicate potential problems. One issue always present in health care situations is truth telling. At a minimum, from the health care professional's side of the case, there is a question of whether all the requested information is given out and whether the information given is accurate. However, there is always a question about whether the patient is giving all the necessary information and whether the information being given is accurate. The following case gives an excellent example of truth-telling issues in combination with confidentiality issues.

CASE 3.3

Steve B. is brought to the emergency room by ambulance after an automobile accident. He is unconscious and in critical condition with multiple injuries. After his clothes are removed, several plastic bags of white powder are found taped to his abdomen. These are placed in a bag with his other personal articles, and treatment is continued. When Steve's condition is stabilized, the unit clerk goes to find more information about the accident. In talking with the police officer she learns that the accident was the result of a high-speed chase—the police were trying to arrest Steve because he is a known drug dealer who was seen selling a bag of white powder. The officer asks whether any more bags were found when he was undressed. The clerk knows that they were, since she did the personal-posessions inventory, but she wonders whether to tell the officer.

As the case stands, confidence is clearly an issue. Also, since the bags probably contain illegal drugs, there is the *issue* of whether health care professionals have a moral obligation to report suspected drug dealers. Finally, since the police officer asked a question, the issue of truth telling (in the response to the officer) is also present.

The clerk, however, is also facing ethical problems in this situation. She must make a choice between ethical alternatives which are competing and cannot both be chosen; she is faced with an ethical dilemma. To act, she must choose between maintaining privacy, which could require lying to the police officer, or telling the truth and compromising Steve's privacy. And all this is compounded by the problem of fulfilling her duties as a citizen (whatever they may be). Also, the specific *problem* the clerk sees in this case will depend on her values. For instance, if she operates on a value system which approves of drug dealing, then her response might be different from that of a person whose value is that drug dealing is the worst possible offense anyone can commit. The first person might then see no problem in maintaining privacy, while the second person most likely will see a serious problem.

Yet another issue almost always found in health care situations is that of consent. In the strictest sense, we need to have consent for anything done to a person, be it amputating a leg or taking a temperature. Thus, whenever something is being done to a person, consent is an issue. Once again, however, there will be a problem only in some cases, such as those situations where appropriate consent is not obtained or obtaining consent conflicts with some other action also seen as morally correct.

As part of your skills for looking at ethical situations, you need to recognize these issues (and others) and learn how problems arise from them. Note, however, that identifying a problem (or potential problem) does *not* involve making a judgment about the moral correctness of an act; it is simply the identification of a certain type of situation.

The importance of spending time sorting out the issues and problems cannot be stressed enough. Issues are complex and appear in many different ways. Certainly it is easy to make a snap judgment about an issue, but there is an important correlation between how long you spend trying to understand an issue *before* trying to deal with it and the quality of your thinking. By paying careful attention to the questions—What is the issue here? What are the hidden issues? What exactly are the complexities of this situation? Am I overlooking anything?—you will be much better equipped to deal with the issues. Similarly, identification of the problem in a careful way will enable you to deal with it effectively and adequately. Don't be afraid to take time; *do* be afraid of snap judgments.

In this way of looking at cases, every health care situation involves some ethical issues, but not every situation involves ethical problems. The job in doing ethics is to distinguish those two things as they actually occur, which is easier said than done. The case data rarely lead you directly to that distinction. Instead, you will have to learn some basic questions that you can ask yourself about a case, so that you can uncover issues and problems. The following list of questions is incomplete; but you can develop still more questions by using this list as a beginning and a model.

Assessment Questions

1 Are there values which may conflict?

2 Are there aspects of the case which do not seem to depend on the medical facts? Is there still a question about the case, even after all the medical facts are known?

3 Is there a disagreement over patient care?

   a Is there a patient-staff disagreement? Is there a family-staff or family-patient disagreement?

   b Does the family interaction help, hinder, or threaten care?

   c What is the patient's reaction to care? Does the patient have a normal reaction to care? Does the patient want care?

   d If there is staff disagreement, is it over the technical dimensions of care, e.g., a disagreement over diagnosis or prognosis? Or is the disagreement over how care should be given, the patient's role in care, consent, etc.?

4 How has the decision making been accomplished? Has there been complete involvement of the patient, family, and staff? If not, why not?

5 Are there uncomfortable choices to be made? Does it appear that no choice of action is really a good one? Does it appear that it might be impossible to do what you think is right?

6 Are there specific issues easily identified, e.g., confidentiality, truth telling, paternalism, etc.?

Once you learn to use these questions, and others that you will develop as you go along, it will be much easier to recognize ethical issues and thus to identify ethical problems. In fact, many people find it helpful to use these questions as a type of ethical history taking, a way of gathering information pertinent to identifying the issues and problems in a case.

Identifying Alternatives for Action

Once the data base has been established for a situation and the problem(s) identified, you need to develop a set of alternatives for action. An *alternative for action* is a possible way to resolve the problem. For each problem you ought to be able to develop a list of several possible resolutions. What is a "possible" resolution? It is one for which reasons may be given and which actually can be taken, with the proposed result. An action does not, at this point, cease to count as an alternative simply because you would probably not choose it for your solution.

This last point is important enough to deserve added comment. The purpose of alternative listing is to help make your resolution of the problem a *choice,* not simply a reaction. You cannot choose if you only have one option for action. Since our personal values tend to set up conditions for snap judgments and standard reactions to similar cases, we often exclude good options simply by not looking for them. How many times, after you have done something, do you find you could have done it better in another way? If you are like most people, this happens quite often. Identification of alternatives as a conscious part of the assessment procedure is an effort to overcome that problem and develop better choices.

Developing a set of alternatives is not easy, since you must learn to look at the situation from different perspectives. You must also develop a spirit of creativity, for finding good solutions to problems is not easy and does not work like a cookbook. To help you develop alternatives you might consider the following four areas of questions:

1 *What are the reasonable possibilities for action?* One of the hardest things to learn is that it is possible to come up with different alternatives to the resolution of a problem. Sometimes there is a great difference, e.g., have an abortion or not have an abortion. At the same time, there may be subtle differences, e.g., talk to the doctor versus talk to the spouse versus talk to the brother of a patient. When determining alternatives, you want to consider not only the ways different people might solve the problem, but also the action constraints that you have discovered in your situation assessment. Keep in mind that you want to have as many reasonable courses of action as possible. One important question that always needs to be asked, but which people often overlook, is this: How do the different affected parties want to resolve the problem?

2 *What ethical principles are required for each alternative?* This question is necessary because you need to understand what each alternative requires in terms of ethical presuppositions. In answering it, you will need to use your knowledge of ethical theories, since they are the ultimate base for ethical principles. For example, an alternative for an abortion case that suggests having an abortion presupposes an ethical principle which allows abortion. Or, an alternative which proposes talking to members of a patient's family to resolve a problem presupposes an understanding of confidentiality which makes this possible. Or, an alternative which suggests discontinuing treatment presupposes a principle allowing such action. As part of this principle identification, you need to ask yourself whether there are conflicting principles in different options. Conflict indicates difficulty with the alternative.

3 *What assumptions are required for each alternative, and what are their implications for future action?* What unstated facts, principles, or values must you accept as true if you take the alternative as correct? These unstated elements, which are called *assumptions,* are particularly important if the alternative depends on them. Because assumptions are unstated, they are frequently overlooked. Yet, if the assumption is necessary for the alternative, the assumption must be examined along with the stated elements. It is important to identify those things which are built into the option so that if you choose the option, you will know what you are committed to as part of that option.

In health care situations, there are almost always unstated assumptions about the purpose of health care. For example, some people believe that the goal of health care is to preserve life at all costs, while others believe that health care should preserve life only when there is good quality of life. Obviously, decisions based on these two goals can be radically different; what is more important, though, is that one will "see" health care differently depending on which goal is assumed to be proper.

4 *What, if any, are the additional ethical problems which the alternatives raise?* Would you cause additional problems by choosing this alternative? This is a crucial consideration if you do not want to create more problems than you resolve. Sometimes additional problems cannot be avoided because there are too many things at issue, and often the choice involves dealing with a lesser problem. But usually, if you are careful in developing your alternatives and are aware of the problems that the alternatives raise, you can successfully resolve an ethical problem.

Once you have a range of alternatives from which to choose, you are ready to begin the two final stages of the process, selection and justification of your action.

Selecting and Justifying an Alternative

Selecting an alternative for action, at least in our model, requires thought and care. You could select in a number of ways which are not thoughtful, e.g., throwing darts at a list, flipping a coin, rolling dice, closing your eyes and pointing, etc. But none of those actions will yield a *reasoned* selection. Since the ethical process requires a reasoned selection among alternatives, none of these means of selection is acceptable for the process. When an alternative is selected without reasoning, it is not part of the ethical process and so is only coincidentally ethical.

A justified alternative is one for which you can give reasons showing why the decision was correct. This means that you need to be able to answer the questions, Why did you decide to do *that?* and Why did you decide to do it that *way?* Normally these questions are applied to lots of different situations and are, in effect, requests for explanation of your reasons for action. Since explanations are always in order for other actions, there is no reason why they cannot be expected for ethical situations as well. This is particularly true since, as we saw in Chapter 2, relativism (understood as being one's own authority) is simply not acceptable.

Justification is essentially a logical process in which you present the resolution for the problem and your reasons why that is the best resolution. In logical terms, you are presenting an argument. Your resolution is the *conclusion* of your argument, while the reasons are the *premises* which are intended to show why that conclusion is correct. Presenting your justification via argument is very important in doing ethics. While examination of values, theories, etc., allows us to uncover our beliefs, argument allows us to go beyond that and say *why* we believe.

If you claim that something is correct, then you are obliged to give reasons why. Simply saying "I believe this is correct" is worth nothing alone. "Because I say so" is not a reason for correctness, although it may be a reason for obedience. Here the "Who are you to say?" point raised in Chapter 2 really does apply. However, the fact that this question is appropriate in these circumstances does not mean that we can never know what is right. The question is appropriate because what is true, or right, or correct, is established on the basis of argument (reasons), not authority. The truth (rightness, or correctness) of a claim is *never* determined on the basis of who makes the claim. No one, by virtue of position, degree, or experience, is, on that basis alone, automatically correct. Rational discourse, upon which the ethical process depends, is rooted in the willingness to engage in the reasoning process, not in blind acceptance of other people's views.

When you formulate your justification, the arguments you use need to answer the essential "Why?" questions raised by your resolution. To do this, the reasons which you present in support of your view must meet two criteria: they must be relevant, and they must be sufficient. A reason is *relevant* to the point at issue if it gives information about that issue. For example, were someone to say, "Abortion is wrong" and you asked "Why?" the response "Because roses are red and violets are blue" would not be a relevant reason. Irrelevant reasons are essentially worthless, because they are not reasons which support the claim you are making. A relevant reason for the abortion claim might be "Because it is wrong to kill." This would be relevant, although without clarification and expansion it is not in itself sufficient to show your claim is true.

The second requirement, that the set of reasons given be *sufficient,* means simply that you must have enough relevant reasons to make your case. Again, in the abortion example, the response "Because my mother told me" may be relevant, but it is not sufficient. Why is your mother correct? What makes her a good source of information or an authority on the matter? How do you know what she says is reliable? The more difficult the argument, the more relevant premises are needed to have a sufficient number. For example, the claim "It is morally wrong to throw babies off the Empire State Building in order to see how much noise they make when they hit the ground" would not require many reasons to show its correctness. However, the claim "Abortion is wrong" would take more reasons to back up because it is a much more complicated question.

Another dimension of the sufficiency requirement is that the reasons given must be true (or accepted as true). An argument is of little practical value if the reasons are false, because then it is not a sound argument. Moreover, false reasons, like irrelevant reasons, are not supporting evidence for the point at issue; and our task must always be directed toward the point at issue, or it is a waste of time. False reasons are a waste of time.

In sum, the justification for your resolution to an ethical problem is really an argument wherein you present relevant and sufficient reasons for the correctness of that resolution.

One question that people usually ask is, How do I know what reasons are needed? The answer is that you must learn from the experience of case analysis. There is no rule which says you need a certain number of reasons to support a given type of argument. You simply have to try and make your argument as complete as possible without being trivial.

Completeness is aided by two specific considerations. First, you need to be careful to present material that will *clarify the key concepts* of your discussion. We have discussed concept clarification earlier, so we do no more with it here. Second, you need to *anticipate objections* to your views and include as much as possible in your argument to respond to those objections. In fact, a main element in learning to do ethics is developing the skills necessary to anticipate objections. That is, you need to learn how to figure out ahead of time what faults other people might find with your argument. Then, by adequately speaking to those objections you can effectively deal with them. When an ethical argument is constructed, this is extremely important because premises are not sufficient if they are rejected or if they cannot be accepted for some reason. You can prevent their rejection by obviating the reasons for that rejection. You can also present a better, more detailed argument if you anticipate objections. Psychologically, your position is also made stronger by concern for this factor, since your position will be more acceptable to people if they are unable to find anything serious to criticize.

The anticipation of objections has another important role in doing ethics; it helps you become more familiar with the views of others. You cannot know how people will object to your argument if you do not know how they think about things. Since ethical discourse requires understanding other people's views, this is a means for accomplishing that task. You might ask yourself, then, "Given what I have said, what could someone else say to try to convince me that I am wrong?" and "How will I respond?"

As with other dimensions of the situation assessment procedure, it is not easy to use argument and reasoning skills in presenting your views. You will have to work at it, striving for improvement and understanding of the process itself. In the remainder of the book, as we look at specific ethical problems, our discussion of sample cases cites many examples of this process. You can begin developing your skills, however, by working through the case studies at the end of this chapter.

CONCLUDING THOUGHTS

This chapter has described the elements in ethical decision making, both to familiarize you with them and to help you begin to see the complexity of such decisions. In the following chapters we continue with this effort by looking in more detail at specific ethical problems in health care. Remember, however, that a book can only raise awareness; true understanding and expansion of knowledge depend on what you do with that awareness. Thus you have to make a conscious effort to recognize situations involving ethical problems and to work through the decision elements until you understand them clearly. This activity is *not* limited to health care cases which you encounter. You can do this, for example, when you read the newspaper or weekly news magazines, since there are always ethical issues in the news.

The key to progress in ethics is that you must recognize *your* responsibility. No one can do ethics for you; it is a thinking activity, and only you can do your thinking. What you get out of it depends on you; how you handle ethical problems in your life is your responsibility, not anyone else's. If you don't know what you are doing, neither will anyone else. The burden is yours. What you choose to do about it is up to you.

SITUATION ASSESSMENT PROCEDURE: SUMMARY OUTLINE

1 *Identify the problem.*
  a *Establish the essential data.* What are the technical facts? What are the relevant nontechnical facts? Are there necessary facts which are unknown? What more do you need to know, and why do you need to know it? Are the key concepts clear?
  b *Isolate the significant human elements.* Investigate age, social and economic situation, family situation, etc.
  c *Identify and sort the value elements.* What are the different values operative in the situation, e.g., religious, economic, social, moral, and legal?
  d *Determine what values are influencing or causing the problem.* Within each type of value, which particular values are affecting the situation? Once the problematic values are identified, is more than one problem apparent? Are there different problems depending on how the identified facts of the case are considered in relation to the key values?
2 *Develop alternatives for action.*
  a *Establish the reasonable possibilities for action.* What things is it possible to do? What restraints on action are relevant? What means might different people utilize to resolve the problem? How do the affected parties want to resolve the problem?
  b *Determine the ethical principles required for each alternative.* What ethical principle(s) must be accepted as true for each alternative to be chosen? What effect would an alternative principle have on the choice of an option?

Are there conflicting principles operative in any one alternative? Are there conflicting principles when different alternatives are compared?

c *Determine the ethical assumptions necessary for each alternative.* What things must be accepted as correct in order for an action to be considered acceptable? Are there conflicting assumptions in any option? Are there conflicting assumptions between different options?

d *Determine what additional ethical problems the alternatives raise.* Would you create more problems by choosing this alternative? Can these additional problems be avoided? Do they allow the choice of a lesser problem than the primary problem?

3 *Resolve the problem by selecting one of the alternatives.*

4 *Formulate a justification for your selection.*

a *Specify your reasons for the action.* What reasons can you give to support (show the correctness of) your decision? Are your reasons stated in as systematic and logical a way as possible? Are your reasons clear and precise? Do you have sufficient, relevant reasons? Why were the other alternatives rejected?

b *Clearly present the ethical basis for your reasons.* What ethical principles, rules, or codes support your reasons? What set of ethical values have you incorporated into your decision? Why have you used those particular values? Are the important ethical assumptions stated and made clear?

c *Understand the shortcomings of your justification.* Why were the other alternatives rejected? How is your justification still "tentative"? Are there ethical problems which will be caused by your solution?

d *Anticipate objections to your justification.* How might someone criticize your justification by using a different ethical theory for the decision? How might your justification be faulty? Are there criticisms to which a response would help make your justification stronger?

STUDY GUIDE

READINGS

M. Aroskar, "Are Nurses' Mind Sets Compatible with Ethical Practice?" p. 157.
D. Thomasma, "The Context as a Moral Rule in Medical Ethics," p. 142.

QUESTIONS FOR REFLECTION

1 Normal everyday experiences consistently involve us in decision making. Compare the situation assessment procedure with that process. How is it similar, and how does it differ?

2 Using the situation assessment procedure, return to the case studies of Chapters 1 and 2. Would you analyze any of them differently? What new features of each case do you see now that you did not see before? Is your resolution of any case different? Can you justify your previous resolution?

3 Try applying the situation assessment procedure to your daily decision making. How does it improve the process? How must it be modified, if at all, to your situation?

CASE STUDIES FOR ANALYSIS

Case Study 1   Mr. Fontanez is an 82-year-old who has been admitted to the medical service with a diagnosis of cancer of the pancreas which has metastasized (spread) to the liver, spleen, and bone. Upon admission, it is noted that Mr. Fontanez has gangrene of the foot and has already lost two toes. He is in considerable pain, with the daily cleaning and care of the foot causing more pain.

A surgeon is consulted and agrees with the attending physician that a partial amputation of the foot is the only hope for stopping the spread of gangrene. Since the surgeon is the one who will do the procedure, he approaches Mr. Fontanez for consent. He explains the procedure, tells Mr. Fontanez why it is necessary, and then asks him to sign the form consenting to the operation. Mr. Fontanez refuses to sign. The surgeon carefully explains the consequences of not having the operation (continued pain, spread of the disease, etc.). However, Mr. Fontanez still refuses, saying, "No, leave me alone and let me die in peace."

The medical staff meets to discuss the case and determine a way to handle his refusal for surgery. The primary care nurse suggests bringing Mr. Fontanez' daughter into the matter, since the daughter visits regularly and she and her father seem to have good rapport. The idea is that she might be able to convince him to have the surgery. Another suggestion is that the doctor have Mr. Fontanez' daughter appointed his guardian so that she can consent even if he won't. The attending physician does not agree with either suggestion. She believes that Mr. Fontanez is rational and making an informed choice, and thus his wishes should be honored. The surgeon disagrees, arguing that if Mr. Fontanez will not consent to the surgery, then he does not, in fact, understand the situation and thus his refusal is not informed.

As a member of the medical team, you are asked for suggestions as to how they might proceed. What would you suggest and why?

Analysis Questions   Can you identify the different values and ethical principles which are affecting this situation? Have all the reasonable alternatives been presented? What basic ethical principles are assumed in each suggested alternative? In formulating your answer, be sure to present an argument which gives supporting evidence for your solution.

Case Study 2 Willa is a 32-year-old mother of three children who is suffereing from advanced bone cancer. She has recently entered an experimental drug program which consists of giving the patient a large dose of a highly toxic substance, followed in 48 hours by a neutralizing agent. The treatment is given on an outpatient basis, since there are no side effects to the drug within the first 50 to 55 hours. At the beginning of the program, participants sign an agreement for the procedure, consenting to the risks (of which they are fully informed) and absolving the center of any responsibility should they not return for the neutralizing agent within the appropriate time.

One day Willa does not show up for the neutralizing agent. The physician for the program becomes concerned and has the secretary try to contact her. She does and reports that Willa said she will not be coming in, she has made her peace, and she plans to let the drug end her life.

As a member of the care team, the physician asks you to go with him to see Willa and help convince her to come in for the treatment. Should you go?

Analysis Questions Can you identify the values Willa is using? Can you identify the values the physician is using? How does analysis from different ethical perspectives change the outcome? What is the key assumption the physician is using? What would your alternatives be if you went to Willa's house? What additional facts would be helpful in resolving this case? Why would *those* facts be important?

BIBLIOGRAPHY

Aroskar, Mila: "Anatomy of an Ethical Dilemma," *American Journal of Nursing,* April 1980, pp. 658–660.

Brett, Allan S.: "Hidden Ethical Issues in Clinical Decision Analysis," *New England Journal of Medicine,* vol. 305, no. 19, November 1981, pp. 1150–1152.

Burke, Gary: "Ethics and Medical Decision-Making," *Primary Care,* vol. 7, no. 4, December 1980, pp. 615–624.

Fromer, Margot J.: "Solving Ethical Dilemmas in Nursing Practice," *Topics in Clinical Nursing,* vol. 4, no. 1, April 1982, pp. 15–22.

Kassirer, Jerome: "The Principles of Clinical Decision Making: An Introduction to Decision Analysis," *Yale Journal of Biology and Medicine,* vol. 49, 1976, pp. 149–164.

Veatch, Robert M.: *Case Studies in Medical Ethics,* Harvard University Press, Cambridge, MA, 1978.

CHAPTER 4

PRIVACY AND CONFIDENTIALITY

. . . ye shall not disclose secrets confided unto you. . . .

Seter Asaph ha-Rofe*

In protecting a patient's secrets, [the professional] must be more insistent than the patient himself.

Haly Abbas**

A LOOK AT THE BASIC ISSUES

From the time we are children, we seem to have an intuitive sense of privacy; that is, we seem hesitant to let others know *everything* about us. We have some secrets, things we do not tell to anyone, except our therapist perhaps, because they help form a part of our lives which is uniquely our own. Similarly, we come to expect that others will keep secrets for us, at least if we ask them to, thus allowing us to share something of our private selves yet maintain a level of privacy. And the most devastating thing a friend can do is to fail to keep secret what was shared. Privacy is also firmly established in law, with 34 states currently protecting the confidence of information gained by a physician while

---

Book of Asaph The Physician, Warren T. Reich (ed.) *Encyclopedia of Bioethics*, Free Press, NY, 1978, vol. 4, p. 1733
**Kamel Al Sanaah al Tildoa*, Warren T. Reich (ed.) *Encyclopedia of Bioethics*, Free Press, NY, 1978, vol. 4, p. 1734

caring for a patient.[1] At the federal level, the Privacy Act of 1975 (Public Law 93-579), passed following the Watergate disclosures, established a range of federal laws relative to privacy and disclosure of confidential information. Constitutional law has been especially concerned with privacy. In fact, privacy served as the basis for the famous Supreme Court decision allowing abortion, in the case of *Roe v. Wade*, in 1973.

Given this general social concern with privacy and the fact that privacy and confidentiality are closely connected, it is not surprising that keeping patient information confidential is an important aspect of health care—so important that nearly every health care profession requires confidentiality of its members in its professional code of conduct.[2] Although the wording may differ for other groups, the code for nurses of the American Nurses' Association is a good example of such a requirement:

> The nurse safeguards the client's right to privacy by judiciously protecting information of a confidential nature. . . . The right of privacy is an inalienable right of all persons, and the nurse has a clear obligation to safeguard confidential information about the client acquired from any source.[3]

Because this statement is an element of the code under which nurses are expected to practice, it imposes on nurses a professional duty to respect the privacy, thus confidence, of each individual with whom they work. This duty has its counterpart in the Patient's Bill of Rights (reproduced in the Appendix), which says

> The patient has the right to every consideration of his privacy. . . . Case discussion, consultation, examination and treatment are confidential and records pertaining to his care should be treated as confidential.

If there seems to be such universal recognition of the need for privacy and the requirement for confidentiality, why do we devote a chapter to the topic? There are two important reasons. First, we need to understand what *confidentiality* means and how requirements for confidence may be justified. Second, we need to examine problems which arise in practice and involve confidential information.

The first concern arises because the simple fact that we see a need for privacy and have professional codes and laws which protect privacy does not give us a justification (in the sense discussed in Chapter 3) for accepting as true the claim that privacy is morally required. We will need to spend time trying to discover what such a justification would involve because, without it, appeals to confidentiality have no serious basis. Moreover, the professional codes and laws are

---

[1]Health Law Center, *Hospital-Law Manual*, vol. IIA, Appendix A, Aspen Systems Corp., Aspen CO, 1982, p.97.

[2]Compare the different statements on confidentiality contained in the professional codes reproduced in the Appendix. How do they differ? How are they the same? Do they seem to serve the same basic purpose?

[3]American Nurses' Association, *Code for Nurses with Interpretive Statements*, American Nurses' Association, Washington, pp. 6–7.

not clear; for example, what does it mean to give someone "every consideration of his privacy"? Does that mean we never break a confidence? Does it mean that only caregivers should have access to patient information? What of the fact that the health care process cannot function without patients giving up a good deal of their privacy? What, in fact, do we mean by *confidentiality?* A close examination will help us develop the conceptual clarity to deal effectively with practical problems.

The second reason for considering confidentiality in detail arises from two facets of information sharing in health care. On one hand, necessary practices of health care professionals often seem to require the breaking of a strict confidence, since many people are engaged in caring for a patient and they must discuss the case with one another. Moreover, the health care system must be primarily aimed at gathering and analyzing the most intimate of personal information if its goal of care is to be met. On the other hand, there often appears to be a general disregard for confidentiality among many health care professionals; cases are often discussed at break, at meals, in the halls and elevators, and so on. When there is an "interesting" patient on a unit, it is not unheard of for staff from other units to stop by and read the chart; if the patient is *very* interesting, it is not long before many people in the hospital know about the case. Such activity, however, is overshadowed by a more pressing concern: Increasing use of computer data bases for storing personal information (e.g., credit agencies, health insurers, educational institutions, etc.) presents a serious threat to privacy because such data bases are not secure. And our elaborate health insurance system guarantees that a large amount of health care related personal information will pass through the hands of countless people who play no role in the health care itself. When all that is added to the fact that health care is at least in part science, and science relies on shared information for progress, maintaining privacy seems a hopeless cause. In fact, one writer has argued, "The principle of medical confidentiality described in medical codes of ethics and still believed in by patients no longer exists."[4] But what of our codes and laws?

It would seem that we have a double standard; we extol privacy and confidence in theory, law, and professional codes, but we do not uphold it in practice. Do we have, then, "privacy in theory" and "privacy in practice," in the same way that we have equality of women and men and yet a woman and a man may be paid different wages for doing the same job? Do the two not always go together? If we do believe (as we seem to) that privacy is so important, then our study in this chapter is necessary to sort out this double standard and to try to determine how privacy *ought* to be understood. By doing this we will be able to enhance our basic feeling for privacy with some good solid reasoning. And we will come to understand more clearly the privacy and confidentiality issues so that we may

---

[4]Mark Siegler, "Confidentiality in Medicine—A Decrepit Concept," *New England Journal of Medicine,* vol. 307, no. 24, December 1982, p.1520.

work toward resolution of those issues and perhaps lessen the theory-practice gap. To accomplish that task, we will look carefully at basic justifications for upholding privacy via confidentiality, and then examine a set of cases to sharpen our understanding of the issues.

Before we begin that task, one last point should be made. We must carefully define the scope of our investigation, because confidence can be seen in both a broad and a narrow way. The broad sense of the word *confidence* covers all types of secrecy, including, for example, the cover-up of professional errors or the membership rites to a secret society. The narrow sense, and that on which we want to focus, restricts the term *confidence* to protecting the privacy of a patient or client, relative to the care and treatment of that person.

JUSTIFYING PRIVACY AND CONFIDENTIALITY

Whenever people are asked to explain why privacy and confidence should be maintained, they usually give some version of one or more of the following reasons:

1 Every person has a right to privacy, thus confidentiality, since confidence maintains privacy.

2 Privacy is the foundation of a person's dignity and autonomy; confidentiality is thus needed for a person to maintain dignity and autonomy.

3 Sharing of private information with a professional creates a relationship which includes an implicit promise of protection, thus a requirement for confidentiality.

4 Without the bond of confidence, people who need help would not seek it because of threatened disclosure, thus causing them harm.[5]

Before we discuss these reasons, notice that they run the range of ethical theories (as discussed in Chapter 2). Reason 1 is clearly rights-based. Reason 2 is probably rights-based because of the reference to the basic elements of personhood, while reason 3 is duty-based (the making of a promise imposes a duty to keep the promise), and reason 4 is based on consequences. As we discuss these reasons in detail, it will help to keep these theoretical positions in mind.

Whether privacy is a right is not really an issue, for, as Ian Thompson points out,

(O)n logical grounds, if we concede the existence of individual human rights of any kind, then it is . . . self-evident that there must be a "right to privacy" for without it there would be no private individuals to have or exercise those rights.[6]

---

[5]For a full discussion of these factors see Sissela Bok, "The Limits of Confidentiality," *Hastings Center Report,* vol. 13, no. 1, February 1983, pp. 24–31.

[6]Ian E. Thompson, "The Nature of Confidentiality," *Journal of Medical Ethics,* vol. 5, 1979, p. 59.

The problem, then, is not to determine that there is a right to privacy, but rather to determine what *sort* of right it is, what justification may be given for its exercise, and when, if ever, that right may be overridden.

Conflicting Claims for Information

Because confidentiality is so firmly established as a part of the health care relationship, professionals are often placed in problematic situations because the person for whom they are caring expects them to keep information private while others expect that information to be disclosed.

CASE 4.1

Following the birth of her daughter, Julia Keetes had a tubal ligation performed, at her request, because she did not want to have any more children. Julia and her physician had agreed beforehand that Julia's husband, Warren, would not be told of the ligation, since he strongly disapproved for religious reasons. Julia and her physician were in agreement that Julia had a right to the procedure if she wished, and the secrecy was needed, they believed, to prevent marital difficulties between Julia and Warren. Because of an inadvertent comment by Julia, Warren calls the physician and asks her directly whether Julia has "had her tubes tied." Warren claims that, as Julia's husband, he has a right to know, and she won't tell him.

Normally we would think that one spouse has a right to information about the other, but why do we think that? Is it because marriage is taken to involve sharing and caring, thus mutual knowledge? The problem here is the specific request by Julia that Warren not be told. Julia's physician wonders what to tell him. If she says, "I'm sorry, but you have to ask Julia," might he interpret that as a positive answer, so she would be indirectly breaking confidence? Perhaps she should tell Warren that Julia has not had the procedure, to preserve Julia's secret and prevent difficulty with her husband; but does the code of confidence also require lying?[7] Although our values might differ, would not Julia, as a competent adult, have as much right to her privacy as anyone else? The physician is certainly not required to lie for the patient; there is also no requirement for the physician to give the requested information. The physician could thus act on her agreement with Julia, her patient, and refuse to answer Warren's question, on the grounds of Julia's right to privacy.

[7]How should Julia's physician respond to an insurance company's request for information? If you think she should give information to the company, why not to her husband? After all, would he not have more right to know the intimate details of his wife's medical history than a total stranger? What if her mother asked?

Whenever anyone talks about a person having a "right," we must ask ourselves where that right comes from and how it is justified. Some people might claim that rights come from laws and cite as support for their claim the U.S. Constitution and the Bill of Rights, both of which specifically list numerous rights, including privacy. But since laws are made by people who have ideas about what is a right *before* they make the law, that does not get us very far. Moreover, as we saw in Chapter 3, law is not a source of moral information because no law is, by virtue of its legality alone, morally binding.

In the case of rights, we also need to distinguish between two different sorts of rights, *bestowed* rights and *natural* rights. Bestowed rights are those which may be given (or taken away) by an act of authority, while natural rights are those which a person has regardless of action by anyone. A bestowed right is in effect only when the authority is in effect, while a natural right is always in effect. On this basis, if privacy is a bestowed right, for example, via the Constitution, then a change in the law could take away that right. This has occurred in states where "sunshine" laws were passed—laws which require open meetings of government agencies, thereby abolishing privacy and secrecy for those agencies. The question is whether individual privacy is *legitimately* subject to the same treatment. It *is* often taken to be legitimately applied to individual privacy in the case of minors.

CASE 4.2

Kay Prince is a 16-year-old who has gone to the family planning clinic to obtain birth control pills. The clinic receptionist tells her that she can be seen at the clinic but that her parents will have to be informed of her visit. She asks why and is told that this is the law in that state. Since Kay does not want her parents to know this, she decides not to be seen at the clinic and subsequently becomes pregnant.[8]

This case presents a confrontation between a request for privacy and a legal requirement for disclosure. On what basis could we argue that Kay has a right to her privacy? One way would be to argue that because the consequences of denying Kay's privacy were so severe, she should have been allowed a right to privacy so that she could receive the protective measures she requested. That would be a shaky argument, however, because it could not be known for sure that those consequences would result; so allowing privacy on the basis of those consequences would not cover all cases. A better argument would be that those

---

[8]What if the case had one of these added features: (1) she is afraid of rape, but does not want to worry her parents; (2) she wants to experiment with sex, but does not want her parents to know. How, if at all, would each of these added elements change the moral considerations in this case?

consequences were probable, and since we don't want them to occur, we should allow privacy. As noted in Chapter 2, though, it is so difficult to predict consequences that we do not have a solid basis in that argument.

We could instead argue for privacy on the basis of reason 1, that Kay, as does any other person, has a right to privacy. Usually, however, laws such as the one invoked here either reject that claim in relation to minors or invoke a principle of parental control. This does not remove the physician's responsibility to the patient; it simply attempts to transfer that responsibility via the parents. Notice, however, that such laws require two assumptions: first, privacy, as a right, is under legislative control; second, parents are *always* the guardians of their children's rights. Both assumptions are questionable, of course, especially in connection with someone 16 years old (in a way that they are not questionable for a 16-month-old). There is also an important issue of values here, since one value upon which the law is based, namely that teenagers should be discouraged from sexual activity, is not of necessity properly reflected in the law. As such, the law binds the clinic to certain actions while morally we would want to consider other options.

One way of explaining this is to make a further distinction within the categories of bestowed and natural rights, namely, between *absolute* and *contingent* rights. According to this distinction, some rights are always in force, i.e., are absolute, while others are in force only on the basis of certain conditions having been met. For example, to be allowed to drive a car, you must meet certain criteria of age, eyesight, dexterity, etc., or you will not obtain a license. It is well recognized that privacy is not absolute because there might be some instances when control of information is not proper. An example would be when keeping a confidence was covering up a crime, or when the patient was not competent. For example, in Case 4.1, if Julia were judged incompetent, her husband (or some other person acting as her guardian) *would* have a need for information and Julia's request for privacy could be overruled. In the same vein, it might be argued that Kay, in Case 4.2, was being protected by the law because she is 16 years old and thus not competent to make her own decisions. Privacy is then seen as contingent on the patient's competence.

Privacy and the Prevention of Harm

Another basis for the contingency of a right is the *prevention of harm,* where divulging of information is required in cases such as child abuse, gunshot wounds, and communicable diseases, as in the case of Lorraine Williams (Case 1.6). Lorraine was told of child abuse but specifically asked by the child's mother not to say anything. As we saw, it was possible to argue for breaking confidence in three different ways: (1) the child 's right to protection overrides the parent's right to confidence; (2) prevention of harm to the child promotes more good than maintaining the mother's confidence; or (3) everyone has an obligation to obey the law, and thus the abuse must be reported. These three approaches to the problem reflect the rights-, consequences-, and duty-based approaches to solving ethical problems, respectively, and reflect the basic reasons for confidence given earlier in this chapter. Notice that the appeal is basically to prevention of harm, but only the third appeals to the requirement of law and, compared to the others, does not seem very forceful. More importantly, the other two would serve as justification for the law. Although prevention of harm seems an easy way to justify breaking confidence, it can be incredibly difficult to determine what is harmful and how much harm is too much and thus subject to prevention. In fact, how difficult this is became quite clear in a recent case:

CASE 4.3

During a therapy session with Mr. P, a university student, the university psychologist learned that Mr. P had threatened the life of Ms. T, also a student. The psychologist notified the campus police; the campus police decided the threat was not serious, released Mr. P, and said nothing to Ms. T . The psychologist also said nothing to Ms. T. Two months later, without additional contact with the psychologist, Mr. P killed Ms. T.[9]

Determination of harm, however, while helping to encourage our willingness to violate confidence, is not easily made. The matter is made particularly difficult by determination of potential harm. The California court gave the family of the victim a large damage settlement because their daughter was not warned that Mr. P had told his psychiatrist that he planned to kill her. The psychiatrist held to a defense of confidentiality and inability to accurately predict potential harm. The judges disagreed, and wrote

> In this risk-infested society, we can hardly tolerate the further exposure to danger that would result from a concealed knowledge of the therapist that his patient was lethal. If the exercise of reasonable care to protect the threatened victim requires the therapist to warn the endangered party or those who can reasonably be expected to notify him, we see no sufficient societal interest that would protect and justify concealment. . . . The protective privilege ends where the public peril begins.[10]

Although the judges were primarily using a consequence-based approach to resolving this moral issue and connecting cases such as this to the established precedent of reporting abuse and communicable diseases, there is also a question of third-party rights. The serious question which remains is whether the rights of the patient to privacy override the right of a third party to protection. In this

---

[9]*Tarasoff v. Regents of the University of California,* Opinion 551, 1.2d 334,131 CAL RPTR. 14 (1976).
[10]Ibid.

case, based on the consequential argument, the judges ruled in favor of the third party. However, that is a position which needs more extensive thought before it is fully acceptable, since the determination of potential harm is so difficult. It is easy for the others, looking at all the information, to fault the doctor. Since the doctor did not have a crucial piece of information—that Mr. P would in fact kill Ms. T—*should* he be faulted?

We really cannot begin to deal with the question of harm until we look more carefully at the basic justification for maintaining privacy. So let's leave that question for the moment and move on to further inquiry aimed at justifying privacy, thus confidentiality.

Even in the best of circumstances, there is still a question of who should have access to what patient information. In the cases discussed up to this point, there was difficulty because of unusual circumstances. The following case gives us a basis for discussing this problem from a different perspective.

CASE 4.4

Andy Tromin has been an inpatient at the Medical School Hospital for 2 months, suffering from an as yet undiagnosed digestive problem complicated by pneumonia. He has been cared for by countless medical students, residents, and staff physicians, not to mention specialists, therapists, and nurses. Recently, he has been cared for by student nurses, a different group twice a week, and respiratory therapy students. At this point he does not know whether to complain; he does not mind the students, because they give him good care, but he does not like being a "specimen," and is tired of giving his history over and over. Since this is a teaching hospital, he wonders if he must simply put up with all this as part of his care.

From one perspective, Andy has probably received outstanding treatment from the various teams caring for him, and he would probably admit as much. The problem lies in the number of people giving that care and his view that he is a specimen, a view that is not exaggerated. The *New England Journal of Medicine* reports that for someone such as Andy, in one teaching hospital which is quite representative of others, care is normally given by

> . . . 6 attending physicians (the primary physician, the surgeon, the pulmonary consultant, and others); 12 house officers (residents and interns); 20 nursing staff (on three shifts) 6 respiratory therapists; 3 nutritionists, 2 clinical pharmacists, 15 students (from medicine, nursing, respiratory therapy, and clinical pharmacy); 4 unit secretaries; 4 hospital finance officers; and 4 chart reviewers. . . . And all of them had a legitimate need, indeed professional responsibility, to open and use (the patient's) chart.[11]

[11]Siegler, "Confidentiality in Medicine—A Decrepit Concept," p. 1519.

With that number of people involved in a case, in what sense is the information about the patient confidential? In what sense has his privacy been maintained?

We might argue that as long as the caregiving teams do not use information about Andy for means other than his direct care, his privacy has been maintained. Such an argument, however, supposes that this technical sense of privacy is all that matters. If we were to consider this case from the ethical framework of utilitarianism, we might also say that although Andy's discomfort was regrettable and should be minimized, it is essential to the students that they care for him. On the basis of overall good, given that the students will learn from Andy and be able to help many people during their professional careers, the bad that Andy suffers will be greatly outweighed by the good that the students will do. Even if we take this position, which of course, is debatable, clearly a major problem remains—balancing the information requirements of good care with the information requirements of a health professional's educational experience.[12]

Privacy, Dignity, and Autonomy

One approach to the moral justification of privacy, which involves a correlated justification for confidentiality, is reason 2, that privacy is essential to a person's sense of dignity and autonomy.[13] From that approach, this technical sense of privacy is not enough, as Richard Wassertrom has forcefully argued. Strict privacy, he says, is an important component in these cases precisely because it is crucial to Andy's self-esteem. While in the health care system, a person's privacy is most vulnerable. It is the business of health care professionals to discover and act on information to which no one other than the patient has access but which, if made public, would at least cause embarrassment or social injury to the patient. If a person's privacy is compromised by having so many people doing so much, it is difficult for an individual to see himself or herself *as a person* instead of as an object. As a result,

> (I)t will be difficult for the individuals (such as Andy) who are the objects of such scrutiny to continue to retain a sense of their own individuality and autonomy. Concomitantly, it will be difficult for the individuals who are conducting and maintaining the scrutiny to continue to retain a sense of the subjects as persons rather than objects.[14]

This is not just a psychological argument, however; privacy is not required simply because it helps patients maintain their perspective and maintaining perspective is somehow healthy. Rather, it is an argument for treating the patient

[12]We must also raise the question about education: When is patient care really student care, and how can invasion of privacy be justified?

[13]Of course, this assumes that dignity and autonomy are morally valuable; since that is a well-accepted assumption, however, we do not question it at this time.

[14]Richard Wasserstrom, "The Legal and Philosophical Foundations of the Right to Privacy," in T. Mappes and J. Zembatty (eds.), *Biomedical Ethics*, McGraw-Hill, New York, 1981, p. 111.

as a *person,* not as an object, which makes it an argument for respect of humanness. Put in different terms, if it were only a psychological argument, then it would be directed toward helping patients see themselves in a certain way; but, instead, it is an argument directed toward the health care professional's seeing the patient in a different way. Helping to maintain dignity and a sense of personhood in the health care setting is then extremely important to the professional as well as to the patient. Confidentiality is crucial to that task because it is through confidence that the dignity and autonomy of a person are maintained in a setting where strict privacy is not possible.[15] This understanding of confidentiality is derived from views of privacy which are in turn derived from a philosophy of personhood.

The third reason for privacy comes from a different source, namely, an understanding of *professional duty* (noted earlier) and the basic elements of making promises. According to this argument, confidentiality is a matter of professional duty which arises because of the contractual arrangement between health care professionals and patients. When a person goes to a health care professional and utilizes those services, a contractual bond has been formed between the person and the professional, one aspect of which is the implicit promise by the professional to maintain confidence. Because contracts are morally binding and promising is morally binding, the patient is said to have a right to expect confidence, and the professional has a duty to uphold that expectation of confidence.[16] This duty is heightened by the continued use of professional codes which reinforce for the public the profession's commitment to confidentiality.

As this continues, "Clients divulge information with an understanding that it will be kept confidential. Allowing such an understanding to develop and persist amounts to an implicit promise (of continuing confidence)."[17] Here we see the reliance on promises as crucial to the argument. To make a promise in normal circumstances is to make a vow or pledge, backed by the strength of one's character. Because a professional is seen to be someone of good character, the promise is seen to be more important. This implicit promise, together with the professional code requirements, forms only a partial basis for confidentiality from this perspective. Also active here is the idea that by acting in the capacity of a consultant, the professional is taking an extra burden of confidence precisely because of his or her role. Historically, this burden is linked to such things as confession, and its importance is demonstrated by, for example, the ceremony of blood brothers or the tradition of accepting something "on your word." The

---

[15]Note in this context that degrading remarks, humiliation, and insults have the same effect as violations of privacy—they reduce the person's dignity. Action of this sort, as well as the failure to maintain privacy, can be devastating to any person.

[16]The reasons we saw above for why someone might break confidence apply here as well.

[17]Alan H. Goldman, *The Moral Foundations of Professional Ethics,* Rowman and Littlefield, Totowa, NJ, 1980, p. 99.

professional requirement does not gain its strength from such history; however, the history demonstrates the precedence for the practice. The basis is deeper: it is

> The contractual relation between patient and doctor, and the patient's right to privacy, both contained within our common moral framework, (which) explain the full force of the duty to keep in confidence information about the patient.[18]

There are two important difficulties with using duty alone as a justification for confidentiality. First, in those cases where duties conflict, we may be unable to decide which is more important. The obvious conflict of duties, already discussed, is between one's moral duty to the patient and one's legal duty to society. Another example is the conflict in Case 4.1, where the physician may see a duty both to Julia and to helping resolve the family problem. Or, in the same case, the physician may be caught between a duty to tell the truth and a duty to maintain confidence. The conflict could also occur between a duty to maintain confidence and a professional duty to give good care, as in Case 4.5.

CASE 4.5

Carl Jungweitz is a respiratory therapist doing prescribed treatments on Lucy Bristol, a 25-year-old with a diagnosis of lung cancer. Lucy tells Carl that she is really feeling badly as a result of her chemotherapy. Carl explains that some lessening of symptoms is possible with altered doses and asks Lucy if she has mentioned this to her doctor. Lucy says, "No, the doctor knows what she is doing, so there is no need to mention it." At that point the doctor comes into the room and asks Lucy whether she is having any problems, and Lucy replies, "No, I feel quite good, so the treatments must be working." Carl wonders whether to confront Lucy regarding her earlier statement, to talk to the doctor privately afterwards, or to say nothing at all.

To whom does Carl owe his loyalty here? Does Lucy's quality of care take precedence over the confidentiality inherent in the circumstances under which Lucy and Carl were talking? How we sort out such conflicts will depend on the basic ethical position we hold. If rights are primary, then it will depend on whether Lucy is seen as having a right to make her own decisions. If duty is primary, it will depend on whether confidence or quality care is more important. If consequences are primary, it will depend on which alternative is judged to produce the best possible consequences.

The second difficulty with using duty to justify confidentiality is that it is quite hard to get at the underlying justification for the duty. Put differently, what

[18]Ibid., p. 221.

are the preconditions for the duty? Is the duty itself somehow basic, or is there an underlying reason for the duty? One obvious candidate for underlying reasons is rights, as discussed earlier. That is, we have a duty to confidentiality because the patient has an independently determined right to privacy. Another alternative is that we have a duty to confidentiality because otherwise we could not prevent undesirable consequences. The underlying reason is then prevention of undesirable consequences, which brings us to the fourth and final reason given for maintaining confidence—the consequences of not doing so are worse than the consequences of maintaining confidence. Sissela Bok describes this position quite well when she says that professional confidence is required

> . . . because of its utility to persons and society. . . . Individuals benefit from such confidentiality because it allows them to seek help they might otherwise fear to ask for; those more vulnerable or at risk might otherwise not go for help to doctors or lawyers or others trained to provide for it.[19]

One problem with this line of reasoning is that, as we saw in Chapter 2, it is not easy to determine relative weights of good against bad. That problem is compounded here, however, because there are various ways in which benefit may be established, and they are not all in the patient's favor.

> Normally, keeping such a set of pledges (of confidence) is, on balance, in the interests of each party. If the lay person does not reveal the necessary information, he or she may not benefit as much from the relationship; the lay person's interest is in disclosure. On the other hand, if the professional breaks the confidence, relatively little is gained and much could be lost. The professional's reputation could be harmed and further clients lost.[20]

If confidence were not maintained, according to this argument more harm than good would be done because people would not seek the help they need and thus could become worse off. There is also a social good to be gained here, in that society is better off if there can be relationships of mutual trust, not just between professionals and their clients, but between citizens in general. The professional-client relationship is then just one of those relationships of good citizenship.

There is a serious drawback to this approach, however. The same "more harm than good" argument may be used to justify *breaking* confidence. Put differently, using consequences to justify keeping confidence also puts us in a position to allow breaking confidence. This was seen in Case 4.3 in connection with preventing harm and is also seen in connection with Andy in Case 4.4. When discussing Andy earlier, we noted that there was a question about students working with patient information. At the time, it seemed to be all right because the students were caring for Andy; thus their knowledge of him and his problems was directed toward him as well as their own education. After all, it might be

---

[19]Bok, "The Limits of Confidentiality," p. 26.
[20]Robert M. Veatch, *A Theory of Medical Ethics,* Basic Books, New York, 1981, p. 185.

argued, the students are able to learn only by working with real patients. Deny students that access and their future patients will suffer since students will have to learn anyhow but later will not have instructors to help. The present system is thus really the best alternative. On this basis, the health professional's instructors like to have their students care for patients such as Andy because the students can learn a great deal from that care. At the same time, there is a serious question, even from the utilitarian framework, as to how far the education argument should be carried. The following case brings out this problem, compounded in the teaching situation which does not include patient care.

CASE 4.6

Carrie Maxwell is a pharmacy intern working on a term paper about the effects on the body of taking many different drugs over a long time. As part of the requirements for the paper, she must interview patients and include their comments in her report. Her instructor has told her of a patient in their hospital who has been taking 13 different drugs for a period of 4 years. Carrie would like to interview the patient but is worried because nothing she learns from the interview will be used in caring for the patient; it will only help advance her education, and she questions whether she has a right to do that.[21]

For the sake of argument, let us assume that, from a strictly technical perspective, the confidentiality of information from both cases is not an issue in the sense that no one caring for Andy has discussed his case outside the group rendering care and no one but Carrie's instructor will see her paper. But with that number of persons knowing about the factors in Andy's case, in what sense is the information confidential? Although Carrie might use her own education as justification for knowing about the multidrug patient, she is directly confronting the problem which Kant raised—treating persons as a means to something, rather than an end in themselves. Although Carrie might use the knowledge gained during the interview to help other patients, nothing of it will help the patient she interviews.[22] She is thus using the patient as a means to her own education. Moreover, since her instructor will read the paper, another person will have access to the information, again without benefit to the patient. In what sense has the patient's privacy been maintained? In what sense would Carrie have maintained confidentiality?

Each of the four viewpoints could be greatly expanded, and we have not reached a resolution on any of the cases. Yet we have enough here to understand the key issues of confidentiality in health care and go on to consider more detailed

---

[21] If you were the patient, would you mind if Carrie did her project on you? Why or why not?
[22] The same problem arises with experimentation.

arguments for the different ethical perspectives on the issues. Before doing that, however, let's review the major points of this discussion.

CONCLUDING THOUGHTS

Our discussion of privacy and confidentiality has shown that the primary focus for ethical consideration is how the disclosure of or access to personal information will be handled. In trying to deal with issues of confidentiality, the basic concerns are, first, what information is to count as confidential; second, who should have access to personal information; and, third, under what circumstances confidence may be broken. Understanding these three matters requires that we also understand how privacy and confidentiality are related and how both relate to such other concepts as trust, respect, professional conduct, and the nature of personhood.

The basic understanding of confidentiality developed here is that it is derived from our views of privacy. If we did not already value privacy, there would be no need for confidentiality, for rules of confidence serve only to protect privacy. Whether or not (if ever) it really is all right to break confidence and divulge information about a person's health is not easily settled. As a first step toward resolving the issue, we looked at the four basic reasons for maintaining confidentiality, and then we considered cases which expanded upon and raised issues about those reasons. From the perspective of ethics, there are different ways in which the concern for privacy, thus confidentiality, may be justified. The readings which follow were selected to help develop these matters further, thereby expanding your understanding of the basic ethical positions on confidentiality.

We have discussed matters of the law in this chapter in more detail than we will in others, because confidentiality is so universally treated in the law of so many states. No other ethical concept relative to health care receives as much attention (although informed consent runs a close second). Do not misunderstand; this has *not* been an argument for the legal basis of ethics. To the contrary, the cases showed that the law does not resolve the issues, even though it settles particular cases. The California court ruled against the university in Case 4.3, but that does not give us the answer to the question of when *particular* information must be disclosed; nor does it give us moral guidelines for that disclosure—that is the providence of ethics. The law was also brought in for another reason— to begin raising the issue of legal compliance versus moral action. A theme of this book is that the law does not describe or dictate moral action. As a result, it is quite possible that moral values may require civil action, as Socrates, Christ, Gandhi, Martin Luther King, and others have shown us. An important part of thinking about ethical questions is to think about principles of justice, especially where they may require failure to adhere to the law. Morally responsible persons must think through the basis for their actions and decide what gives the best support for their position; then they must act on the basis of *moral* judgment.

As a final note, clearly we have not been working toward a view of universal honesty, whereby the morally proper thing would be for everything to be openly known about everyone. This cannot be our position because no matter which ethical justification one might use, a basic, crucial element of that justification must be the presupposition of privacy as a fundamental element of being a person.

In a world such as that depicted by George Orwell's *1984* (updated to include more sophisticated technological monitoring and eavesdropping devices),

> Fear, suspicion, and insecurity would prevail even among persons of goodwill. The context of human interaction would be so threatening that . . . (it) would preclude the possibility of certain desirable forms of human interaction.[23]

We must be honest, or we will have the result just described; it does not follow from that truism, however, that we (or someone, e.g., the government) must know all that can be known about an individual.

With these ideas in mind, turn now to the reading, then the case studies, working all the while for a fuller, deeper understanding of privacy and confidentiality.

STUDY GUIDE

READINGS

R. Wasserstrom, "The Legal and Philosophical Foundations of the Right to Privacy." p. 169.

QUESTIONS FOR REFLECTION

1 For each case in this chapter, try to determine how, if at all, the different ethical theories would require you to consider each case.

2 What is the ethical position taken in the reading? Would the author's position change if a different ethical theory were used?

3 What suggestions would you make to help alleviate some of the problems of confidentiality discussed in the chapter?

4 What is your moral reponsibility regarding information which someone else would consider private? Can you make a general statement, or does it depend on circumstances? Why?

---

[23]William J. Winslade, "Confidentiality," in Warren T. Reich (ed.), *Encyclopedia of Bioethics*, Free Press, New York, 1978, vol. 1, p. 196.

CASE STUDIES FOR ANALYSIS

Case Study 1   Juanetta is a 23-year-old in end-stage renal disease. Because of complex medical problems, Juanetta is not a candidate to receive a transplant, from either a cadaver or a relative. Presently on dialysis, Juanetta comes to the clinic several days a week; as the receptionist in the clinic, you have come to know Juanetta quite well and have even gone to lunch with her on occasion. One day, during dialysis, Juanetta is talking to you and indicates that she is not really feeling well; the dialysis is becoming less effective (as is often true with this disease). You ask whether she has mentioned this to the nurses or to her doctor, and she says, "No, there is no need to trouble them, because this is the last time I will be in for dialysis." You ask her why, and she explains that she is going to let the disease end her life.

Analysis Questions   Below are three different conclusions for this case. Using each separately, decide, for each set of circumstances, what you would do if you were faced with this situation. Be sure to identify the moral problem and sufficiently justify your answers. Remember, simply being sincere about your response is not enough; you need to give adequate reasons in support of your decision.

1 After a bit of discussion you discover that Juanetta has thought this out carefully and discussed it with her parents, who leave the choice up to her. She asks you not to tell anyone and thanks you for taking good care of her.

2 After a bit of discussion you discover that Juanetta has thought this out carefully but not discussed it with anyone. She asks you not to tell anyone and thanks you for taking good care of her.

3 After a bit of discussion you discover that Juanetta has not given much thought to this idea; and in fact, she admits that she just started thinking about it while sitting there that day. She asks you not to tell anyone and thanks you for taking good care of her.

Now rethink the case but put yourself in Juanetta's position. How would you expect someone to respond in each of the situations above if *you* were the one stopping dialysis? Do your expectations as the patient differ from your expectations as the professional? Why or Why not?

Case Study 2   As a community member of a hospital ethics committee, you are present at a meeting called to discuss the following matter.

Two months ago a surgical technician was notified that a person whose case she had worked on had been diagnosed as having AIDS. She and others who assisted with the surgery were asked to have the screening tests done for AIDS, to see whether they had contracted the disease. The technician tested positive for the AIDS antibody, although she did not have symptoms of the disease.

Because surgery personnel often are stuck by needles during surgery and because AIDS can be transmitted in that way, 82 percent of the surgical staff signed a petition asking that the hospital do two things to protect them from AIDS. First, they asked that the hospital require a question about sexual preference on the admission form of all persons admitted for surgery, to identify homosexual persons; second, they asked that the hospital routinely perform the screening tests for AIDS on all those who identify themselves as homosexuals.

When the medical laboratory staff learned of the petition, they joined in asking for its adoption, since they too must handle possibly contaminated needles and blood products.

After presentation of the petition, the hospital administration has asked the ethics committee to consider whether the two requests on the petition should be granted. There are no known laws which would prohibit such action, but the administration is concerned about the moral implications and has asked the committee for a recommendation.

Analysis Questions   What exactly is the ethical dilemma in this case? Is there more than one? What alternatives have the surgical staff overlooked? What moral problems would be caused by the adoption of the two requests? What would be your recommendation to the administration? Why?

Case Study 3   You are a nurse who has witnessed a procedure in which a physician made a mistake. The mistake caused the patient to need additional treatment and spend additional time in the hospital, although the mistake will not have residual health effects.

Analysis Questions   What, if any, is your moral responsibility? What moral problems must you solve?

Case Study 4   You are a general practitioner who has had two young people as patients for a number of years. You have treated each on many occasions, and they come to you for their premarital blood tests. The results show that the young man has herpes and probably syphilis as well. You contact him and explain the results. He steadfastly refuses to tell his fiancée of his problem.

Analysis Questions   What, if any, ethical problem do you, as a physician, face?

Case Study 5   Dr. Samuels discovers that his patient, Antonio Sciapelli, is suffering from an aortic aneurysm which is so extensive that it cannot be repaired. There is nothing for Antonio to do but wait for it to burst, at which time he will die almost instantly. The problem is that Antonio has asked Dr. Samuels not to tell anyone of his diagnosis—he doesn't want anyone feeling sorry for him, he says. But Antonio makes his living driving a taxicab. Were the aneurysm to burst while he was driving, his passengers might be killed or seriously injured, since the cab would surely crash. Dr. Samuels tells Antonio that he should not drive anymore, and Antonio says that he will not. But Dr. Samuels wonders whether he should call the cab company and report Antonio as unfit or at least follow up in a few days to see whether Antonio has quit his job.

Analysis Questions   What should Dr. Samuels do? Would Dr. Samuels have the same problem if Antonio earned his living as a clerk in the bank? If we abide by a strict understanding of confidentiality, is there any set of circumstances in which Dr. Samuels may break Antonio's confidence? Must we give consideration to the well-being of others? Who has that responsibility?

Case Study 6   Wu Chen is a 19-year-old cystic fibrosis (CF) patient who has been a regular on your service for his periodic "clean-out." You have come to know Wu and Wu has come to trust you and rely on you for his care. As is usual with CF, Wu's visits have become more and more frequent, with today being his most recent admission. While you are helping Wu to settle in, he tells you that this is the last time he will be in for care. Upon questioning him you discover that he plans to let his next attack go untreated so that he will die. He asks you not to tell anyone and says that it is "our secret."

Analysis Questions   What should you do? Suppose, instead of Wu saying that he does not want to come back for treatment, he says that he wants a no-code and a good stiff dose of morphine. You ask whether he has discussed the matter with his physician, and he says "No, he wouldn't understand." What should you do?

BIBLIOGRAPHY

Abrams, Natalie, Michael D. Buckner, and Richard I. Levine: "The Urban Emergency Department: The Issue of Professional Responsibility," *Annals of Emergency Medicine,* vol. 11, no. 2, February 1982, pp. 86–90.

Bok, Sissela, *Secrets,* Pantheon Books, New York, 1982.

Donovan, John: "An Experiment in Privacy Protection," *Medical Journal of Australia,* vol. 141, November 1984, pp. 648–649.

Francis, H. W.: "Of Gossips, Eavesdroppers, and Peeping Toms," *Journal of Medical Ethics,* vol. 8, no 3, September 1982, pp. 134–143.

Goldman, Brian, "Professional Misconduct: Does the Public Have a Right to Know?" *Canadian Medical Association Journal,* vol. 131, no. 6, September 1984, pp. 637–644.

Harvard, John: "Confidentiality—A Major Issue in Medical Ethics," *Journal of Medical Ethics,* vol. 11, no. 1, March 1985, pp. 8–11.

Kenney, A. M., J. D. Forrest, and A. Torres,: "Storm over Washington: The Parental Notification Proposal," *Family Planning Perspectives,* vol. 14, no. 4, July 1982, pp. 185ff.

Lansing, Paul: "The Conflict of Patient Privacy and the Freedom of Information Act," *Journal of Health Politics, Policy and Law,* vol. 9, no. 2, 1984, pp. 315–324.

Meissner, William: "Threats to Confidentiality," *Psychiatric Annals,* vol 2, 1979, pp. 54–71.

Morreim, Haavi, Jeanne Brimigion, Alice Donovan, Ruth Huey, and Eleanor Fine: "The Patient's Right to Privacy," *Nursing Life,* vol. 2, no. 3, May/June 1982, pp. 35–38.

Paul, R. E.: "Tarsoff and the Duty to Warn: Toward a Standard of Conduct that Balances the Rights of Clients against the Rights of Third Parties," *Professional Psychiatry,* vol. 8, 1977, pp. 125–128.

Pheby, D. F. H.: "Changing Practice on Confidentiality. A Cause for Concern," *Journal of Medical Ethics,* vol. 8, 1982, pp. 12–18.

Purtilo, Ruth, Joseph Sonnabend, and David T. Purtilo: "Confidentiality, Informed Consent, and Untoward Social Consequences in Research on a New Killer Disease, AIDS," *Clinical Research,* vol. 31, no. 4, October 1983, pp. 462–472.

Rosner, Bennett: "Psychiatrists, Confidentiality, and Insurance Claims," *Hastings Center Report,* vol. 10, no. 6, December 1980, pp. 5–7.

Schechter, D.: "Medical Records Access: Who Shall See What and When?" *Occupational Health and Safety,* vol. 51, no. 7, July 1982, pp. 23–26.

Sheldon, M. G.: "The Doctor, the Patient and the Computer," *Practitioner,* vol. 228, December 1984, pp. 1121–1124.

Siegel, Max: "Privacy, Ethics, and Confidentiality," *Professional Psychiatry,* vol. 10, no. 2, April 1979, pp. 249–257.

Siegler, Mark: "Confidentiality in Medicine—A Decrepit Concept," *New England Journal of Medicine,* vol. 307, no. 24, December 1982, pp. 1518–1521.

Tiemann, William: *The Right to Silence: Privileged Communication and the Pastor,* John Knox Press, Richmond, VA, 1964.

Wilson, Susanna J.: *Confidentiality in Social Work,* Free Press, New York, 1978.

CHAPTER 5

COMMUNICATION IN HEALTH CARE: INFORMATION, DECEPTION, AND INFORMED CONSENT

To be truthful in all declarations, therefore, is a sacred and absolutely commanding decree of reason, limited by no expediency.

Immanuel Kant*

. . . the art of medicine consists largely in skillfully mixing falsehood and truth. . . . [Thus] every physician should cultivate lying as a fine art.

Joseph Collins**

TRUTH, THE BASIS FOR COMMUNICATION

It only takes a bit of thinking to recognize that the expectation of truth telling is one of the foundations of any meaningful exchange of information. Were we unable to expect truth in our exchange of information, that exchange would be nearly impossible and certainly useless. What good is exchanging information which cannot have a known truth value? Even learning would be severely restricted, since only what people found out on their own could be trusted. Truth is thus a prerequisite for meaningful communication, and telling the truth is a basic requirement of informative language usage. In fact, truth is so basic, and

Critique of Pure Reason, L. W. Beck, (trans.), University of Chicago Press, Chicago, 1949.
**"Should Doctors Tell the Truth?" *Harper's Magazine*, August 1927.

so necessary, that in legal affairs one must swear to "tell the truth, the whole truth, and nothing but the truth," and perjury is a serious crime.

Without communication, health care as we know it would not be possible. The persons receiving care must communicate with the professional, and the professional with the care recipients as well as colleagues. Patients must give information relative to their concerns, and the professional must ask questions and give information relative to diagnosis, treatment, and prognosis.

All communication situations have the potential for being misleading, because the possibility of communicating false information always exists. In addition, information may be misunderstood, misinterpreted, or incomprehensible to the listener for a variety of reasons. The ethical problems of communication arise, however, only when there is *intended deception*. That is, we must distinguish between those cases where false or misleading information is communicated by accident and those in which there is a purposeful action aimed at manipulating the information.

Although we clearly understand lying as a means of deception, it is important to recognize that there are many other ways of deceiving through information. For example, gestures and false clues, and even silence in a situation where information is called for, contribute to deception. Note that intended deception always involves the manipulation of information so that beliefs will be altered and intentions will be hidden.

Generally speaking, in our normal, everyday lives, if two people are in a situation which requires information giving, then intended deception is considered morally wrong. Despite this fact, persons seeking health care are often not truthful when giving a professional the information needed for their care. Since complete, correct information is needed for adequate diagnosis and treatment, professionals complain loudly about this practice. At the same time, by long tradition a double standard of truth telling exists in health care:

> The [professional] requires his patient to respond truthfully to questions; at the same time, the [professional], in some instances, does not feel bound to respond completely truthfully to the patient's queries.[1]

The reasons for this double standard are varied, from "They wouldn't understand anyhow" to "They are better off not knowing," and have a historical basis going back at least to Hippocrates. Following this tradition, health care professionals generally believe that they have the right, perhaps even the duty, to decide what people should know about themselves and what they should not know. In addition, they often engage in what they believe is justified deception. Since this is contrary to normal information communication, we must take time to examine this viewpoint.

Clearly the issue of truth telling is not all there is of moral concern in matters

---

[1]S. Reiser (ed.), *Ethics in Medicine,* M.I.T. Press, Cambridge, MA, 1977, p. 201.

of communication, since communication cannot be reduced to issues of truth alone.

> Too often, texts reduce the "issue" in communication to the decision whether to tell the truth about a particular diagnosis or procedural outcome. Although [truth] is a focal moral problem, it cannot be separated from the general mode of communication with patients throughout the whole range of information sharing. . . . [We] must never forget that it is never a matter of simply telling the truth about a fact and leaving a patient with it. . . . [Truth] is communicated as part of an emotional interaction that must also be understood for its messages and for the way in which it supports the therapeutic process itself.[2]

Our goal in this chapter is to better understand this issue by dealing with different cases of deception. Throughout, however, our discussion presupposes competent persons on both ends of the communication process. In Chapter 6 we examine how these issues affect the care of incompetent persons.

TRUTH IN THE PROFESSIONAL-PATIENT RELATIONSHIP

A number of different arguments are given for professionals not to tell people the truth about their condition, diagnosis, or prognosis; instead, it is argued, the health care professional should be free to suppress or distort information, despite the patient's expressed or implied wishes. Three basic reasons have traditionally been given to support such action: people do not really want to know about their illnesses; telling the truth would cause the person significant harm; and it is up to the professional to determine what is in the person's best interest and what should be known.[3] There are, in addition, three primary means for keeping the truth from a person: by giving false information, by not correcting mistaken ideas or misunderstanding, and by simply withholding information. Let us briefly examine these reasons by looking at illustrations of their application.

The Person Doesn't Want to Know

The belief that people do not really want to know about their conditions is often used as a reason for deception in communication, particularly when the medical problem is severe or fatal, as in the following case.

CASE 5.1

Barbara Wainright, a 57-year-old mother of two, was admitted to the hospital for tests to rule out obstructive cancer of the colon. While the tests are being

---

[2]Natalie Abrams and Michael D. Bucker, *Medical Ethics: A Clinical Textbook,* M.I.T. Press, Cambridge, MA, 1983, p. 172.
[3]For a detailed discussion see Sissela Bok, *Lying: Moral Choice in Public and Private Life,* Pantheon Books, New York, 1978.

processed, Barbara's husband and children meet with the doctor and ask her not to tell Barbara if the results are positive. "She doesn't like to hear bad news," they say, "so let's keep this from her and keep her happy." The physician is unhappy with this request because she believes in giving patients information about their diagnoses, and Barbara has not asked her to withhold information. The family insists that Barbara not be told, because "she takes bad news so hard." The physician reluctantly agrees. The tests come back positive; but when Barbara asks about them, the physician says, "The tests are inconclusive, but don't worry, you'll do just fine."

Clearly the family members are trying to protect Barbara from bad news which they believe she will find very upsetting. However, the decision to deceive is *not* based on the request of the person affected, but on the request of others which is unknown to the affected person.

This position is frequently supported by the "experience" of health care professionals. Joseph Collins makes a typical argument:

> . . . in forty years of contact with the sick, the patients I have met who [say they want to know] could be counted on the fingers of one hand. The vast majority who demand the truth really [have no serious disorder]. . . . Many experiences show that patients do not want the truth about the maladies.[4]

Despite the fact that Collins gives no statistics and the arguments are not based on any sort of recognized, reproducible research, his position has become that most often used to justify deception. At the same time, recent research shows that large numbers, up to 80 percent, of the patients, when asked if they want to know the truth about their illness, say that they do.[5] This reason for withholding information is thus not well established and should not be taken seriously.

"The patient doesn't want to know" also falls short as a reason for withholding information if we compare normal situations to the medical situation. Under normal circumstances, our basic assumption is that people *do* want information. Moreover, we often give people bad news, whether or not they want it. For example, suppose that a person's checking account is overdrawn. Is there any question that the banker would tell the person, despite the fact that no one likes to receive such news?[6] That the person does not want to know seems, then, of little consequence.

Usually this sort of action stems from a consequentialist position, where being upset counts as a "bad" consequence to be avoided but being happily ignorant counts as a "good" consequence. At the same time, an important factor is that the *patient* has not requested that she be deceived. The importance of the con-

---

[4]Joseph Collins, "Should Doctors Tell the Truth?" *Harper's Magazine,* August 1927.
[5]For further discussion see Sissela Bok, *Secrets: On the Ethics of Concealment and Revelation,* Vintage Books, New York, 1983, pp. 241ff, and *Making Health Care Decisions,* a report by the President's Commission for the Study of Ethical Problems in Medicine (cited in Bibliography).
[6]This analogy was suggested to me by Patty Beach.

sequences is thus being assessed on the basis of *someone else's values*. If Barbara had told the doctor, before the tests, "Don't tell me if there is cancer; I just couldn't bear to know that," there would seem to be better reason for not telling her. Yet, this is not what has happened; instead, she may very well *want* to know, but the information is being kept from her by well-meaning, but misguided relatives.

The Truth May be Harmful

The next common reason for withholding the truth, namely that the patient may be harmed by the information, initially seems to allow a much more forceful argument. Case 5.2, which is a revised version of Case 5.1 (the changed portion is italicized), presents a situation in which the patient is deceived *to protect her from herself*.

CASE 5.2

Barbara Wainright, a 57-year-old mother of two, was admitted to the hospital for tests to rule out obstructive cancer of the colon. While the tests are being processed, Barbara's husband and children meet with the doctor and ask her not to tell Barbara if the results are positive. *They tell the doctor that Barbara fears cancer very much, and they believe she would become extremely upset and very depressed, and give up all desire to live. "Don't tell her," they say. "It will be too hard on her."* The physician is unhappy with this request because she believes in giving patients information about their diagnoses, and Barbara has not asked her to withhold information. The family insists that Barbara not be told, so the physician reluctantly agrees. The tests come back positive; but when Barbara asks about them, the physician says, "The tests are inconclusive, but don't worry, you'll do just fine."

This reason has the support of a long tradition, dating at least back to the Hippocratic Oath, that a physician must "so far as possible, do no harm." By using the "do no harm" principle, two different sorts of argument can be made to support the nontruthfulness of this case.

One argument is that the trauma of receiving bad news would be so significant that it would constitute harm, so lying is allowed to prevent that harm. In fact, this seems to be the substantive point in most arguments favoring nontruthfulness:

> . . . comfort with solicitude and attention, revealing nothing of the patient's future or present condition. For many patients through this cause have taken a turn for the worse.[7]

---

[7]Hippocrates, "Decorum," from W. H. S. Jones (trans.), *Hippocrates,* Harvard University Press, Cambridge, MA, 1923.

Two issues arise here. First, what constitutes harm? It might be argued that Hippocrates was asking for protection from physical harm, while we are now arguing for protection from psychological harm. Second, there is only anecdotal evidence that telling the truth is, in fact, harmful. We may find reference to cases where a patient died or committed suicide after being told of grave illness, but we have no proof that there is a causal connection between the two or that this is the usual outcome such that it is always potentially harmful to tell the truth. To put it differently, that the truth should be withheld because the consequences of truthfulness are harmful is a claim subject to the same sort of proof as the claim that patients do not want to receive bad news.

If we look more carefully at this sort of reason and relate it to nonmedical events, we also see its flawed nature. For example, if you take your car in for repairs and the mechanic finds a major problem, such as bad brakes, would you expect the mechanic to decide whether to tell you about the problem, depending on whether she thought you would become upset by the news? Of course not. So why, then, do that very thing in health care? Some people argue that preventing this sort of harm makes the person's life easier. Even if that were true (many would argue that it is not), we would also need a good argument to prove that we should always do what makes life easier—and no such argument is presently available.

There is an interesting additional consideration when the harm reason also shows up in situations where the patient is not told but family members are, as in Cases 5.1 and 5.2. The basic reasoning is that this saves the patient from harm. But then why tell the family members? Why not keep them from harm, too? Also, telling family, but not the patient, makes little sense when the same logic is compared to nonmedical events. Consider again the car repair situation. If the mechanic finds your brakes faulty, does she first notify your family, asking them whether you should be told of the problem? Or does the banker call your family to tell them of your overdraft and ask whether you should be told? The answer to both questions is no, because our normal procedure is to give the information to the person affected. So why not do the same in medical situations? There seems no overwhelmingly strong reason. In fact, as we will see, there is a very strong reason to tell, despite the potential harm.

Sometimes the harm argument is also based on the fact that a health care professional can never be certain of any conclusion reached through diagnostic analysis, since errors can be made and knowledge is always limited. Thus, it is argued, the health care professional never really knows that a conclusion is correct, but knows only that it is correct "as far as I can tell." Prognosis, especially in terminal illness, is then seen as prediction, which could be wrong. To give the patient information which is uncertain could, if it proves wrong, be significantly harmful to the patient, by both undermining trust in the professional and causing unnecessary psychological trauma to the patient. Thus, the argument goes, it is better not to tell the patient and to avoid the harm of potential error.

Aside from the need for justification by research, this argument seems easily set aside by simply enjoining health care professionals to be sure the patient understands the nature of the information, i.e., that it is prediction, not absolute fact. Moreover, it is simply silly to say that because absolutely accurate information is not available, distorted or known false information can be given. By that logic, if your TV repairer were not sure whether the problem with your set was the picture tube or the video driver, he would be justified in telling you that the set was OK!

Misunderstanding and Deception

Deception does not always occur just by withholding information or giving false information. There are many ways to deceive by manipulating information. One very common means is to allow a person's mistaken ideas to go uncorrected.

CASE 5.3

Karen Rebikov, a 16-year-old high school senior, was diagnosed as having an oat-cell cancer of the leg. (Oat-cell cancers spread very rapidly and have one of the highest mortality rates known.) Although chemotherapy may be of some help, amputation plus chemotherapy would give Karen a good chance of survival but by no means guarantee a cure. Karen agrees to the chemotherapy; however, she refuses the surgery because, she says, "I would rather die than lose my leg." Her family is very upset by her refusal, and the members of the health care team are concerned because they see Karen's refusal as unreasonable. As a means of helping Karen change her mind, her family arranges for Sybil Freneau to visit, since Sybil had an amputation, although not for cancer. Sybil comes and talks with Karen. As a result, Karen changes her mind and agrees to the surgery. Her comment as she consents for the surgery is, "Well, if the amputation can cure Sybil's cancer, so she can still do everything she did before, then I guess it's dumb for me to refuse." Her comment is not challenged, and she has the surgery the next day.

Here we see an uncorrected mistaken impression lead a patient to make the decision that her family and health care team desired, even though it is questionable whether she would have consented if she knew Sybil did not have cancer and understood that her own surgery did not offer a guaranteed cure.

As in the previous cases, the primary arguments in support of such actions are based on an assessment that the good consequences produced by the deception, namely not wasting an otherwise valuable life, outweigh the bad character of the deception. Or, in this case, they may be based on a notion of duty which requires one to preserve life. The primary assumption, however, must be that it is more important for Karen to have the surgery than for her to make a decision based on correct information.

When someone clearly misunderstands and that misunderstanding is not corrected, she believes she has true information when it is, in fact, false. Often we do not correct misunderstanding if it is seen as an alternative to specifically giving false information and true information is to be kept from the patient. In reality, however, this action is no different from giving false information. Allowing recognized misunderstanding has exactly the same result as giving false information, since in both situations a person is making decisions on the basis of incorrect information.

Manipulation of information is not always intended to influence a person's decisions; instead, its aim is often to prevent harm.

CASE 5.4

Max Chambers and his family were all seriously injured in a car accident on the turnpike. Max's wife, Irene, is nearly dead from serious head injuries, while the children, Joyce and Bryan, are in stable condition with a good chance for complete recovery. Max has a broken back with severed spinal cord as well as internal injuries, but he is not near death and will probably recover, although he will be paraplegic. When Max asks about himself and his family, the emergency room doctor tells him, "Your children were injured, but they are doing very well, and we expect a complete recovery. Your wife has a head injury, but she is in stable condition. You have a broken back, and may lose the use of your legs, but we cannot be certain about that yet. The children are already being moved to the pediatric floor; you will be moved to the orthopedic floor, and your wife to the neurologic intensive care unit. If you have any questions or want to get messages to your family, just ask the nurse. Now, I have to go take care of the admission forms for your family. You just lie back and relax; everything will be OK." Max responds, "Well, I'm glad to hear we're all going to be all right. Thank you, doctor. I appreciate knowing about everything. I was really worried."

In addition to withholding information from Max about his wife's condition, the physician has not corrected his mistaken understanding of the seriousness of everyone's injuries. He has simply allowed Max to formulate his own images of everyone's condition. Because Max is himself critically injured, the complete news of his family is seen as quite liable to seriously affect his condition. So he is not told everything, and his mistaken impression is not corrected.

This is a classic example of a health care professional manipulating information "in the patient's best interest." Notice, however, that it is unlike Case 5.3 in one important respect, namely, Max is not making a decision based on the deceptive information. Karen, however, decided to have the surgery on the basis of the information she received, thus raising questions about informed consent, which we will discuss soon. But first, let us look at one last situation involving deceptive information giving.

The use of placebos also raises questions both about giving false information and about withholding information for the patient's "best interest." With placebo therapy, patients are told they are receiving medicine while they are actually receiving a nonmedicinal substance, such as a sterile saline injection or a sugar pill. Moreover, the patients are usually not told the underlying reason for the placebo.[8] Again, an example will clarify the issues.

CASE 5.5

K'ai Liang is a 17-year-old who is in the hospital recovering from abdominal surgery to repair a gunshot wound. K'ai is recovering nicely but continues to ask for his pain shot every 4 hours. The nurses do not see evidence of pain, but K'ai claims he is "in terrible pain" and needs the shot. The doctor believes that K'ai is becoming addicted to the pain medication and so orders the medication to be gradually diluted with normal saline solution. K'ai will receive the same size shot each time, but the amount of medication in each injection will decrease. When the nurse goes in to give the third diluted injection, K'ai asks her, "Is that my usual medicine? It doesn't seem to work as well." The nurse replies that it is his usual medicine.

The basic reason for not telling persons about the placebo they are receiving is that what they know may have an effect on how the drug works. It is not that patients don't want to know or don't have a right to know, but rather that their knowing will produce harm because a "cure" will be impossible. The primary reason is that placebo therapy is essentially psychological therapy. To work, patients must *think* they are receiving medicinal therapy, although they are not; otherwise, the "placebo effect"—the fact that the nondrug works as a real drug— probably would not occur. Thus the resulting alleviation of the problem could not be achieved. For example, if K'ai were to no longer complain of pain after receiving the sterile saline injection, which he *thought* was medication, then it would be clear that he was not really in pain but was dependent on the medication. However, if K'ai were told, "We are giving you a shot of sterile saline to see if you really have pain," chances are that he would perceive no pain relief because he would know that it was not medication and so would not expect it to ease his pain.

[8]For a full discussion see Howard Brody, *Placebos and the Philosophy of Medicine*, University of Chicago Press, Chicago, 1980.

Placebo therapy is controversial for several reasons: the psychological factors are not clearly understood; there is a potential for serious harm if a person is not receiving medication that is really needed; and if the deception is discovered, the person may feel cheated and lose faith in the health care professions. Yet the basic underlying ethical principle—that concealing information from a person because otherwise an effect which is good for the person might not be achieved—is widely accepted.

In a broader context, this argument frequently permits deception whenever it would enable the health care professionals to do what they think is best for the patient. Accepting such a position as correct would certainly permit health care professionals much greater control in health care situations. Whether that control is *morally* justified remains to be seen, however, and is our concern in the next chapter.

IS SILENCE GOLDEN?

Sometimes it is tempting to think that there is a significant moral difference between telling an outright lie and withholding information. Telling a lie is seen as an action, while withholding information is seen as an omission, but not an action. At the moral level, withholding information is then thought to be less troublesome, because remaining silent prevents deception, since deception is a function of communication. Yet we have just seen several situations in which a person *is* deceived by excluded information as well as by uncorrected misinterpretations of information. To really grasp the problem, though, think about the following examples and decide whether you think the silence argument holds. Then consider each example from the perspective of the "prevent harm" and "they don't want to know" arguments.

1 A physician uses a new, experimental drug on a patient without telling her that it is experimental or asking her consent to use the drug.

2 The management of a company which makes electronics parts does not tell the employees that chemicals used in the manufacturing process can cause lung cancer and brain damage.

3 The administration of a college fails to tell students that the college has lost its accreditation and thus their credits will not be accepted at other colleges.

4 The selection committee of a nursing school does not tell applicants that preference is given to students between the ages of 18 and 22.

5 A woman is not told that by refusing a test for cervical cancer she is exposing herself to significant risk of having undetected cancer.[9]

Stop for a moment and assess these five cases before going on. What are the issues in each and how would you resolve the problems?

---

[9]Each of these examples summarizes a court case in which a person sued, and won, on the basis that he or she was improperly deceived.

TRUTH OR CONSEQUENCES?

Our discussion of deception in information giving so far has focused primarily on an analysis of consequences as justification for not being truthful. As it is most often used, a consequence-based justification could allow a person not to be truthful if so doing would ensure being able to do what is thought best for another person. Widespread use of this justification overlooks another very important point, namely, that outside of the health care situation, our normal assumption is that a person has an *obligation* to tell the truth. In fact, one reason that manipulation of information works so well in the health care situation is that people do not expect it. Put differently, in normal communication situations, the expectation is that information exchanged will be truthful. Thus, when people enter the health care situation, they expect to be told the truth. Moreover, because the recipients of health care services are usually not knowledgeable about most of what goes on, it is easy for them to believe that they are being told the truth. The health care professional's obligation to tell the truth, then, comes from recognizing the vulnerability of persons in the health care situation and not using that vulnerability to take advantage of them.

Another major reason for telling a person the truth, a reason obscured by the consequences arguments, is that having true information available to make choices is a *right* which may not be violated. As such, this argument goes, the professional has neither a right nor a duty to take the decision making away from a competent person. This argument, however, raises an important issue concerning patient autonomy, which we must examine now, because the issue of truth telling cannot be understood otherwise.

Understanding autonomy as roughly equivalent to free will or freedom of choice, we see two major areas of concern. First, if autonomy means freedom to choose and if patients have autonomy, then interference with the patient's decision making violates autonomy. Not telling a patient the truth or withholding information is then morally problematic, since freedom of choice is compromised if correct and adequate information is not available. Because informed consent is so important in health care and because truth telling affects informed consent, autonomy, as a key feature of both, becomes a primary concern.

A person who is not able or not allowed to decide how to act cannot perform actions which are freely chosen; similarly, being forced to act in a certain way results in an action that is not freely chosen. Autonomy of judgment (decisions) requires both the freedom and the capacity to utilize reason in making choices; autonomy of action requires both the freedom and the capacity to act on those choices. If either autonomy of judgment or autonomy of action is interfered with, the person involved cannot choose freely. Four factors for autonomy were introduced in Chapter 2; let's see now how they apply to the situations described so far in this chapter.

1 *Capacity for deliberation and action.* An absence of truth, or a lack of complete information, does not have an effect on a person's competence, since competence is a function of ability, not information. A person may be fully competent to make a decision, but if not given the chance to decide, no decision can be made. Deceptive information may limit choices, but it does not limit the capacity for choice.

2 *Adequate information.* For autonomous decisions, the person deciding must have all the available relevant information. Since a choice is a function of its situation, and since information defines a situation, information defines choice. A person considering one set of facts will make different choices than if considering a different set of facts. Deceptive information manipulates choices by making a person believe the decision concerns one matter when, in fact, it concerns another. Moreover, it is doubly deceptive, because that person is lead to believe that she *does* have adequate information and thus is making a legitimate choice. In each case except 5.4 (Max), decisions are affected by the adequacy of information and thus are not autonomous in that regard.

3 *Alternatives for action.* By definition, one cannot make a choice if there are no alternatives, for *choose* means "to pick among options." Since available alternatives are a function of the situational information, adequate information is required for proper consideration of alternatives. Insofar as truthful information is not complete, the decision maker's alternatives for action may be severely restricted. This would then add to the reduction of autonomy in the decision situation of each case except 5.4.

4 *Absence of coercive factors.* It is very difficult not to be coercive when one gives incorrect information or withholds information. If information is withheld from people in order to force them to decide in a certain way, they are being manipulated; if we leave their mistaken ideas uncorrected, they are being deceived. For example, Karen misunderstood an explanation, but that misunderstanding aided the goal of obtaining consent for surgery, so the misunderstanding was not corrected. In this way, Karen was operating on false information, because her misunderstanding was not corrected. She was tricked into consenting to the surgery. Similarly, in the placebo incident, K'ai Liang was deceived in an effort to make him think the medication was really a pain killer. In both instances the deception is intentional but covert, allowing the deceiver to appear as a friend, not a manipulator, while being a manipulator nonetheless. Perhaps this is what makes deception so morally problematic; the patient is fully trusting, and health care professionals try to build and encourage that trust but then use it to deceive.

There is no question that our social and legal values support the autonomy of a competent person. Accordingly, not telling the truth or limiting available information is unacceptable. We may be able to give reasons justifying such action in some situations, but the norm is nondeceptive information giving, with the burden of proof on the person who intends to deceive. To do otherwise is to deny the basic autonomy of the competent person.

The seriousness of deceptive information and denial of autonomy becomes much clearer in health care, however, if we notice that such action has a direct influence on informed consent. Without correct information a person is not adequately informed, so that any consent given on the basis of deceptive information is deceptive, uninformed consent, not informed consent.

INFORMED CONSENT

Obtaining informed consent is extremely important in health care today. However, this concern for informed consent is relatively recent, having developed primarily within the last 40 to 50 years, from two different directions—research and clinical practice. The research concern with consent arose in the early 1950s, following the discovery, through the Nuremberg trials, of Nazi medical "experiments" in the death camps. Because the world was outraged at the atrocities, requirements for consent were instituted as a means of protecting people from a recurrence. As medical sciences began their meteoric advancement and human experimentation became both necessary and common, informed consent for research grew in importance as a means for protecting people from unwilling or unknowing participation in experiments. In addition, through federal law, committees called *Institutional Review Boards* were established to oversee the protection of human subjects in research, both by ensuring informed consent and by assessing the risks to persons participating in experiments.

Application of informed consent to clinical practices actually preceded concern with research, although from the law, not the medical community. Traditionally, principles of medical practice required physicians to do what they thought best for the patient, without concern for the patient's views. It was not until 1914 that Judge Benjamin Cardozo applied the force of law to the principles of individuality and autonomy in medical practices, when he ruled that

> . . . every human being of adult years and sound mind has a right to determine what shall be done with his own body; and a surgeon who performs an operation without his patient's consent commits an assault, for which he is liable in damages.[10]

Although this statement was directed toward surgery because the case being tried was a surgical case, it nonetheless formed the basis for several other cases, expanding the concept to nonsurgeons as well. Notice, however, that the judge is not bestowing a right to self-determination; rather, he is recognizing an existing natural right and applying the force of law to uphold that right. Recent rulings consistently uphold a person's specific right to informed consent and have expanded the application of that right to refusal of treatment, including life support.[11]

---

[10]*Scholendorff v. Society of N.Y. Hospital*, 211 N.Y. 125, 105 N.E. 92 (1914).

[11]*Nathanson v. Kline*, 186 KAN. 393, 350 P.2d 1093, 1104 (1960), expanded application of the right to refusal of treatment, while *Truman v. Thomas*, 27 CAL. 3d 285 (1980), applied the basic concepts of consent to *informed* refusal. *Bartling v. Glendale Adventist Medical Center*, 209 CAL.

The Patient's Bill of Rights (reproduced in the Appendix), presented by the American Hospital Association in 1972, had a significant influence on the development of our current views toward consent. Although it only has twelve stipulated rights, eight of those relate to the patient's right to knowledge and informed consent. Perhaps of more importance than its stipulations was the fact that the Patient's Bill of Rights motivated similar documents for other persons, including the disabled, the mentally ill, the handicapped, the pregnant, the elderly, children, and the dying. Coupled with a growing consumerism and increasing education of persons about their rights in health care, consent has become an important factor not only in health care but also in malpractice suits. As a result of this increased concern for consent, nearly half the states now have laws regarding informed consent in health care, although only Texas has specific requirements about the information that must be given in clinical medicine.[12]

The clinical emphasis on informed consent was not received with open arms, and many health care professionals resented what they saw as the interference of the law in matters of clinical (i.e., professional) judgment. Most health care professionals today willingly go along with some form of consent, but generally because it reduces their legal liability. However, they often reserve for themselves the decision of what will be disclosed, depending on how they believe the information will affect the patient, and what they believe a person needs to know in order to make a decision. Unfortunately, the recognition of individual autonomy is missing; the patient takes the risks, the patient suffers the consequences, but there is reluctance to accept the patient's right to a decision which is free and uncoerced.[13] Moreover, because most legal action concerns physicians and because physicians usually bear the legal burden of ensuring consent, other health care professionals, especially nurses, mistakenly regard consent as none of their concern and are reluctant to intervene, even when they are the witness for consent and do not believe the patient is really giving informed consent.

ELEMENTS OF CONSENT

Consent is properly understood as a free, rational act by a competent person, based on accurate information which that person is able to understand. Over the years, five basic components of the consent process have become generally accepted:

RPTR. 220 (Cal. App. 2 dist. 1984), and *Leach v. Shapiro*, 13 Ohio App. 3d 393 (October 1984), extended the application to refusal of life-support equipment. *In the Matter of Claire C. Conroy*, 98 N.J. 321, 486 A.2d 1209 (1985), the application was further expanded to include removal of nasogastric feeding.

[12]6 Texas Reg. 4669 (Dec. 15, 1981). This regulation stipulates specific information which must be given in 120 different instances of consent.

[13]For an in-depth discussion of this viewpoint see A. Meisel, Loren H. Roth, and Charles W. Lidz, "Toward a Model of the Legal Doctrine of Informed Consent," *American Journal of Psychiatry*, vol. 134, March 1977, pp. 285–289.

1 An explanation of the person's condition, in terms understandable to the person receiving the explanation

2 An explanation of the procedures to be used and the risks and benefits of those procedures, in noncoercive terms understandable to the person receiving the explanation

3 A fair (i.e., noncoercive) description of alternatives to the suggested procedures, including nontreatment options

4 Adequate allowance for questions and assurance that the person has understood the information in items 1, 2, and 3

5 Adequate allowance for persons to change their mind and withdraw consent, without penalty

Certainly, the basic right which necessitates consent also allows a competent person to waive such an explanation and give consent in ignorance. In such a case, however, the person obtaining consent still has the obligation to ensure that the consent is valid, i.e., that the person giving consent is competent, and to note on the consent that the person refused to allow an explanation. Moreover, in an effort to promote autonomy, some effort should be made to help the consenter understand the importance of fully informed consent. Yet if the explanations are still refused, there is not much choice but to accept the consenter's decision.

Of particular concern, in any consent situation, is how much information should be conveyed to the person consenting. On one hand, it is unnecessary and unreasonable to go into every minute detail, since that will only confuse or, worse, scare the person. Yet there is still the need to present a "reasonable" amount of information, including details which are important to making an informed decision. For example, it is not necessary for a person to know that the opening surgical incision will be made with a number 21 blade, followed by the use of a Bovie to stem the bleeding, blunt dissection of the muscles, etc. It *is* necessary to know the potential for dying during the surgery; whether the surgery is an emergency, life-saving procedure or a cosmetic elective; how likely the procedure is to succeed; and so forth.

On the other hand, many people want to know, and believe they have a right to know, whatever *they,* not the health professional, think is important. The opportunity to ask questions and discuss alternatives is then an important element of the consent procedure, because it allows the individual to obtain such information.

It is important to remember that consent is what makes health care practices acceptable. As Sam Gorovits has so aptly noted, professional behavior which is allowable with consent becomes unacceptable without consent:

Sometimes [professional] behavior involves cutting people, sometimes even taking parts of them that you do not like and discarding them. Now, on the face of it, that would seem not best described as medical practice, but as felonious assault. The kinds of things that [health care professionals] do day in and day out are just the kinds of things that, but for very special justification [via informed consent], would in fact *be* felonious assault.[14]

No consent can ever be completely free or fully informed, however, simply because no one can ever have all the information relevant to a decision or all the knowledge needed to completely understand everything. The ethical problem with consent is thus not whether totally free and absolutely informed consent is possible, for it is not; rather, the problem is to determine when consent is reasonable and sufficient. To put it differently, are the information and voluntarism in this situation such that a reasonable person would consider them adequate for informed consent? This is clearly an important, though difficult, question to answer. The moral issue is not whether a person consented, but whether the consent was based on an informed, autonomous decision.

TRUTH RECONSIDERED

When a competent person is not told the truth, choices have been restricted (thus interfered with), because the person's information base is not adquate. Since interfering with a person's choice is a violation of his autonomy, not being truthful in the ways discussed violates a person's autonomy. Moreover, the person has also been deceived and manipulated, since he expects to be told the truth, and so he is operating as if he had true information on which to base a decision. For both these reasons, the "choice" which results from the patient's decision is not a true choice. The patient's freedom has been significantly restricted. Again, there may be good reasons for doing this, but the burden of proof is on the health care professional, and the instances requiring it will be rare indeed. As noted earlier, the basis for ethics is autonomy; thus the basis for treating a patient as a person, as a fellow human being, is to respect autonomy. Any arguments supporting other actions will then have to take autonomy into account and show, in effect, that violating the person's autonomy in this instance actually enhances his autonomy overall.

Notice that because autonomy is fundamental to ethics, each of the basic ethical theories must carry a commitment to the view that since people have a right to choose (if they are competent), they have a right to information, since choice is not possible without information. Different theoretical considerations will determine whether, in that theoretical context, it is morally correct to violate autonomy. However, the basic premise of moral behavior in any case must be to uphold autonomy if at all possible.

[14]Samuel Gorovits, "Can Physicians Mind Their Own Business and Still Practice Medicine?" in Nora K. Bell (ed.), *Who Decides: Conflicts of Rights in Health Care*, Humana Press, Clifton, NJ, 1982, p. 85.

The more that one comes to view patients as free agents, the more one will be pressed to see the medical professions as ways of reestablishing patient autonomy over their bodies and minds. In fact, insofar as one sees the ethical community as one bound together on the basis not of force, but of respect for the freedom of others, one will come to envision the relationship among medicine, society, and individuals as one of a more or less formal negotiation about goals.[15]

Since the choice affects the chooser, it is the chooser's prerogative to make the choice; it is thus the health care professional's duty to help make the circumstances for that choice the best possible. A conscious regard for the patient's autonomy, by preserving the freedom of choice if at all possible, must then be achieved by giving truthful, complete information, information to which the competent patient, as an autonomous person, has a right.

STUDY GUIDE

READINGS

D. French, "Nurse, Am I Going to Live?" p. 186.
F. Ingelfinger, "Informed (but Uneducated) Consent," p. 200.
R. Goldberg, "Disclosure of Information to Adult Cancer Patients: Issues and Update," p. 188.
D. Ost, "The 'Right' Not to Know," p. 225.

QUESTIONS FOR REFLECTION

1 Each case in this chapter is presented with the health care professional's resolution of the ethical dilemma. For each case, first identify the ethical dilemma and then assess the given resolution. Would you have done the same thing? What would you have done differently? Why would you have done this?
2 Assess each case presented in this chapter by using the five criteria for informed consent. Does informed consent apply equally to each case? How are the cases different? How might a change in circumstances alter the assessment of consent for each person?

CASE STUDIES FOR ANALYSIS

Case Study 1   You are the primary nurse caring for Barbara (Case 5.1). While you are caring for her, she says to you, "I have the feeling the doctor and my family are not telling me the truth. Am I really OK, or do I have cancer and they are not telling me?"

---

[15]H. Tristram Englehardt, Jr., "Goals of Medical Care: A Reappraisal," in Nora Bell, *Who Decides: Conflicts of Rights in Health Care*, Humana Press, Clifton, NJ, 1982, p. 62.

You know that the family and physician have not told Barbara the truth. Should you tell her now?

Analysis Questions   What is the ethical dilemma in this case? Is there more than one? One alternative is to contact the physician and ask what to tell Barbara; but what will you tell her in the meanwhile? If you tell her, "I really don't know. You must ask your doctor," you are lying; but if you say "I'm sorry, but I am not allowed to give you that information. You must ask your doctor," won't you have really answered her question?

Case Study 2   Rita Kynard is the shift nurse responsible for medications in a team nursing situation. In the process of giving medications, she accidentally gives Mr. Updike the medication intended for his roommate, Mr. Evans. When she discovers the mistake, she checks the drug book and decides that the medication will probably not hurt Mr. Updike; so she does nothing about it. However, since the hospital pharmacy works on a unit-dose basis, she has no medication to give Mr. Evans. If she calls pharmacy for another dose, she will have to explain what happened to the first one, and she knows she could be fired for the drug error. Should she simply write on the chart that Mr. Evans received his medication as ordered?

Case Study 3   Kareem Mofolo is a surgical physician's assistant who is called in to assist with emergency surgery. Prior to the case, while helping to set up the instruments, Kareem notices that Frank Samson, the perfusionist, is behaving erratically, dropping instruments, bumping into equipment, and leaving the room frequently without completing the setup. When Kareem leaves the room to notify the emergency room that the team is ready for the patient, he finds the perfusionist standing in the hallway, just staring at the floor. Kareem approaches him, to see what is wrong. Startled, Frank yells at Kareem to leave him alone and then walks off down the hall, away from the operating room. During the outburst, Kareem smells the unmistakable odor of alcohol on Frank's breath.

When the surgeon comes, Kareem tells her of his concern that the perfusionist is drunk and unable to perform properly. The surgeon goes to find the perfusionist. Agreeing with Kareem's assessment, she sends Frank home, delaying the surgery until another perfusionist can come in.

After surgery, as Kareem is entering postoperative notes, he reads the surgeon's note which says, "F. Samson was taken ill and went home; procedure delayed 25 minutes until G. Allen could come in to take over perfusion." When Kareem asks the surgeon about the note, she replies, "Look, the guy has a drinking problem; let's not crucify him professionally on top of that." What, if anything, should Kareem do?

Analysis Questions for Cases 2 and 3   How do these cases differ from those discussed so far? What is the difference of deception here, as opposed to the other cases in this chapter? Does it matter to the resolution in each case who is being deceived by the misinformation? Would you resolve these cases differently if you took a duty-based approach or a rights-based approach?

Case Study 4   You are a judge who has been asked to intervene in the following case.

A 31-year-old man, father of four children, has been brought into the emergency room of Boston City Hospital, having been seriously injured in an automobile accident. His injuries include both a ruptured spleen and a lacerated liver. The resulting hemorrhage requires both surgical intervention and blood replacement. Because of religious beliefs, the patient has refused the blood replacement; on hope of reversal, the hospital asked the patient's wife to consent to the procedure, and she, too, has refused.

Under the law of the state, you, the judge, may appoint the hospital as guardian for the patient, thus allowing administration of the blood despite the patient's wishes. The hospital is asking for this appointment.

Analysis Questions   What is your decision? Why? What are the moral questions which arise in this case? On what grounds did you resolve them?

Suppose the case is the same but the patient is a 7-year-old girl. How should this case be handled and why? Are there different moral questions in this instance? If so, what are they and how do they affect the decision?

Case Study 5   As a medical laboratory technician, you are asked to participate in a research project intended to show a correlation between renal function and antibiotic therapy. The project involves chemical analysis of urine samples obtained from patients treated by the three physicians engaged in the research.

After agreeing to the project, you discover that the patients do not know that their urine samples are being used in the research. Instead, they are only being told of the standard urinalysis which is necessary for their treatment. So the additional tests you are running are being done without the patients' knowledge or consent.

Analysis Questions   What, if any, are the ethical problems raised here? What should you do about it? Why?

Suppose you also discover that the patients are being billed for the extra tests, with the billing only showing the fee for routine urinalysis. How does this change the situation? What are the new ethical problems?

Case Study 6   Your doctor has completed a series of tests which conclusively indicate an inoperable malignant tumor of the brain. The prognosis is poor, and it is known that neither chemotherapy nor radiotherapy is of any value. Should your doctor tell you of your condition? Should she tell you the prognosis? Justify your answer.

Analysis Questions Take the same case, but now argue for the opposite viewpoint (if you said she should tell you, now argue that she should not, or vice versa).

BIBLIOGRAPHY

Baram, Michael S.: "The Right to Know and the Duty to Disclose Hazard Information," *American Journal of Public Health,* vol. 74, no.4, April 1984, pp. 385–390.

Berg, Robert N.: "The Great "Informed Consent" Debate: Should Disclosure Risks and Alternatives by Physicians Be Standard Preoperating Procedure?" *Journal of the Medical Association of Georgia,* vol. 72, April 1983, pp. 285–288.

Bok, Sissela: *Secrets: On the Ethics of Concealment and Revelation,* Vintage Books, New York, 1983.

Curran, William: "AIDS Research and the Window of Opportunity," *New England Journal of Medicine,* vol. 312, no. 14, April 1985, pp. 903–904.

Davies, Lord Edmund: "The Patient's Right to Know the Truth," *Proceedings of the Royal Society of Medicine,* vol. 66, June 1973, pp. 533–536.

Davis, Anne J.: "To Tell or Not," *American Journal of Nursing,* January 1981, pp. 156–158.

Ellin, Joseph S.: "Lying and Deception: The Solution to a Dilemma in Medical Ethics," *Westminister Institute Review,* vol. 1, no. 2, May 1981, pp. 3–6.

Freedman, B.: "A Moral Theory of Informed Consent," *Hastings Center Report,* vol. 5, no. 4, 1975, pp. 32–39.

Goldie, L.: "The Ethics of Telling the Patient," *Journal of Medical Ethics,* vol. 8, 1982, pp. 128–133.

Green, Richard S. "Why Schizophrenic Patients Should Be Told Their Diagnosis," *Hospital and Community Psychiatry,* vol. 35, no. 1, January 1984, pp. 76–77.

Helm, Ann: "Truth Telling, Placebos, and Deception: Ethical and Legal Issues in Practice," *Aviation, Space and Environmental Medicine,* January 1985, pp. 69–72.

Kelly, Lucie Y.: "The Patient's Right to Know," *Nursing Outlook,* vol. 24, no. 1, January 1974, pp. 26–32.

Kelly, William D., and Stanley R. Friesen: "Do Cancer Patients Want to Be Told?" *Surgery,* vol. 27, 1950, pp. 822–826.

Lipkin, Mack: "On Lying to Patients," *Newsweek,* June 4, 1984, p. 13.

Payton, Rita J.: "Nurses Share Ethical Responsibility for Informed Consent," *AORN Journal,* vol. 39, no. 5, 1984, pp. 755–758.

President's Commission for the Study of Ethical Problems in Medicine and Biomedical and Behavioral Research: *Making Health Care Decisions: A Report on the Ethical and Legal Implications of Informed Consent in the Patient-Practitioner Relationship,* Government Printing Office, Washington, 1984.

Sheldon, Mark: "Truth Telling in Medicine," *Journal of the American Medical Association,* vol. 247, no. 5, February 5, 1982, pp. 651–654.

Vanderpool, Harold Y., and Gary B. Weiss: "Patient Truthfulness: A Test of Models of the Physician-Patient Relationship," *Journal of Medicine and Philosophy,* vol. 9, 1984, pp. 353–372.

"What Should the Doctor Tell?" *British Medical Journal,* vol. 289, August 1984, pp. 325–326.

Yearling, Roland R.: "Ethical Analysis of a Nursing Problem: The Scope of Nursing Practice in Disclosing the Truth to Terminal Patients," *Supervisor Nurse,* pt. I, May 1978; pt. II, June 1978.

CHAPTER 6

DECISIONS FOR OTHERS: PROXY CONSENT AND PATERNALISM

Medicine is not geared to passive observation and the allowance of self-destructive behavior. This compassionate interventionism is a key feature of the medical model, and is not to be lightly discounted

Colleen Clements*

CONSENT FOR THE INCOMPETENT

We saw in the last chapter that the predominant arguments in favor of being untruthful are based on analysis of consequences (doing what is best for the patient) or duties (either to do what is best for the patient or to protect the patient from harm), while the primary arguments in favor of being truthful are based on recognizing a person's right to self-determination and informed consent. Up to this point, however, we have only considered consent by competent adults. The problems become even more complicated in decisions for persons whose autonomy is limited, e.g., incompetent adults, children, or persons in institutions such as prisons, mental hospitals, or long-term care facilities. In such cases the issue is one of *proxy consent,* that is, who should consent and how the decision to consent should be made.

The problem, of course, is that competence is not easily determined. To see

Medical Genetics Casebook, Humana Press, Clifton, N.J., 1982, p. 28.

this and work with the concept, let's return to Mr. Fontanez, whose case was presented as Case Study 1 at the end of Chapter 3:

CASE 6.1

Mr. Fontanez is an 82-year-old who has been admitted to the medical service with a diagnosis of cancer of the pancreas which has metastasized (spread) to the liver, spleen, and bone. Upon admission, it is noted that Mr. Fontanez has gangrene of the foot and has already lost two toes. He is in considerable pain, with the daily cleaning and care of the foot causing more pain.

A surgeon is consulted and agrees with the attending physician that a partial amputation of the foot is the only hope for stopping the spread of the gangrene. Since the surgeon is the one who will do the procedure, he approaches Mr. Fontanez for consent. He explains the procedure, tells Mr. Fontanez why it is necessary, and then asks him to sign the form consenting to the operation. Mr. Fontanez refuses to sign. The surgeon carefully explains the consequences of not having the operation (continued pain and spread of the disease). However, Mr. Fontanez still refuses, saying, "No, leave me alone and let me die in peace."

Clearly, Mr. Fontanez' competence is a crucial issue here, since the exercise of autonomy depends on competence. How do we determine his competence?

TESTING FOR COMPETENCE

Traditionally three types of test have been used (separately and in combination) to determine competence:

1 *Outcome test.* If the decision a person makes is not the one others think is best, that is evidence of incompetence.

2 *Status test.* If a person's mental and/or physical status would impair decisions, that is evidence of incompetence. (This status could be determined by the situation, e.g., prisoners; by law, e.g., minors; or by health-related factors, e.g., diagnosis, use of pain medication, etc.)

3 *Function test.* If you are unable to function as a decision maker, that is evidence of incompetence.[1]

Each of these "tests" has characteristics which distinguish its use. To understand them better, we briefly apply each to Mr. Fontanez.

As the case was originally presented, the surgeon used *the outcome test* to argue that, since Mr. Fontanez had not consented to the surgery, it was clear

---

[1]For a full discussion of this problem, see George Annas and Joan Densberger, "Competence to Refuse Medical Treatment: Autonomy v. Paternalism," *Toledo Law Review,* vol 15, 1984.

he was not competent. If the staff and family all agreed that Mr. Fontanez' choice was inappropriate, that would still be the outcome test. The crucial element of that test is the idea that agreement certifies correctness: "If we don't agree with you, you are wrong." At the same time, the fact that there is substantive disagreement with a decision can indicate that the decision is questionable. The outcome test, however, relies solely on assessment of the choice made, without taking other things into account.

The classic example of applying the outcome test is the view of suicide which says, "No person in his right mind would want to kill himself; thus anyone who tries to kill himself must be incompetent." On the basis of this version of the outcome test, for many years attempting suicide was sufficient grounds for involuntary commitment to a mental health facility.

The status test could apply to Mr. Fontanez in a number of ways. Because he is 82 years old, we might argue that he is most likely confused, thus not competent; because he is in a lot of pain, we could say that his reasoning is affected; because his cancer is widely spread and he knows he is dying, we could say that he is too depressed to make a reasonable decision; and so on. The point is that when the status test is used, specific factors are identified as interfering with competent decision making, and when those factors are present, the decision is not accepted.

Age is a frequently used status indicator, especially when the decision maker is under the legal age (usually 18 years) or late in life (e.g., over 65). Thus it could be argued that in Case 5.4 Karen should not have been involved in the decision to amputate her leg, since she was only 16 years old. Another frequently used status indicator is education. In fact, one long-standing argument against allowing patient autonomy in health care is that most people do not have enough education in health care matters to make a competent decision. Autonomy is also related to the status test whenever the argument for autonomy rests on the fact that each person has a right to autonomy. In that case, one's status as a person is the determining factor for one's right to autonomy.

Although the outcome and status tests are, on the surface, easy to use, they both incorporate a serious flaw—the criteria selected are arbitrary. In addition, both tests assume that competence is an all-or-nothing determination; a person is either competent or incompetent, period. *The function test,* which is a fairly recent development, attempts to overcome both problems by using outcome and status as only part of a much more comprehensive assessment. Using this test, we would need to determine whether Mr. Fontanez understood his situation and the information given to him; whether his choice was reflective; whether his consideration of alternatives showed understanding; whether he reasonably understood the consequences of his decision; whether his decision was in character for him; what his intentions were in making the decision; and so on.

The function test is quite different from the other two because it takes competence to be a matter of degree, such that a person could be competent for some decisions but not for others. The result is a much fairer assessment, which recognizes a need to protect autonomy. Another difference is that the outcome and status tests are more frequently used from a framework of assumed incompetence, while the function test more frequently assumes competence and tests for the accuracy of that assumption.

Take a moment now and look back on your handling of Mr. Fontanez' case. How did you deal with the competence problem? If you used the outcome test, what outcome was most important—his death? If you used the status test, what indicators of status did you consider? If you used the function test, what considerations of function were important? Now that you understand the tests, do you want to change or reject your earlier decision about Mr. Fontanez?

A great deal more could be said about testing for competence, but that would take more space than we have. We continue to work with these tests, though, as we continue our discussion. Now, however, we need to look at what happens once the decision of incompetence is made and the proxy decision process comes into effect.

PROXY CONSENT AND SUBSTITUTED JUDGMENT

When thinking about consent in cases of diminished competence, thus restricted autonomy, we must recognize the difference between the primary and the secondary consenter. The *primary consenter* is always the person who is affected by the consent decision, while the *secondary consenter* is the person who makes a decision on behalf of the primary consenter. For example, a newborn infant is the primary consenter, and his parents are the secondary consenters; a comatose 60-year-old is the primary consenter, and her spouse is the secondary consenter.

Proxy consent is the consent which is given by a secondary consenter on behalf of the primary consenter. The question of consent then divides into two parts: When is there a need for the proxy consent of a secondary consenter? and On what basis should the secondary consenter make decisions?

Since the Karen Quinlan case in 1976, courts around the country have been taking their task to be the determination and implementation of the rights of incompetent persons. The basic principle of these cases is that incompetent persons have as much right to self-determination as competent persons; the only problem is determining how to ensure the exercise of that right. In the 1977 case of Joseph Saikewicz,[2] the court articulated for the first time a principle of *substituted judgment,* which has now become a common element in our understanding of informed consent for incompetent persons. The idea behind substituted judgment is that the secondary consenter should, as much as possible, attempt to utilize the values of the primary consenter when making a proxy

---

[2]*Superintendent of Belchertown State School v. Saikewicz* 373 Mass. 728, 370 N.E. 2d 417 (1977).

decision. Obviously this is a problem in the case of persons who were never competent, such as babies, the severely mentally handicapped, etc.; but the basic principle—when you are deciding for others, use their values, not your own—is sound.

The case of Bill Anderson (Case 1.6), the Jehovah's Witness, is a good example of how substituted judgment could be used. Once Bill was unconscious, he was no longer competent to make his own decisions. On the basis of substituted judgment, the secondary consenter should refuse consent for the transfusion, because that is the decision Bill would have reached if he were making the decision himself.

How is it possible to utilize substituted judgment? First, the secondary consenter may know enough about the person, her values, and her beliefs to make reasonable assumptions about her wishes. Second, the primary consenter could have prepared a *living will* or a *durable power of attorney,* documents describing the person's wishes for treatment if she becomes incompetent.

Although living wills and durable powers of attorney are growing in their acceptance, the primary means for substituted judgment is knowledge of the person, as shown in the case of Brother Fox.

CASE 6.2

A member of a religious order, Brother Fox, was admitted to the hospital for surgical repair of a hernia. During surgery, for unknown reasons, Brother Fox suffered a severe stroke, which left him irreversibly comatose, with his life supported by mechanical ventilation.

When it was determined that Brother Fox's situation was medically hopeless, the superior of his order asked that life support be withdrawn, a request with which the family agreed. The hospital and doctors refused, however, so the matter was taken to court.

On behalf of Brother Fox, the superior argued that he was requesting only what Brother Fox would request, if he could. As evidence, he cited numerous public discussions of the Karen Quinlan case, where Brother Fox had consistently maintained that if the same thing happened to him, he hoped they would not prolong his life. In addition, Brother Fox's religious beliefs were used to support the view that he would not be afraid of dying and did not deem it necessary that his life be prolonged at all costs.[3]

Here the superior is engaging in substituted judgment, trying to ensure a decision that is in keeping with the beliefs and values of the primary consenter.

[3]*Eichner v. Dillon,* 73 A.D. 2d 431, 426 N.Y.S. 517 (1980).

PERSONAL BELIEFS AND DECISIONS FOR OTHERS

Often it is hard for secondary consenters to utilize substituted judgment, because the primary consenter's beliefs either cannot be known or are at odds with their own. The first instance does not present an ethical problem, because the secondary consenter's only option is to use his own beliefs and values as a basis for the proxy decision. The second instance does present an ethical problem, both because there is a conflict of beliefs and because that conflict may cause the secondary consenter to rely on his own beliefs instead of those of the primary consenter. An even more serious problem arises when someone assumes the role of secondary consenter based on such disagreement, for then there is a serious problem of *paternalism*. Before considering paternalism, however, we need to look at how it arises through secondary consent.

CASE 6.3

Wesley Marshall, a 56-year-old smoker who suffers from chronic lung disease, was admitted to the hospital for severe rectal bleeding. The diagnostic workup showed the cause of the bleeding to be a rectal fissure (a split in the wall of the rectum) which could be repaired only by surgery. As part of the consent procedure, the surgeon discussed with Wesley and his family the possibility that, because of the lung disease, Wesley could become dependent on mechanical ventilation following the surgery. Wesley made his wishes quite clear: "I don't want to live my life hooked up to a machine. If I can't live without the machine breathing for me, pull the plug and be done with it."

Following surgery Wesley became dependent on the machine. Every known effort was made to wean him from the machine, but he simply could not breathe on his own. After several weeks on life support, Wesley slipped into a coma. The doctor then asked Wesley's wife for permission to remove the machine, as Wesley had requested before surgery. His wife refused, saying, "I know he said that, and I know that is what he wanted; but I don't think it's right not to do everything possible. If he dies on the machine, fine, but I'm not allowing you to disconnect him." As a result, Wesley stayed on life support until he was brain-dead 2 months later.

This case presents a common example of disagreement between the primary and secondary consenter. If Wesley's wife had utilized substituted judgment, she would have given permission to remove the machine even though she disagreed with his decision. As it was, she used her own values to make the decision for Wesley.

The problem is that substituted judgment may put a person in the position of giving consent for something she considers morally wrong, simply because it is what the other person wanted. At issue is the basic principle that it is generally unacceptable to force a person to do something which she considers to be morally wrong. The conflict is with the basic principle of freedom and self-determination, for if the primary consenter is autonomous, so, too, is the secondary consenter.

This conflict may be partially resolved by recognizing that the secondary consenter is not the one making the decision, because the primary consenter has already made the decision. To use substituted judgment means to ensure that the primary consenter's wishes are granted, so that the responsibility for the decision lies with the primary consenter, not the secondary. Thus there is no difference between allowing a primary consenter's decision and allowing anyone else's decision. If the secondary consenter would not normally interfere with the decision, then there is little ground for interfering at the point of proxy consent. In the context of autonomy, if a person would not normally interfere with the autonomous decision of another, then there is no reason to interfere when acting as the secondary consenter.

However, if the secondary consenter truly believes that the decision is not in the best interest of the primary consenter, is there a moral obligation *not* to abide by that decision? In the context of Case 6.3, if Wesley's wife believes that it is really not in his best interest to withdraw life support, is she then justified in not utilizing substituted judgment and acting instead upon her own values and beliefs? An understanding of paternalism[4] will help clarify this problem.

PATERNALISM IN HEALTH CARE DECISIONS

A look at the literature of ethics in health care shows that the word *paternalism* is ambiguous between three different applications: as a label for an action which is right or wrong; as a label for a type of action, but without a connotation of value; and as a label for an attitude, but without connotation of value. Because we are attempting to understand and apply the term, we consider it in the second and third ways, since the first presupposes the questions of value that we are exploring. Our task, then, is to establish an understanding of the concept so that it will be possible to assess an action or an attitude to determine whether it is paternalistic, without making a judgment as to whether the action is correct. For ease of discussion, we begin with action and then discuss attitude.

The key to understanding paternalism is to see that a parent generally tries to act *on behalf of* his or her children. The children are not given the opportunity to agree or disagree, and if they are allowed to act on their own, it is usually

---

[4]The word *paternalism* means "acting toward others as a father would act toward his children." Because the term has sexist implications and because women can act just as paternalistically as men, some people prefer the term *parentalism*. The word *parentalism* is not as well known, however, and the literature consistently uses *paternalism,* so we stick with that term with the understanding that it includes men and women.

within the confines of family rules: "Yes, you may date, but only on Friday and Saturday nights." The parent consequently holds veto power over the child's decisions and stands ready to impose his or her will upon the child. As such, the child is seen as having limited autonomy of action, usually because the child is seen as having limited competence.

The health care application of paternalism involves someone other than the patient (usually the health care professional) assuming decision-making responsibility for the patient, assuming veto power over the patient's decisions, or being ready to impose her will on the patient. The paternalistic person then limits the autonomous action (or decision) of another person and treats that person as if his competence were limited. The significant point is that the parental relationship does not exist, and the patient would, for any other purposes, be considered competent to make and act upon his own decisions.

Since such action would, under normal circumstances, not be considered proper, what makes people think it is OK in the context of health care? The primary reason used is that the action is taken "in the patient's best interest."

IN THE PERSON'S BEST INTEREST

Although the most frequent reason given for acting paternalistically is that it is in someone's "best interest," the term *best interest* has many different meanings. This is because *best interest* is a relative term, depending for its meaning on a subjective determination of what is "best" for a person. However, the relative nature of best interest also means that the primary responsibility for determining best interest belongs to the person whose interest is being affected. It also means that best interest will be determined by analyzing consequences, since that is how we determine which choice is best. How, then, do people justify paternalism on the grounds of best interest?

Two arguments are frequently used to justify interfering with the decision of a person: the welfare argument and the harm argument. The *welfare argument* says that the best interest of persons is promoted when their welfare or the welfare of others is promoted. The *harm argument* says that the best interest of persons is promoted when they are prevented from doing harm either to themselves or others. By either argument, it would be acceptable to interfere with the decision of another if the appropriate aim could be promoted.

The first problem is how to determine what constitutes harm and welfare. That done, there remains the question of degree; that is, how much harm, or welfare, must be at stake before it is legitimate to interfere? As a correlative, there is consideration of how to evaluate harm to oneself versus harm to others.

The issue is *not* whether it is ever right to interfere with the decision of another person, for when someone is acting incompetently and harmfully, we usually see an obligation to interfere, to help the person protect himself. Thus, for example, there would be no objection to preventing someone under the influence of LSD from jumping off a building if he thought he could fly. Similarly, it would make little moral sense to say that a person has an absolute right to do whatever he wants, for then a terrorist would have a "right" to shoot passengers in an airport and we would not be justified in interfering, i.e., in trying to stop him. The issue, then, is to determine what constitutes reasonable *moral* grounds for interfering with the decisions and actions of another person.

In any given situation, the harm or welfare determination may apply to different persons, in different ways. To see how these arguments work and to better understand the problems, we consider a number of cases from previous chapters in addition to several new ones.

The typical case of paternalism involves withholding or manipulating information in order to "protect" a person from harm, without the affected person's knowledge that they are being "protected."

CASE 6.4

Darryl, a 7-year-old, was born with spina bifida (a birth defect which causes serious damage to the spinal cord) and is in the hospital for additional corrective surgery. Angie Reynolds, a physical therapist, is checking the chart prior to giving Darryl exercise therapy, when she notes that Darryl has been quite uncooperative with others giving care. The physician has thus ordered that if Darryl is uncooperative, playroom privileges are to be withdrawn until Darryl cooperates.

When Angie visits Darryl and tries to do his therapy, he is quite uncooperative, refusing to assist Angie and fighting her efforts to force the exercises. Instead of continuing with the exercises, Angie tries to talk to Darryl and find out why he is being uncooperative, but without recording his lack of cooperation and revoking his playroom privileges. From the conversation she learns that Darryl's family has taken a vacation while he is in the hospital, and he has not seen them in 5 days. She believes this is the cause of his lack of cooperation, and so she talks to Darryl's primary nurse, relating her conversation; however, the nurse claims the doctor knows that and still wants the privileges withdrawn. Because Angie believes that the doctor's order is inappropriate, she does not record the lack of cooperation because she does not want Darryl to have to stay alone in his room all day, since she believes that would only add to the problem. She thus simply records the exercises accomplished, adding a note that Darryl seems very lonely and misses not having his parents visit.

Normally, failure to record accurate, complete information is a serious professional error. Not only is correct information needed to care for the person properly, but also it is needed in the event that later problems (or questions) arise. In this instance, however, Angie appears to regard Darryl's lack of cooperation as an exception to the rule of charting. Why? Angie sees in the situation not simply a lack of cooperation, but a lonely child, probably acting out in order to gain the attention that is not being given by his family. Regardless of her reasons though, she has not reported truthfully and is thus deceiving the physician or anyone else reading the chart. Notice, however, that there is no intended deception of the *patient*, only of other health care professionals, with the intention of protecting the patient from what she sees as harmful actions of others.

The next case is different because emotional, not physical, harm is involved.

CASE 6.5

Barbara Wainright, a 57-year-old mother of two, was admitted to the hospital for tests to rule out obstructive cancer of the colon. While the tests are being processed, Barbara's husband and children meet with the doctor and ask her not to tell Barbara if the results are positive. They tell the doctor that Barbara fears cancer very much, and they believe she would become extremely upset and very depressed, and give up all desire to live. "Don't tell her," they say. "It will be too hard on her." The physician is unhappy with this request because she believes in giving patients information about their diagnoses. The family insists, however, that Barbara not be told, so the physician reluctantly agrees. The tests come back positive; but when Barbara asks about them, the physician says, "The tests are inconclusive, but don't worry, you'll do just fine."

The harm in this case is primarily emotional, with the family and physician *assuming* that from Barbara's values it is in her best interest to protect her from becoming upset. The situation would be entirely different had Barbara *requested* that she not be told if her diagnosis was cancer. In that instance there is no paternalism, but instead an explicit following of the patient's wishes. Since she has *not* made such a request, however, there *is* paternalism.

Even when a person does make an explicit request, there may be consideration of whether to honor that request.

CASE 6.6

Carl Jungweitz is a respiratory therapist doing prescribed treatments on Lucy Bristol, a 25-year-old with a diagnosis of lung cancer. Lucy tells Carl that she is really feeling badly as a result of her chemotherapy. Carl explains that some lessening of symptoms is possible with altered doses and asks Lucy if she has mentioned this to her doctor. Lucy says, "No, the doctor knows what she is doing, so there is no need to mention it." At that point the doctor comes into the room and asks Lucy whether she is having any problems, and Lucy replies, "No, I feel quite good, so the treatments must be working." Carl wonders whether to confront Lucy regarding her earlier statement, to talk to the doctor privately afterward, or to say nothing at all.

Should Carl take action, he would be interfering with Lucy's decision to simply go along with the doctor's orders. Carl, when deciding what to do, is actually considering two questions: Is Lucy wrong (for whatever reasons) in not telling her doctor how she feels? and Is the harm to Lucy sufficient to justify interference? Even if Carl decides that Lucy is wrong, based on the harm-welfare arguments, he is still not justified in interfering if the harm is not sufficient. Thus, if Lucy is uncomfortable and she chooses to remain that way, even when the discomfort could be alleviated, there is little ground for interference. However, if the discomfort were a known indicator of life-threatening harm, Carl should certainly inform Lucy of that and try to get her to discuss it with the physician. If she refused, then he would be faced with the problem of whether to interfere to preserve her life or to respect her wishes.

The following case presents a specific problem of harm, although not to the person requesting noninterference.

CASE 6.7

As Helen Jones is preparing to leave the hospital, she is talking with Lorraine Williams, her primary care nurse, and tells Lorraine that she dreads going home because she knows that her husband has been physically abusing their 14-year-old daughter. She says that she has already decided not to make an issue of the matter, but to accept it, since "parents have a right to do as they wish with their children." She says, "I don't like what he is doing, but he says she needs the discipline. I don't agree, but then we don't see eye to eye on a lot of things." Helen then says, "Please don't tell anyone about this; I just told you because I needed to talk to someone about it."

If Lorraine does anything, she will be going against the wishes of the parent, thus interfering with the decision of the parent. At the same time, if Lorraine does nothing, she will not interfere with the parent but will also not prevent further harm to the daughter. Unlike the previous cases, whatever is done will be known to the parent, so no deception is involved. There is still the judgment, however, as to whether the prevention of harm or the decision of the parent is of primary importance.

The problem of interference becomes particularly troublesome when a person's decision will affect whether she lives.

CASE 6.8

Karen Rebikov, a 16-year-old high school senior, was diagnosed as having an oat-cell cancer of the leg. (Oat-cell cancers spread very rapidly and have one of the highest mortality rates known.) Although chemotherapy may be of some help, amputation plus chemotherapy would give Karen a good chance of survival, but would by no means guarantee a cure. Karen agrees to the chemotherapy; however, she refuses the surgery because, she says, "I would rather die than lose my leg." Her family is very upset by her refusal, and the members of the health care team are concerned because they see Karen's refusal as unreasonable. As a means of helping Karen change her mind, her family arranges for Sybil Freneau to visit, since Sybil had an amputation, although not for cancer. Sybil comes and talks with Karen. As a result, Karen changes her mind and agrees to the surgery. Her comment as she consents for the surgery is, "Well, if the amputation can cure Sybil's cancer, so she can still do everything she did before, then I guess it's dumb for me to refuse." Her comment is not challenged, and she has the surgery the next day.

Some people might argue that there is no paternalism here as long as Karen's parents want the surgery, since she is a minor and thus it is not her decision. This argument utilizes a status test for competence, which overlooks the fact that a 16-year-old is nearly at legal majority and so is most probably functionally competent (unless there is some other reason for her incompetence). The real problem here is whether paternalism is justified when the person's choice will end or shorten her life.

CASE 6.9

Willa is a 32-year-old mother of three children who is suffering from advanced bone cancer. She has recently entered an experimental drug program which consists of giving the patient a large dose of a highly toxic substance, followed in 48 hours by a neutralizing agent. The treatment is given on an outpatient basis, since there are no side effects to the drug within the first 50 to 55 hours. At the beginning of the program, all participants sign an agreement for the procedure, consenting to the risks (of which they are fully informed) and absolving the center of any responsibility should they not return for the neutralizing agent within the appropriate time.

One day Willa does not show up for the neutralizing agent. The physician for the program becomes concerned and has the secretary try to contact her. She does and reports that Willa said she will not be coming in, she has made her peace, and she plans to let the drug end her life.

As a member of the care team, the physician asks you to go with him to see Willa to help convince her to come in for the treatment. If that fails, he wants you to help him give her the treatment anyhow.

If we are going to assess consequences and to count dying as a very bad consequence, an argument can be made for interfering. However, if we are going to support the right of autonomous decision making, whether we interfere will depend on the way it is seen. If autonomy is an absolute value which must be preserved, then preserving life preserves autonomy, and it is correct to prevent actions which will end life. At the same time, if autonomy is an absolute value which must be preserved, an equally strong argument can be made for allowing the decision, as long as it is autonomous, since to do otherwise is to violate autonomy.

This case also raises serious questions about competence, since it is not known whether the toxic drug could have an effect on Willa's ability to think clearly. In Case 6.10, which involves dialysis, that is also a problem, since a person in need of dialysis is often severely depressed and feeling badly because of toxic levels in the blood.

CASE 6.10

Juanetta is a 23-year-old in end-stage renal disease. Because of complex medical problems, Juanetta is not a candidate to receive a transplant, from either a cadaver or a relative. Presently on dialysis, Juanetta comes to the clinic several days a week. As a nurse in the clinic, you have come to know Juanetta quite well and have even gone to lunch with her on occasion. One day, during dialysis, Juanetta is talking to you and indicates that she is not really feeling well because the dialysis is becoming less effective (as is often the case with this disease). You ask whether she has mentioned this to her doctor, and she says, "No, there is no need to trouble her with that, because this is the last time I will be in for dialysis." You ask her why, and she explains that she is going to let the disease end her life.

If we are to take autonomy seriously and make an effort to carefully analyze situations which are paternalistic, this case is quite troublesome as it stands. First, we know nothing about Juanetta, her state of competence, and the thoughtfulness of her decision. Second, if it is argued that her life is of poor quality, thus her decision will be her way of escaping that poor quality, we would need to be concerned with the criteria for "quality," and the basis for its determination. In either case, though, how would the consideration of the paternalistic nature of the situation be changed if one of the following facts were true?

1 After a bit of discussion, you discover that Juanetta has thought this out carefully and discussed it with her parents, who leave the choice up to her. She asks you not to tell anyone and thanks you for taking good care of her.

2 After a bit of discussion, you discover that Juanetta has thought this out carefully but not discussed it with anyone. She asks you not to tell anyone and thanks you for taking good care of her.

3 After a bit of discussion, you discover that Juanetta has not given much thought to this idea. In fact, she admits that she just started thinking about it while sitting there that day. She asks you not to tell anyone and thanks you for taking good care of her.

AUTONOMY OF THE INCOMPETENT PERSON

Before we conclude our discussion of paternalism, it is vital to note that a person does not have to be currently autonomous for action to be paternalistic. In a derivative sense, we can violate at least the spirit of autonomy by not utilizing substituted judgment. If someone was at one time competent but is no longer, or if someone who was fully competent is now partially competent, insofar as we ignore or fail to determine his wishes, we have not respected his autonomy.

To argue that the formerly competent have "lost" their autonomy shows a failure to recognize both autonomy of decision and autonomy of action. The previously competent but now incompetent certainly lose autonomy of action, but not autonomy of decision. We cannot pretend that such persons had no thoughts, desires, or wishes while they were still competent, for to do so is to diminish their dignity as persons. It is to impose upon such situations the principle that once someone becomes incompetent, we can do with her whatever we want, within the limits perhaps of what society will allow. But how can that be recognizing the now incompetent person as a person?

As noted earlier, increasing numbers of people are using a living will or a durable power of attorney to transmit their wishes to others. But why should the existence of a document make a difference? Does a person's autonomous decision stay autonomous if it is written down but cease to be autonomous if it is not written down? If you make a living will, then you have a right to expect others to honor it, because in accepting the notion of wills, the duty of society is to grant your wishes. Once a person becomes incompetent, of course, his or her right to make such decisions ceases; however, the moral obligation to carry out the prior decision does not cease. If you do not make a living will but do make your wishes known, then reason dictates that the same considerations hold.

There is no moral problem of autonomy if the person has never been competent. In that case secondary consenters have no choice but to use their own values and to make a sincere effort to do what they think will be best for the person receiving care. A problem arises only when the autonomous decision of the person who was formerly competent is not treated with the same respect as it would be if the person were still competent.

CARING FOR OTHERS

Up to now we have been looking at cases where paternalism arose in making a decision for others. In those cases there was always an element of moral disagreement about what should be done, and someone intervened in order to resolve the disagreement in terms acceptable to himself. As a final point, we need to examine the problems caused when moral disagreement is substantial yet the disagreeing parties are in a health care relationship. Although a health care professional, as a person, should not be forced to violate her own moral principles, she may find herself in a position of caring for someone who has acted in a way that the caretaker finds morally wrong. Must the health care professional then care for that person? A case will sharpen our focus on this problem.

CASE 6.11

Melissa Morgan is an obstetrical nurse at a small town hospital. She has, on the basis of moral conviction, consistently refused to participate in abortions. Although she has worked at the hospital for 2 years, this is the first time she has been asked to care for a person who has had an abortion, since other staff usually take those patients. This time, however, several nurses are on vacation, and there are a higher number of patients than normal.

The patient Melissa has been asked to care for is a 26-year-old married attorney who had planned the pregnancy. She now has an opportunity to handle a big case which will be very important to her career. Even though she is 18 weeks pregnant, she has elected for termination because "it is simply inconvenient to be pregnant right now."

Melissa believes that every person has a right to good nursing care, yet she does not want to care for this person, since she believes that the abortion was not morally justified.

Notice that Melissa is not being asked to participate in the abortion, although a similar problem would arise if she were the only nurse available and were asked to participate. Is she being inappropriately judgmental? As a nurse, does she have an obligation to care for this patient? If she refuses to care for the woman, will Melissa be acting paternalistically?

PATERNALISTIC ATTITUDES

Paternalism arises out of the removal of control from its legitimate source, the individual affected by the action, and giving control to another, the individual effecting the action. Paternalism sits on a fine line between moral acceptability and nonacceptability. If the paternalistic person is mistaken about the diminished capacity, then the interference is not acceptable. If the action takes control over more than a specific domain, it is unacceptable. And if the control remains beyond the time necessitated by the original justifying condition, it is unacceptable.

The cases we have considered clearly illustrate paternalistic actions. Although there is certainly a good deal of discussion needed for the justification of each one, the primary problem is *not* whether paternalism is justified. Rather, the basic question is, When is paternalism justified, and how can that justification be supported? Those occasions when the person's best interest, *as determined by himself* either directly or through substituted judgment, requires action on his behalf are not the predominant situations of health care. What is more common is paternalistic action taken as a result of a paternalistic *attitude*.

The paternalistic attitude presupposes that someone other than the person receiving care has ultimate responsibility for determining what is in the recipient's best interest. Health care professionals are the ones who most often have this attitude, with families of the care recipient close behind. Although laws and the assertiveness of individuals may come between this attitude and its full implementation, it remains nonetheless. The health care professional who adopts this attitude functions in the care context from the viewpoint that *he* is in charge. As much as possible, he will direct and control the activities of the care recipient in the health care relationship.

Even though someone may not fully act on a paternalistic attitude, it cannot help but influence the interpersonal relationship. Someone who sees himself in charge will also see other persons as subordinate. This subordination of the other then easily leads to objectification of the other, with subsequent reduction of her status as a person in the eyes of the health care professional.

The problem of objectification has been covered in several other contexts. However, the paternalistic attitude may represent the most morally problematic for several reasons. First, our paternalistic attitudes may easily remain hidden to us and to others. We may then have a "hidden agenda" in all that we do. Second, attitudes reflect values; if the attitude is unrecognized, so, too, will be the values. If we do not recognize these values, then we will not recognize when these attitudes create conflict or when they cause actions which are morally unacceptable. Third, a person who has a paternalistic attitude is most liable to be opinionated, for, after all, his *own* judgment is the pinnacle of evaluation. This rigidity and narrow-mindedness can lead not only to increased conflict with others but also to increasingly paternalistic *actions* toward others. After all, if I know what is best for you and you are too stupid to know it yourself, then what option do I have but to help you, for your own good?

CONCLUDING THOUGHTS

A great deal has been written about paternalism, primarily as a result of the increased awareness of autonomy as a factor in health care decisions. Whether in action or as an attitude, paternalism is not morally unproblematic. We must be careful in its use, however, making it the exception rather than the rule. For without such care, the autonomy which is so highly prized will surely be lost.

The responsibility for avoiding paternalism lies not with the health care professional alone, but with all who participate in health care relations. Recipients of care must be unwilling to accept paternalistic action, because it reduces their autonomy. Health care professionals and others must be unwilling to act paternalistically, because that reduces the autonomy of the person receiving care.

STUDY GUIDE

READINGS

M. Benjamin and J. Curtis, "Parentalism," p. 203.
E. Cohen, "Autonomy and Paternalism: Two Goals in Conflict," p. 213.
S. Gadow, "Allocating Autonomy: Can Patients and Practitioners Share?" p. 235.

QUESTIONS FOR REFLECTION

1 Carefully review the case studies of previous chapters to determine how paternalism might be an issue.
2 Some people say that the justification for paternalism is different depending on the profession. Is that a reasonable statement? Why or why not?
3 Find five examples of paternalism in your life experience. How are they different from or the same as the cases discussed in this chapter? Are those examples, in your view, justified? Why or why not?

CASE STUDIES FOR ANALYSIS

Case Study 1 Sarah is a 12-year-old who was diagnosed as having cystic fibrosis (CF) at 8 years of age. Following diagnosis the patient was lost to follow-up for a period of 4 years. When she finally returned to the CF center, it was because of severe, extensive pulmonary disease. After treatment and subsequent release, the patient had recurrent hospitalizations over the next 8 months; however, each time, it was clear the admission was the result of her parents not carrying out prescribed therapy. They were, in fact, using the CF center for crisis intervention and maintenance of the patient's life, while making little or no effort on their own (the child's medicine was given irregularly and postural drainage treatments were rarely performed). Sarah is again an inpatient, having been brought to the emergency room in severe distress (an x-ray score of 8 and obvious cor pulmonale). Treatment has stabilized her condition, and the physician has asked social services if they can be of any assistance in dealing with the case before Sarah is sent home again.

You are the responding social service worker. What problem are you facing? What alternatives of action are open to you? How would you solve the problem that you have identified? What are your reasons for this resolution?

Case Study 2   A 54-year-old woman has been admitted following a cardiac arrest. She was resuscitated after 30 minutes; during most of this time she had no pulse or respirations. Admitted to the intensive care unit, the patient remains stable on the respirator. She is in a coma, however, and her electroencephalogram is nearly flat. The physician consults with the members of the family about removing life support, and they reject that proposal. After 2 days, the physician calls the family and asks again: again the family refuses. He then writes an order to discontinue the respirator, although he leaves the patient with oxygen through a nasal cannula. You are a nurse on the unit and pick up the order sheet. When you read it, you know that the family has refused and does not know of the order. What should you do?

Case Study 3   You are a pharmacist in the drugstore where Mr. Williams (age 67) is a regular customer. You know Mr. Williams because he usually comes in during your shift for his refills. From the prescriptions you have filled you know that Mr. Williams suffers from congestive heart failure, and rather badly at that, given the dosages the physician has ordered. The past few times Mr. Williams has been in the store, you have noticed that he buys several different packages of salted nuts. This time is no exception.

When you fill the prescription, you review the records and note that the physician has an open refill (may be refilled as often as needed) and that Mr. Williams has been filling it more and more frequently. As Mr. Williams is picking up the medicine, you ask him whether he has been back to the doctor recently and had his medication dosage increased. He replies that he has been increasing it himself because he doesn't think it has been working as well as it used to—he needs more to feel better. Since increasing dosages helps, he sees no need to go to the doctor.

What, if any, ethical problems do you face, and how would you handle this situation?

Case Study 4   John and Sarah are both 23 years old and have been married for 5 years. Although Sarah has been pregnant several times, she had been previously unable to maintain a pregnancy, with spontaneous abortion occurring in each case. Now she has carried to term and successfully delivered a baby girl; however, the baby is severely affected by Down's syndrome. In addition, it is discovered that the child has a duodenal obstruction which could be easily corrected with surgery. Without surgery, the baby will surely die; with the surgery, there is no question that she will live and be healthy.

You are the pediatrician attending to the baby. Should you recommend the surgery to John and Sarah?

You are a judge and are asked by the hospital for a guardianship order, since John and Sarah have refused to consent to the surgery. Decide whether to issue the order, and justify your decision.

Case Study 5   You are a staff ethicist assigned to the family court. Part of your responsibility is to recommend a resolution for cases raising ethical problems not specifically covered by statute. Judge Wilson has instructed you to prepare recommendations for her on the case below. She particularly instructs you to give a justification for the two possibilities for action and to indicate which you would suggest that she choose.

[*Tringle v. Morrison*, 406 A.2d 1275 (Luc Co Ct, 1983]

Marion Tringle is 15 years old, the daughter of John and Helen Tringle, second oldest of four children, the youngest being 3 years old and the oldest being 17 years old. John Tringle is an architect, and Helen is an elected member of the school board in her community. No member of the family has ever had a proceeding before this or any other court. Cyrus Morrison represents Marion in suit against her parents.

Suit was brought by Marion, through Morrison, to gain an injunction prohibiting her parents from interfering with her pregnancy. Marion is 2 months pregnant and wishes to have the baby, whose father is a 15-year-old whom Marion has been dating for 2 years. The conception was with intent; that is, Marion was trying to become pregnant, and the father was aware of this fact. The pregnancy was discovered by the parents when Marion's pediatrician (whom she consulted when she thought she was pregnant) called to inform them of the pregnancy. When they were told, the parents requested that arrangements be made for an abortion at the earliest possible time. The physician did this; when the parents told Marion of the arrangements, she ran away from home to the house of Sally Morrison, a friend, whose father is bringing suit on Marion's behalf.

When interviewed in court, Marion explained that she wanted to have the baby because she wanted to be a mother, and to have a child she could take care of and raise. She also admitted that she knew of the emancipated minor laws which allowed married minors to be freed from parental control. Marion admitted that she and the baby's father hoped that their parents would let them get married if she were pregnant. She said they were "deeply in love" and wanted to be together and have their own family. She refused to have an abortion, she said, because it wasn't the baby's fault and so she would not kill it for her parents.

When interviewed in court, Marion's parents contended that she should not be allowed to keep the child because she was too young and "immature—a highly imaginative girl who doesn't realize what she is getting into." Marion's father admitted that he thought his daughter's having a baby would "not sit well with my colleagues," while Marion's mother admitted that "if word got out, I could never get reelected."

Court records show that the baby's father's parents would allow the marriage if Marion's parents approved; also, although they would not encourage the marriage, they would help out "as much as we can."

BIBLIOGRAPHY

Bartholome, William G.: "Proxy Consent in the Medical Context: The Infant as Person," *Child Nurturance,* vol. 1, 1982.

Baylin, E.: "Autonomy, Paternalism, Community," *Hastings Center Report,* vol. 14, no. 5, 1984, pp. 5–49.

Buchanan, Alan: "Medical Paternalism," *Philosophy and Public Affairs,* vol. 7, no. 4, summer 1978.

Finkelhor, David: "What's Wrong with Sex between Adults and Children?" *American Journal of the Orthopsychiatric Association,* vol. 49, no. 4, October 1979, pp. 692–697.

Gadow, Sally: "Basis of Nursing Ethics: Paternalism, Consumerism, or Advocacy?" *Hospital Progress,* vol. 64, no. 10, October 1983, pp. 62–78.

Gert, Bernard, and Charles M. Culver: "Paternalistic Behavior," *Philosophy and Public Affairs,* vol. 6, no. 1, Fall 1976.

Halper, Thomas: "The Double-Edged Sword: Paternalism as a Policy in the Problems of Aging." *Health and Society,* vol. 58, no. 3, 1980.

Kilpack, V.: "Ethical Issues and Procedural Dilemmas in Measuring Patient Competence," *Advances in Nursing Science,* vol. 6, no. 4, 1984, pp. 22–33.

O'Neil, Richard: "Determining Proxy Consent," *Journal of Medicine and Philosophy,* vol. 8, 1983, pp. 389–403.

Steinbrook, Robert, and Bernard Lo: "Decision Making for Incompetent Patients by Designated Proxy," *New England Journal of Medicine,* vol. 301, no. 24, June 14, 1984, pp. 1598–1601.

CHAPTER 7

PERSONS, CARING, AND COMMUNITY: THE ETHICAL BASIS FOR HEALTH CARE

Honor those whose words or deeds
Thus help us in our daily needs
And by their overflow
Raise us from what is low!

Henry Wadsworth Longfellow*

In the sufferer let me see only the human being.

Moses Maimonides**

BEYOND THE CONFUSION

Any introductory book about ethics which adequately treats the issues and problems often leaves an impression that ethical problems can never be resolved; i.e., who is to say what's right or wrong anyhow? This is a mistaken impression, however, which usually results from the feeling of uneasiness that goes with discovering new complexity in something we thought was pretty well settled. In particular, ethics is unsettling because serious thinking may ultimately mean

---

*Santa Filomena. In *The Poetical Works of Longfellow*, Houghton Mifflin, Boston. 1975, p. 197.
**Daily Prayer of a Physician*, Warren T. Reach (ed.) *Encyclopedia of Bioethics*, Free Press, New York, 1978, vol. 4, p. 1733.

changing our beliefs, which we want to avoid because it is difficult and uncomfortable. A first encounter with ethics can leave us adrift, not sure what to believe and not sure what to do about it, yet recognizing that something must be done. The "Who's to say anyhow?" response can then become a convenient way out, a way to push aside thinking and do what feels comfortable. Head in the sand, we ignore the problem and keep repeating, "Who's to say anyhow?"

Although the theories may be confusing and the philosophical arguments may appear to be endless, the bottom line is that we must, and do, act. It is simply a fact of life that we must resolve ethical problems and live with the consequences of those resolutions. It is also a fact of life that when someone believes that we have done something wrong and wants an explanation, the "Who's to say anyhow?" response does not go very far. What becomes important, then, is *how* we act and *why* we act as we do; there is a need for personal moral responsibility and a willingness to *decide* how to act, not just to react. At that point frustration can easily set in, because everything seems so confused and it is unclear how to proceed. Yet the thinking about ethics that has gone along with reading this book *can* be of some help, for a great deal has already been done toward developing an understanding of ethical issues and how they might be approached.

Throughout this book ethical issues have been examined from the perspective of consequences, duties, and rights, with an overall concern that autonomy must be recognized as a crucial component of any analysis. The philosophical arguments have yet to settle on the best way to look at things, and the basic concepts, particularly autonomy, need much more work before we fully understand them. But this is by no means a condemnation of the process or a reason to throw up our hands in despair, allowing the legitimacy of the "Who is to say?" position. To do that is to abdicate our responsibility to be moral persons and to pretend that what we do as individuals does not count.

The difficulty, of course, is that something has to serve as a base for our thinking. By nature, people want things to be nice and tidy; we like to have clear-cut rules so that it is easy to justify or criticize someone's action. Clearly, however, we cannot develop a cookbook of moral rules without exception, for that disallows individual needs in special circumstances. What is even worse, the rules become an end in themselves, to be followed simply because they are rules, with no thought of their moral implications. At the same time, there is uncertainty, and often injustice, if we look at only the consequences of our actions, for then calculation, not morality, becomes the focus. Furthermore, the calculations are rarely based on the values of the person affected, which means the decision may easily violate personal autonomy. What, then, of rights? Without some balance, rights can be as much a tyranny as duties; and without a clear recognition of basic rights and some means of identifying those rights, an appeal to rights can be as arbitrary as an appeal to consequences. Similarly, unbridled autonomy can ensure us freedom to do as we wish, but only at the cost of another person's autonomy and a tyranny of the powerful.

So how do we proceed? First, we must recognize that *all* the theoretical bases are important in every ethical decision. We cannot ignore our duties, abridge others' rights, or impose undesirable consequences without moral justification. What is required, then, is a theoretical perspective which, instead of focusing on *one* basis alone, melds them into a coherent unity. But this is not an easy job, and it will be evolving for some time to come. Nonetheless, it must be pursued. Second, we must recognize that being a moral person, regardless of the ethical theory involved, requires attention to three things: (1) a recognition of persons, (2) a commitment to caring, and (3) a sense of moral community. These are not three new theories, but three characteristics which cross the boundaries of ethical theory. As a means of drawing this book to a close and raising the questions which set the stage for future inquiry, let's look at these three requirements.

A RECOGNITION OF PERSONS

Health care is now, and will continue to be, a highly technical enterprise. As knowledge expands and technology develops, it will be increasingly possible to do more. For example, we can now keep a person's body functioning indefinitely through the use of drugs and machines; we can now save lives that even a short time ago would have been lost. Yet in all this it is hard to maintain our perspective, because it is too easy to get caught up in the "Gee whiz!" excitement of science and the high-level skill demands of technology. When these things happen, science and technology become ends in themselves, and the goal of health care, the *person* who receives that care, is forgotten.

Without recognizing the person as the recipient of health care, there is no obvious reason for the care. Without the person for whom developments of science and technology may be utilized, those developments are merely intellectual games, with little to recommend them except perhaps the feeling of accomplishment inherent in discovering or developing something new.

There are very few people who would fail to recognize care for a person as the ultimate goal of health care. Nonetheless, in the application of that care, it is easy to forget and to treat the person receiving care as an object. While being poked, prodded, observed, monitored, checked, and analyzed, the person receiving care becomes more and more an object of attention. Diagnoses classify people, treatments isolate people, and technology disconnects people from the rest of us by making them adjuncts to machines. And the more specialized the care, the more objectification of the person is liable to occur, especially as we develop analogies of plumbing, mechanics, electricity, etc., to aid our understanding.

This is *not* to say, however, that science and technology ought to be abandoned or that the analogies used to understand human physiology should be replaced. Rather, science and technology must not be seen as ends in themselves. Treating a person as an object is inappropriate; yet being objective, i.e., unbiased, knowledgeable, efficient, etc., is certainly important. The balance that must be struck is between objectivity and cold impersonality. To overstep this bound and objectify the person is to overlook the basic respect for dignity which is necessary to being a moral person. In other words, one cannot be a moral person if one fails to treat someone else as a person, instead of as an object.

The necessity for recognizing persons as the focus of health care also becomes apparent when we remember that autonomy is a basic element of ethics. We have said a good deal about autonomy and the need for our conception of health care to make room for a recognition of autonomy. At the same time, there can be no recognition of autonomy without a prior recognition of persons (at least) as harbingers of autonomy. And since *persons* have and exercise autonomy of judgment or of action, they are also moral agents.[1] Our moral perspective must then include recognition of the inherent dignity of persons, based on their autonomy and moral agency. In short, if we are to consider autonomy as fundamental to ethics, then we cannot fail to recognize nonobjectified persons as a primary focus of ethics. Our understanding of moral status in difficult cases, such as infants, comatose adults, animals, and even cybernetic machines, will then be based on that primary focus. No matter what basic ethical position we might take (i.e., consequences, duties, or rights), there must be a commitment to maintaining a framework for recognition of others not as objects, but as persons with a basic level of dignity that must be preserved.

Recognition of others as persons and a respect for their autonomy are both important, but do not alone establish a moral framework for health care. Also needed is a commitment to the basic *relation* between persons, the relation of *caring*. Without caring, there will certainly be health technology and many health problems will be overcome and yet the moral framework of health *care* will be missing. Even if health care values could today be miraculously transformed so that everyone, health care professional or not, would appropriately value autonomy and respect persons, we would still not have a complete moral *context* for health care. Unless the recognition of persons, who have autonomy, is coupled with a sense of caring, the moral interchange, if it can exist at all, will be only superficial.

A COMMITMENT TO CARING

We cannot escape the fact that health care is a person-to-person activity. If I enter into the health care context, either as a provider or recipient of health care, I cannot function in that context without encountering another person. But the

---

[1]This is not intended to be an argument for persons as superior beings or to deny that other entities might be owed moral recognition. See, for example, Justin Leiber, *Can Animals and Machines Be Persons?* Hackett Publishing, Indianapolis, IN, 1985.

moral nature of that encounter will be set quite clearly by the *way* in which I relate to that person, which is how we arrive at the need for caring. Caring is a relationship between persons, such that the recipient of care and the giver of care are involved with each other *as persons*.

It has been pointed out many times that ethics presupposes both interpersonal relations and moral responsibility. Although autonomy is the condition of moral responsibility, simply recognizing another as a person is not sufficient to meet the need for interpersonal relations. We must, in addition, *interact* with others at a level which recognizes not only their nature as persons but their inherent dignity as well. The simple act of doing something to a person does not constitute interacting with that person; instead, the doing must be coupled with an intention to *care* for someone as a person.

When we speak of caring, often a subtle ambiguity creeps into our thinking, for caring can be quite good, in the technical sense of meeting physiological needs and correctly utilizing science and technology, and yet not be caring at all. To understand this ambiguity, think not of the word *caring* but of what is done. If I am seeing to your every physiological need, I am certainly giving you care or *taking care of* you, but I may be doing this without *caring for* you at all. I may be seeing what I do simply as my job, something that must be done to guarantee my paycheck. Although such a view is appropriate for fixing cars or manufacturing spoons, it is not appropriate in dealing with other persons, because then the person is treated as an object. More specifically, the person is treated as an object to be used as a means for achieving my own ends. The person ceases to be important for herself and becomes important only as a means to my paycheck.

A common misconception is that caring for someone involves too much commitment and is psychologically too difficult, especially in areas of health care where people frequently die. However, this is not to say that caring cannot be accomplished or should not be accomplished—just that it is difficult to accomplish. Health care professionals are often portrayed as cool, cold, and calculating people who try not to "get emotionally involved" with the persons for whom they care. Thus the intensive care unit nurse who cries when the person for whom he is caring dies is said to be "too emotional"; the physician who goes to the funeral of the person for whom she was caring is said to be "too close." Is the caring required by moral action demanding this? Are we really required to enter into an intense emotional relationship with everyone?

How each of us defines the personal relationship of caring depends on a number of things, including the ethical theory being used, the basic conception of the nature of health care, and the role of professionals in the life of the person. However the relationship is specifically viewed, several general characteristics are worth noting. First, caring is a function of our interrelatedness as persons. If I cannot see you as a person (instead of as an object), I cannot see an interrelatedness; and if I cannot conceive of you and I as interrelated in any way, then I cannot care for you. Second, caring involves recognition that the moral values of the other person count as much as our own. This does not mean I must accept your values as my own, nor does it mean that I must allow you to do whatever your values dictate. It *does* mean that I must take you seriously and respect your basic right to freedom of both belief and action. Should I see your belief, or action, as inappropriate, the burden lies on me to show that; you are right until I can show that you are wrong. Third, caring necessitates a willingness for some sacrifice of self on behalf of the other person. This does not preclude caring for myself and seeing to my own needs; nonetheless, I must be ready to yield to your needs in appropriate circumstances. Although much needs to be worked out before this sense of caring is complete, much can be done in the meantime. This sketch gives a basic framework that can be built upon as each person develops individual moral character.

We mentioned earlier that the technical and scientific approach causes moral problems because it leads to objectification of the person. That same objectification can also interfere with caring. If health care is seen as a series of technical solutions to scientific problems, then the cause of those problems becomes an abstraction. Caring, and the moral decisions which accompany it, cannot occur in abstraction, however, for caring occurs in situations between persons. A health care problem cannot exist independent of the person who has the problem or of those who must resolve the problem. Resolution of a problem, not just an abstraction, then requires the interaction of persons, during which the potential for caring exists.

Given the complexity of health care today, resolution of problems often involves numerous professionals and, with the growing recognition of holistic care, families and friends of the care recipient. Recognition of persons, for whom we care, thus brings with it a recognition of interrelatedness, a mutual responsibility that goes beyond an individual and into the moral community.

THE MORAL COMMUNITY

Recognition of others as persons and the relationship of caring are both important for the development of a moral perspective. Yet neither can be achieved without a sense of community, for a community gives context to the caring relationship of persons and substance to the moral imperative. The moral responsibility of persons to others, in the caring relationship, is framed by the community within which that relationship occurs. The community does not define that relationship; it gives it a context. Only the persons engaged in the relationship can define it, and only society can give it a context in which to occur. The community is, in this sense, a primary condition for the relationships and moral responsibilities of persons. Despite all else they might be, persons are part of a community.

The days are past in which self-sufficient individuals face the frontiers of life alone, with only their native wit and tenacity to sustain them. We depend on each other for survival and for nurturing. It is simply a myth that we can be completely self-sufficient. As a result, no matter how much we want to be self-sufficient, in reality we must pay attention to the community and support it, so that it may support us. Without persons to care for, health professions cannot exist, and without persons to care for us, we cannot exist either. We have, in this sense, a basic need for each other.

One's community need not be large, and different situations may redescribe our context of community, although never remove it. As the context for our relationships, the community is more than just the sum of individual relationships. Rather, the community uses those relationships, but adds to them the ever-present context for their assessment and support. At the same time, by our actions (or lack thereof), we may separate ourselves from the community as criminals and hermits do. This does not excuse us from our moral responsibility, however; it just isolates us from it.

The impact of the community on health care is also an important moral consideration, given that an increasing burden of health care costs is borne by the community, not the individual. Rarely do health insurance premiums cover the costs of serious illness; thus the payments of others may cover the costs of my care. Furthermore, the tax monies of all are used to support the health care of others, through Medicare, Medicaid, the kidney program, and so on. How those monies are allocated is a problem for the community, not the individual. It is also a serious moral question, because inherent in the allocation are the ethical problems of justice in distribution. Who shall have when not all can have? Who shall live when not everyone can live? How shall the finite resources of society be allocated? How are those decisions to be made?

A moral community is also the basis for determining what may or may not be done. For example, it cannot be left to individuals to decide how new technology should be utilized, because the decision base for any individual is too narrow. Without the give and take of the moral decision process, the result is arbitrarily built on the values and judgment of a single person. If actions affected only the decision maker, that would be acceptable; but since health care decisions *always* affect other persons, it is not acceptable. Thus it should not be up to the implanting surgeon to decide how and on whom the artificial heart will be used; it should not be up to the geneticist to decide how and upon whom new techniques of gene manipulation should be used; it should not be up to an organ procurement administrator to decide who should receive a donated organ; and it should not be up to a researcher to decide how persons should be utilized in experiments. These and other such decisions are based in the community, affect the community, thus need the community as a component of the decision process.

The need for community in the moral decision process, however, is *not* a reason for social relativism. Rather, it is an argument for the need to consider persons, in a caring relation to each other, as members of a moral community, as the driving force in health care decision making. Because the community serves as a context for the exercise of autonomy based on moral values, the community may serve as a sounding board for moral argument, a restraint against excesses, and an encouragement to recognize that it is persons with rights to whom we have a duty to promote well-being. If nothing else, the community serves as a constant reminder of our relation to others and the fact that, to be moral, we must interact with others.

As we each go our separate ways, to deal with situations and problems that are normal for our lives, we will participate in a community. As we relate with each other, trying to solve the problems of our human condition, we must engage each other in the context of the moral community, wherein we are ultimately responsible for each other.

CONCLUDING THOUGHTS

The work we have done in this book is just a beginning. From the first to the last, we have looked at ethical concerns in health care by working with basic, everyday problems. The "big" issues (such as abortion, euthanasia, suicide, genetic experimentation, allocation of resources, and so on) have been set aside, but not because they are unimportant. Instead, we have worked with materials necessary for developing an understanding of issues and concepts needed to deal with those big issues. Put in different terms, this book has been a primer aimed at preparing you to face the everyday problems of health care with a clearer understanding of what is going on and some basic intellectual skills for dealing with those problems. Most important, the focus has been on helping you see more clearly the relevance of different perspectives on ethical issues as well as the complexity of the issues themselves. The "big" issues are not everyday issues and are not faced by every person, while the issues covered in this book *are* everyday issues and *are* faced by every person. As a result of examining those issues, you will be better prepared to deal with the larger issues as they confront or interest you.

Every book must come to an end, and often much is left unsaid. The ethical issues in health care are so extensive and so complex that no single book can adequately deal with them. Every year hundreds of new articles and dozens of new books are published, each presenting new ideas and developments. The aim of this book has been to help you *understand* the basic ethical issues in a reasonable way and develop the skills necessary to *begin* working with those issues. The book also tried to raise questions and make you want to think about answers to those questions. But all this has been *only* the barest beginning; what happens now is up to you. You could drop the whole thing and move on to something else; or you could make a commitment to stick with it and try at least to recognize and deal with ethical issues as they confront you; or you could move ahead, trying to expand both your understanding of the issues and your ability to deal constructively with them. What will you do now? The choice is yours.

STUDY GUIDE

READINGS

D. Callahan, "Competency in Medical Care," p. 137.
D. Benfield, "Two Philosophies of Caring," p. 246.
N. Noddings, "Why Care about Caring?" p. 253.

QUESTIONS FOR REFLECTION

1 How might the notion of caring be differently understood from each of the four types of ethical theory? Would the requirement for caring be the same? Would the justification for caring be the same?
2 Review the cases of Chapter 6 from the perspective of caring. Is there, then, a different perspective for paternalism? Does paternalism become more or less acceptable from the perspective of caring? How would an understanding of caring change the criteria for morally acceptable paternalism?
3 What is the relationship between caring and autonomy? May they be seen as separate, or must they somehow be joined in the process of moral justification? Why or why not?
4 How might a recognition of the need for caring affect public policy decisions about health care and the allocation of resources?

CASE STUDIES FOR ANALYSIS

Case Study 1   Your state legislature is considering a bill which would prohibit the use of any state funds to care for people diagnosed as having AIDS. Because the issue is controversial, the legislature has placed the item on the ballot, so that the people of the state may vote for or against the bill. The argument given in favor of the bill is as follows:

The state is currently at its financial limit in supporting health care, so no new additions to the coverage can be made without eliminating something else or raising taxes. AIDS is a terminal illness for which there is no known cure and from which no one is known to have recovered. Moreover, the cost of caring for someone who is dying from AIDS, especially in the end stages of the disease, is currently running around $200,000 per person. We simply cannot afford that amount of money. Therefore, there is no choice but to eliminate AIDS from coverage so that the money may be used to benefit people who will survive.

Analysis Questions   Despite what you believe to be the appropriateness of this bill, formulate an argument against it as part of your analysis of the argument for it. Is the given argument adequate? Are the relevant alternatives covered? How will you vote on the bill?

Case Study 2   You are an employee not involved in patient care (e.g., receptionist, clerk, pharmacist, laboratory technician, x-ray technician, etc.) at a hospital where the nurses are on strike. The hospital administration has asked you to work part of your shift on a patient care unit, assisting the nursing supervisors in their care of patients. You would not be asked to perform technical nursing functions, such as giving medications, but you would see to patient comfort needs and nontechnical care. How will you respond to the administration's request?

Analysis Questions   The case study does not give a reason for the nurses' strike; does the reason matter in your decision? What if the strike were only for higher wages? What if the strike were for improved quality of patient care through reforms in the structure of hospital nursing practice policies? What if the administration said you would be fired for not doing as it asked?

Case Study 3   You are a member of the organ transplant committee for a local hospital. The committee is asked to decide whether a child with Down's syndrome should be placed on the list of persons to receive a liver transplant. The child is 4 years old and moderately retarded. She is not institutionalized, and the prognosis for her mental retardation is good. Yet some committee members argue that because she cannot be a productive member of society she should either not go on the list at all or go at the end, to receive a transplant only if no one ahead of her on the list can be served. At present, putting her at the end of the list will probably mean that she will not receive a transplant, since her blood type is O positive and her general compatibility is about the same as that of several others on the list.

Committee practice is that each member must vote openly (there is no secret ballot) and give reasons for the vote. How will you vote and why?

Analysis Questions   How does the notion of community fit this case? Does caring enter into the deliberation at any point? How? Should the committee have even known that the child had Down's syndrome? Why or why not?

Case Study 4   An inmate serving his third year of a 15-year sentence for murder has Hodgkin's disease. Chemical therapy has been used but no longer works; thus a bone marrow transplant is needed if there is to be any hope of putting the disease into remission. Because the patient is an inmate of the state prison, the prison system will have to pay the estimated $150,000 cost of the transplant. Led by the family of the victim, an influential group of citizens is trying to block the expenditure of state money for the transplant on the grounds that the inmate, as a murderer, has no right to the potentially lifesaving treatment. What is your view? Should the transplant be allowed?

Analysis Questions   Although the health care question is the transplant, what is the real issue in this case? What sorts of factors need to be considered in determining whether to allow the transplant?

Case Study 5   Melissa Morgan is an obstetrical nurse at a small town hospital. She has, on the basis of moral conviction, consistently refused to participate in abortions. Although she has worked at the hospital for 2 years, this is the first time she has been asked to care for a person who has had an abortion, since other staff usually take those patients. This time, however, several nurses are on vacation, and there are a higher number of patients than normal.

The patient Melissa has been asked to care for is a 26-year-old married attorney who had planned the pregnancy. She now has an opportunity to handle a big case which will be very important to her career. Even though she is 18 weeks pregnant, she has elected for termination because "it is simply inconvenient to be pregnant right now."

Melissa believes that every person has a right to good nursing care, yet she does not want to care for this person, since she believes that the abortion was not morally justified. Does Melissa have a moral obligation to care for the patient, or may she morally refuse to care for her?

Analysis Questions   Notice that Melissa is not being asked to participate in the abortion, although a similar problem would arise if she were the only nurse available and were asked to participate. Is she being inappropriately judgmental? As a nurse does she have an obligation to care for this patient? Where do the moral notions of person, caring, and community come into the resolution of this dilemma? What must be the basis for a decision in such conflict situations?

BIBLIOGRAPHY

Carper, B.: "The Ethics of Caring," *Advances in Nursing Science,* vol. 1, no. 3, 1979, pp. 11–19.

Gadow, Sally: "Existential Advocacy: Philosophical Foundations of Nursing," in S. Spicker (ed.), *Nursing Images and Ideals,* Springer, New York, 1980, pp. 79–101.

Kopelman, Loretta, and John Moskop: "The Holistic Health Movement: A Survey and Critique," *Journal of Medicine and Philosophy,* vol. 6, 1981, pp. 209–235.

Lebacqz, Karen, and Robert J. Levine: "Respect for Persons and Informed Consent in Research," *Clinical Research,* vol. 25, no. 3, 1982, pp. 101–107.

Menzel, Paul T.: *Medical Costs, Moral Choices,* Yale University Press, New Haven, CT, 1983.

Muyskens, James L.: "No Easy Choice: Resolving Everyday Ethical Dilemmas," *Nursing Life,* vol. 4, no. 4, 1984, pp. 28–32.

Noddings, Nel: *Caring: A Feminine Approach to Ethics and Moral Education,* University of California Press, Berkeley, 1984.

Ramsey, Paul: *The Patient as a Person,* Yale University Press, New Haven, CT, 1970.

Thomasma, David C.: *An Apology for the Value of Human Life,* Catholic Health Association, St. Louis, MO, 1983.

Vaux, Kenneth L.: *This Mortal Coil: The Meaning of Health and Disease,* Harper & Row, NY, 1978.

COMPETENCY IN MEDICAL CARE

Daniel Callahan

There can be no doubt that one of the greatest achievements of medicine is the successful application of a scientific methodology to both basic biomedical research and clinical application. The Flexner Report of 1910, and the increasing application of scientific thinking to medical problems that came in its aftermath, are the principal reasons for the success of contemporary medicine. The triumphs of biomedical research are real and obvious, and the radical improvements in mortality and morbidity data since the turn of the century provide all the evidence one could ask for about the efficacy of scientific medicine. Nonetheless, as we move into an era of chronic disease, and apparently past the point where inexpensive vaccines or cures for widespread disease are still likely, we will be forced to reevaluate some aspects of the efficacy of scientific medicine, and also take a fresh look at some of the problems it may have caused.

Among those problems has been a sharp sundering of the technical from the human side of medicine, and in particular on that aspect that bears on the care of human beings as a whole. Competency in medical practice has come to connote almost exclusively the ability of a physician, or other health care worker, to bring to bear on the treatment of illness a rational, analytical method and a careful deployment of scientific skills. To be "competent" means, in effect, to be a good technician. That is the general thrust of contemporary medical education. It is

Reprinted with permission from *The Nebraska Law Review*, vol. 63 (1984), pp. 663–667. © 1984 University of Nebraska Law Review.

a clear message that one can gain by examining medical journals, and a general attitude well in keeping with a society that prizes scientific knowledge and its application to human problems.

Just as the history of much twentieth century philosophical and scientific thought has been marked by an allegedly sharp chasm between the "is" and the "ought," between facts and values, so too there has developed an equally great chasm in medical practice between the supposed empirical solidity of scientific medicine in the diagnosis and treatment of illness, and the far more subjective, relatively intractable side of medicine represented by subjectivity, personal values, and medical ethics. The former are thought to be "hard," and the latter "soft." That phenomenon is hardly unique to medicine, but cuts through much of our contemporary thinking. An important consequence, however, is that it has helped to abet a general tendency to ignore the whole person and to focus instead on particular illnesses or organ systems, and to be relatively indifferent to all of those personal and subjective factors that influence the way patients are actually treated, or at least the way they perceive their treatment.

Viewed crudely, one might well ask just what difference does it make anyway, and why ought one not worry exclusively about the scientific side of medicine? That kind of an attitude might make perfectly good sense if one's aim is to vaccinate people against a plague or a cholera epidemic. There the aim is to save as many lives from a potentially fatal disease as possible, and the personal relationships, or the desires of patients, are relatively unimportant. But in an era of chronic illness, where people are not going to be saved readily or inexpensively, and where death will be for most people a long drawn-out phenomenon, an exclusively technological attitude is not only conducive to professional insensitivity, but is not likely to meet the genuine needs of patients.

If it was ever valid in the past to distinguish sharply between the technical and the human side of medicine, that distinction is no longer tolerable. Put more pointedly, it is impossible to say that a health care worker is competent if that person is not able to grapple effectively with the moral problems involved in medical care, or able to deal with the human dimensions of that care. Every medical decision, either tacitly or explicitly, must find an appropriate blend between the technically correct course of treatment and that which is morally defensible. In almost no case will it be utterly irrelevant to ask for the technically appropriate approach, and in almost no case will it be irrelevant to ask what the best moral course would be. The major difficulty will be to find the right blend between the technical and the moral.

Implicit within this is the assumption that it is of the essence of morality to ask the question: what is the good of human beings? That broad question encompasses such issues as choosing that behavior that most advances the human good, determining how to make decisions in the face of conflicting possibilities of the human good, and in deciding what character traits or virtues are most conducive to a seeking and an achievement of the good for human beings.

Inevitably, any attempt to define an ultimate good will be problematical, and probably controversial, at least in a pluralistic society; but that social reality does not absolve us of a responsibility to make the effort. It also will force us to grapple with such fundamental questions as the nature of human life, the meaning of such concepts as "health" and "illness," and the relationship among physical, psychological, and spiritual or philosophical goods.

In a medical context, moral questions arise both implicitly and explicitly. They arise implicitly when, in making what seems to be an obvious treatment decision, we affirm a set of values that may be widely shared but rarely articulated. No one, for instance, will ordinarily start a moral debate about saving the life of an otherwise perfectly healthy child who is the victim of an accident when it is easy and inexpensive to do so (or even when it is not). It is taken for granted that saving the lives of healthy children is a valid moral enterprise, and anyone involved in such a decision would immediately move to the technical problems in doing so, not pausing for a moment on the underlying ethical conditions that stimulate a decision to treat in the first place.

In those morally obvious cases—"obvious" at least because of a general social agreement—medical competence will be displayed not simply in having the correct values, but much more dominantly in those simple situations involving a choice of the right methods of treatment. The real and only *issue* in such cases is the technically appropriate course of action, not the morally appropriate course. The technical methods chosen simply implement and bear out the basic moral decision, and the technically best decision then becomes the morally best means to achieve the good of a particular individual.

At the other extreme, of course, would be situations in which there was great uncertainty about the appropriate moral goal to be sought (e.g., whether to keep alive a very elderly, debilitated, vegetative patient), and perhaps also about the appropriate technical means to achieve a hazy moral goal. Indeed, when one looks at the wide range of possible medical decisions—on people of different ages, physical conditions, religions, and so on—it makes considerable sense to think in terms of a continuum. At one end of the continuum would be those decisions that command universal, or almost universal, moral agreement, leaving the only important issues those that bear on the best technical care. Saving a life of a dying healthy child, or setting the broken leg of a healthy adult, would fall on one end of the continuum. At the other end of the continuum would be decisions where the moral good was uncertain, and perhaps the technical choices no less uncertain even if one could determine the moral good to be sought. The most difficult ethical dilemmas, of course, are those where one is in doubt about what will genuinely serve the welfare of patients, and the dilemma is made all the more complicated if there are a number of treatment possibilities available as well. A decision, for instance, that would involve some kind of trade-off between the mere extension of life, and a shorter life without the radical disfigurement that might be the result of some life-extending surgery, would pose an enormously difficult choice, blending in an exceedingly complex fashion the technical and moral aspects.

To envision the decisionmaking mix between the technical and moral aspects of medical care as part of a continuum by no means solves the problem of how one ought to determine the extent to which a particular medical problem ought to be seen as essentially moral, or essentially technical. In their enthusiasm to break down a fact-value dichotomy, some commentators like to argue that all medical decisions are essentially nontechnical. Even in the most obvious kinds of situations—that of saving the lives of healthy babies—there is a fundamental moral choice made, even if not stated. All medical decisions, viewed that way, are moral decisions, and the technical always remains secondary. That is probably true enough; but it is not a very interesting truth. For it is no less a fact that the technical does exist, that technical decisions must be made, and that the range of technical options available will in great part determine the possibilities for advancing human welfare. If the moral shapes the technical, we ought to know from contemporary medical practice that the technical possibilities shape the moral choices as well.

The care of the chronically ill, or of the dying, poses some of the most difficult kinds of questions. For in both of those cases one knows that there is nothing that medicine ultimately can do to save the life of a patient, and that it is simply a matter of caring for the patient in the most effective way possible when the eventual outcome—death—is known with certainty. In the case of the chronically ill, death may not be imminent at all, but many months or even years into the future. In the case of those we determine to be terminally ill, death will be more imminent. In either situation, however, the main point will be to choose those technical means that will provide the best comfort and care, and the highest quality of life, compatible with the fact of an inevitable end. That is a particular challenge to medicine, because the ethos of technical medicine is to treat aggressively with the most sophisticated means—means which, in the case of the chronically ill, may be perfectly inappropriate to achieving their moral or spiritual welfare.

A brief commentary of this sort is not conducive of a detailed examination of the myriad problems that confront anyone who tries to find the right balance between moral and technical considerations in the providing of "competent" care. Suffice it to say that medical training that does not introduce students vigorously and rigorously to that issue will be remiss. Since all medical decisions will entail some value commitment or other, the more conscious the understanding of those values the more likely it is that the care given will be appropriate to the patient. In some cases, the choice will be very difficult. Competency, therefore, can be defined not simply as an ability to master and manipulate technological means of providing cures, but also the capacity to relate those technologies to the needs of individual patients, through some view of the good of human beings, and in the light of some method of relating moral and scientific values.

That is an enormously difficult task, and the notion of competency suggested here is not one that is easily achieved. Nonetheless, if we can at least agree that a notion of competency that focuses exclusively on technical skills is an inadequate one, and perhaps as likely to do harm as to do good, we would at least have made a great advance, and set the stage for a different way of treating patients in the future. For all of its services in the past, an excessively technical outlook on medical care is not likely to be appropriate in light of a rapidly aging population, a growing proportion of the chronically ill, and a citizenry that is increasingly conscious that it must make medical decisions in the light of personal and social moral values.

THE CONTEXT AS A MORAL RULE IN MEDICAL ETHICS

David C. Thomasma

ABSTRACT: A purely deductive medical ethics cannot properly account for the varieties of circumstances which arise in medical practice. By contrast, a purely inductive medical ethics lacks sufficient guidance from ethical principles. In resolving ethical dilemmas in medicine, most often an appeal is made to middle-level axioms and methodological rules to mediate between theory and practice. I argue that this appeal must be augmented by considerations of context, such considerations, in effect, constituting a moral rule based on the social structure of medical practice. A contextual grid is proposed which assists the process of weighing values in resolving cases.

Medical ethics currently must face a struggle between abstract and concrete. Much of the theory of medical ethics owes its existence to an attempt to establish moral principles in an era which accepted the view that immutable principles should govern human behavior. But the application of these principles to medicine, which deals with individuals, has been problematic to say the least. For example, Gorovitz and MacIntyre, in their influential paper on medical infallibility, excoriate Aristotle for his presumed lack of attention to the individual. The reason for this attack lies with the authors' recognition that medicine, even if taken as a science, must be a science of individuals (Gorovitz and MacIntyre, 1976).

Even more germane to medical ethics is the challenge put to it by Franz Ingelfinger, a distinguished physician and editor. Ingelfinger charges that phi-

Reprinted with permission from *The Journal of Bioethics*, vol. 2 (1984), pp. 63–78. © 1984 Human Sciences Press, Inc.

losophers and theologians create an absolutist ethic which cannot be employed in particular cases and is of little use to practicing physicians. He notes, "The practitioner appears to prefer the principles of individualism. As there are few atheists in fox holes, there tend to be few absolutists at the bedside." (Ingelfinger, 1973).

My approach in this paper will be first to delineate various attempts to meet the challenge of the individual case in medical ethics. I shall then present a contextual grid for medical ethics which can serve as either an alternative or a supplement to these approaches.

JOUSTING WITH INDIVIDUALISM

Recognizing that medicine deals with concrete, historically existing individuals in specific situations, several thinkers have tried to supply a bridge between abstract moral principles and individual cases. I shall take up each of these in turn and shall provide a brief critique as well. In each category of response I will describe one or two thinkers. I find the following categories of response: 1) Acceptance of Absolutist Principles; 2) Casuistry; and 3) Development of Intermediate Norms.

Before examining each of these positions, it is important to clarify levels of "ought" statements prevalent in the literature to be examined. This clarification will also establish initial definitions for terminology that is often left vague and confusing. The vocabulary proposed is as follows: "principles," "axioms," "policies," and "indicated courses of action."

"Principles" are "ought" statements which describe fundamental and abstract theoretical views, such as Mill's "We ought to maximize the general happiness." or Kant's principle of autonomy. "Axioms" state middle-level "ought" claims, claims which might be jointly recognized by competing ethical theories. Among such axioms might be respect for persons, beneficence, or appeals to the protection of self-determination and autonomy. "Policies" provide "ought" statements which indicate how to resolve conflicts among axioms in certain kinds of situations. An "indicated course of action" describes what ought to be done in a particular situation.

A different catalogue of component stages in moral reasoning is offered by Paul Ramsey, who said in his essay, "The Case of the Curious Exception,"

> Our model of the component stages in moral reasoning can, therefore, be stated as follows: ultimate norm; general principles; defined action principles, or generic terms of approval and generic offense terms; definite-action rules or moral species terms; then the subsumption of cases (Ramsey, 1968, p. 78).

This listing is useful to illustrate both the confusion caused in moral thought by a lack of agreement regarding the terminology of different levels of moral reasoning, and the generally essential agreement that there *are* identifiable levels with different functions. At any rate, Ramsey's ultimate norm is my principle; his general principles are my axioms; his defined action principles which contain generic terms of approval and opprobrium I call policies; and his definite-action rules are my indicated courses of action which are involved in case analysis.

The difference among the three various positions to be examined lies in the role principles, axioms, and policies play in determining what is morally right in particular medical circumstances. In general, accepting principles means that some thinkers propose medical ethics issues be determined by fidelity to one or another principle, or at least look to such a principle which would be always and everywhere applicable. Casuistry, on the other hand, represents a tradition aimed at determining an indicated course of action in a particular circumstance by adjusting different principles. Thus, casuistry would include at least some effort to embody moral policies, axioms, and even a number of principles in suggesting a course of action from a case-specific point of view. Finally, approaches taken to develop intermediate norms, or axioms, determine a course of action by applying a moral principle through more specific rules.

Clearly, some appeal to context is necessary to interpret principles or their applicability to matters at hand. Normally, ethicists regard this appeal as guided by moral rules. Examples of such rules are Kant's categorical imperative, a utilitarian calculus of feelings, or the "principle" of double effect. The categorical imperative "interprets" the principle of autonomy by commanding action in keeping with that autonomy. A calculus of feeling is presented as a way of deciding which values shall be regarded more important in bringing about the greatest good for the greatest number. The double-effect rule is a methodological interpretant of the natural law principle: Do good and avoid evil, in that it helps determine a way to avoid doing evil in a conflict situation.

My suggestion in this paper is that answers to moral quandries in medicine do not rest on principles alone. Only the most rigid deductive ethicist would hold such a position. Rather I argue that the medical context itself functions as a moral rule, aiding the resolution of medical ethics quandries. With these distinctions in hand, I now turn to the three categories of solutions recommended for the problem of linking the abstract with the concrete.

Absolutism

It is quite possible to deny that ethics should develop absolute moral principles, and instead focus on Aristotle's theory of virtue or Dewey's theory of character. Neither accept moral principles the way Kant does, i.e., in some absolute way, but they do accept general guides to moral conduct. This approach requires, however, a very solid reassessment of psychology and sociology upon which the theories have been based. Most medical ethics theorists, instead, seem to adopt the notion that moral principles are, indeed, required for ethics. Otherwise one is left ethically rudderless in a pluralistic society. But these thinkers fall into at least three subcategories.

First, some ethicists may accept without questions the assumption that moral principles are absolutes. Instead, they may countercharge that medicine also makes some assumptions of absolute principles. In a sense this argument takes the form of "your daddy is bigger than mine." James Rachels' response to Ingelfinger is an example.

Ingelfinger's charge, recall, is that moralists tend to be absolutist while physicians abhor absolutism, especially at the bedside. Rachels chooses to question the latter claim. He charges that physicians themselves employ even more dangerous abstract principles than moralists, such as the distinction between active and passive euthanasia (Rachels, 1977). Such an approach, however, fails on three counts. First, the distinction is not just one employed by physicians. Ethicists also employ it. Second, physicians rarely use the distinction when faced with serious life-prolonging decisions (Crane, 1978). Even more telling is the fact that the approach of counustercharging fails to shed much light on the relation between abstract principles and concrete cases because it rests on stereotypes of the physician as opportunist and the ethicist as idealist. This third point has been emphasized in Mark Siegler's response to a similar statement by William Ruddick (Ruddick, 1981; Siegler, 1981).

A second approach to the relation of abstract principles and concrete practice is to deny that such principles can have any real application in medicine, or that philosophy can help medicine in any real fashion. If moral principles are inherently designed to represent consensus on ultimate moral claims, this consensus evaporates in a pluralistic society. Both Alasdair MacIntyre and Daniel Callahan have grappled with this problem.

MacIntyre's earlier articles are illustrative of the problems encountered by those who would apply the abstract to the concrete without attention to cultural and professional determinants. MacIntyre argues that a pluralistic society destroys the moral authority of ethical principles enunciated in a less pluralistic culture and that, therefore, medicine ought not to seek help from philosophy since there is no ultimate moral arbiter (MacIntyre, 1975, and MacIntyre, 1977). In a later article, he has modified this view, arguing that some conclusions may follow from moral principles in a pluralistic society, but consensus and objectivity vanish (MacIntyre, 1979). If one assumes with MacIntyre that ethics must be based on abstract principles, then his logic and conclusions are inescapable. Medical ethics could not help make medical decisions.

Daniel Callahan's recent effort to sketch the future of medical ethics in his Shattuck Lecture sounds the same warning (Callahan, 1980). He excoriates analytic medical ethics which focuses on specific ethical issues in medicine because the real debate lies in the realm of moral principles and public policy. In this realm, Callahan observes, much less consensus occurs than in case studies and specific problems. The lack of agreement about ultimate moral principles signifies an enormous cultural upheaval requiring the development of new ethical norms.

The second approach to the problem of abstract and concrete in ethics can be summarized as follows. Moral principles are absolute only in the context of consensus. Once consensus vanishes, so does the basis of ethics. Application of the principle, while still possible, gains one no real problem-solving advantage because objectivity and agreement no longer occur. Only the development of some new culturally pluralistic principles can help resolve such a dilemma (a difficult process, to say the least).

A possible response to this position is to argue that moral principles, while abstract, are not absolute. There are a number of ultimate moral principles which must be "weighted" in the contexts in which they are to be applied. Weighting or adjusting values can be done acording to intermediate axioms and rules as defined, but can never obtain the objectivity and absoluteness of a science. The contextual norms are then seen as applying *ut in pluribus,* or for the most part.

A third subcategory is that occupied by a whole host of authorities in medical ethics, namely, the application of standard ethical principles to medical problems. Thus, attempts like Paul Ramsey's to rule out non-therapeutic research on children from the standpoint of what he calls a canon of loyalty (itself based on Kantian presuppositions) neglect other values operative in clinical research (Ramsey, 1973).

Hare's paper on abortion also typifies this approach, although he applies a utilitarian principle (Hare, 1977). These attempts succumb to Ingelfinger's challenge on two grounds. First, they ignore the realistic context of the dilemmas, thus appearing to preserve certain ethical principles at the expense of medical and professional ones. Second, they presuppose widespread acceptance of either a Kantian or a utilitarian approach to moral problems, both of which presuppose universal moral principles guiding human behavior. A utilitarian cannot accept Ramsey's conclusions on the latter's grounds. A Kantian certainly cannot accept Hare's (Rachels, 1977).

Casuistry

Casuistic analyses of medical cases without any appeal to norms or standards, which Ingelfinger seems to suggest in his challenge, are not usually successful because they place too much value on the concrete, and fail to develop a consistent and coherent pattern for action. This has been the charge against Situation Ethics from its inception. Deciding on a case-by-case basis without any moral guidelines or policy cannot meet the demand for moral accountability in our society.

But casuistry has some merit. I have argued that the use of a process of moral reasoning (called an Ethical Workup) can produce a consistent theory of moral action if one keeps in mind that the only asbolute in medicine is the professional obligation to make a decision on behalf of a patient or patients (Thomasma, 1978).

Terrence Ackerman has proposed that the proper object of medical ethics providing practical and realistic guides to decision making in medicine ought to be to preserve as many values and interests in the case as possible (Ackerman, 1980). This approach, which admits a pluralism of general, but not absolute, principles is a significant contribution to the arguments by Arthur Dyck for a "moral policy" approach to ethics, which he describes as follows:

> Moral policy refers to that portion of the total ethical enterprise in which whatever is known or believed to be true in normative theory as well as on Methaethical theory is applied to specific moral issues and the methods used to cope with them. Decisions about what is right or wrong . . . are not solely decided, nor ought they be, on the basis of ethical theory per se (Dyck, 1978).

If this approach is not followed, however, too much attention will be paid to individual variants in cases. No pattern of action could be developed from case to case. Thus, Dyck begins his article on the same problem addressed in this paper with these words:

> Whatever their merit, these responses to contemporary moral dilemmas in medicine are inadequate. They are made without explicitly offering the framework for understanding the relationship between ethical standards and medical practice implied by the policies they advocate (Dyck, 1978).

Intermediate Principles

A third response to the challenge of individualism in medical ethics has been the development of intermediate principles, either ethical or professional.

This approach differs from casuistry in that the general principle rather than the case is the starting point. In a casuistic approach, the case or cases introduce the ethical problem. A search for an indicated course of action includes assembling moral rules, axioms, and principles joining these as far as possible. By contrast, the approach of employing intermediate principles, while dovetailing with casuistry, starts with general moral principles and applies these to cases by developing more restrictive axioms and interpretative rules through an analysis of social or medical values.

Beauchamp and Childress address this problem in their excellent volume, *Principles of Biomedical Ethics* (1979). However, the applicability of these principles to the medical situation is not always clear. Less sophisticated but more practical are the principles governing biomedical research found in the *Belmont Report* of the National Commission for the Protection of Human Subjects (Belmont Report, 1978). These principles are clearly drawn from medicine as well as philosophy and have the added benefit of applicability through DHEW (now HHS) policy.

With Edmund Pellegrino, I have argued elsewhere for intermediate axioms developed from within professional obligations and the value of healing (Thomasma and Pellegrino, 1980). I have also made a case for a normative medical ethics less abstract than moral principles (Thomasma, 1980).

Whatever the considerable merits of this approach, the notion of intermediate principles is clearly demanded as one bridge between the abstract and the concrete. Mill himself noted:

> Without such middle principles, a universal principle, either in science or in morals, serves for little but a thesaurus of commonplaces for the discussion of questions, instead of a means of deciding them (Mill, 1965).

Re-establishing a professional code of medical ethics is also a fruitful avenue for providing a bridge between abstract principles and concrete cases. Two recent attempts are especially notable. Veatch argues from professional obligations to a new code of ethics (Veatch, 1979). Pellegrino has constructed the outlines of a new code based on human need, a point which we together develop in a volume on the philosophy of medicine (Pellegrino, 1979; Pellegrino and Thomasma, 1981).

It seems to me that intermediate norms embodied in a revised code of ethics or moral policy, can supply a necessary bridge between abstract principles and concrete cases provided one accepts the notion of a pluralism of relevant moral principles which must be adjusted depending on the context. However, a kind of "map" of contexts is needed, a task to which I now turn.

CONTEXTUAL GRID

A middle course between a generalist application of ethical theory and specialized case-by-case analysis is possible with a contextual grid of medical ethics. It is only an example of work on contexts to which medical ethics must address itself in the future. I hold that neither axioms nor rules are sufficient, although they are necessary, to determine the role of moral theory and ethical principles in resolving medical ethics quandries. Additional rules, or guidelines for applying theory to practice, must be developed. Among these is the context as a formal adjustment to values in concrete circumstances.

As I suggested in the first part of this paper, the root of the difficulty in medical ethics lies in a confrontation between an abstracting tendency in the long and rewarding history of ethics and the concrete, individualized concern of health professionals. The latter must make decisions, sometimes rapidly. On the other hand, care and attention to numerous ethical theories and a minimally decent conceptual analysis takes time and quickly can become quite abstract.

Health professionals rapidly lose interest in these abstractions and theoretical meanderings if they are not at least remotely related to the realities of patient care. They must do ethics on the run.

Ethical principles appear abstract, or better, speculative, because they do not possess the same degree of social legitimacy as the values of everyday life. Moral abstractions are often not seen as active ingredients in the moral life of a people. No doubt they can, and do, seep into that life, but that process is a long and subtle one.

Thus, what is needed is a means by which to locate a moral problem and the likely values and principles at issue within that locus. The context having been established by such a "grid," the discussion can proceed to means of resolving the case by protecting the interests and values of those affected by it.

I shall first lay down the assumption of the grid, then outline a possible grid, then describe some examples of the content of the grid, and close by summarizing some claims made for it.

Assumptions

With respect to the application of abstract principles to medical contexts, I have noticed in over ten years of clinical teaching of medical ethics that the "weighting" of values in cases is dependent on the context. I call this the variability of contexts. It is not so much that the values or moral principles are relative in themselves; rather, the weight they bring to bear on a case is partially determined by the medical speciality involved, the personal values of the patient, family, or social group, the personal and professional values of the health care professionals involved, and the institution in which the problem arises. Bergsma and Duff have also noted this array of variables, further distinguishing micro, macro, and meso levels of value clashes (Bergsma and Duff, 1980).

In a search for "middle principles," as Mill called them, with a view toward uniting the casuistic, moral policy, analytic approach to the resolution of cases, and the intermediate principle approach, one component can be a grid or outline of contexts in which some moral principles and norms are most likely to be given more weights than others. Three points need to be emphasized here. First, such a contextual grid is only one tentatively proposed component of what should be called context variable moral rules. Second, the grid cannot encompass the many varibles which do occur in cases; it is only intended to encapsule *most likely* emphases on some values over others. Thus, the rule of protection of autonomy is more likely to be given prominent focus in a primary care context than in tertiary care, where one's autonomy is virtually destroyed by a serious disease. In that case, restoration, not protection, is a guiding rule (Thomasma, 1983). Furthermore, the rule of protection of autonomy is more likely to be emphasized in cases in which there is no threat to others than in cases wherein the common good must be considered, sometimes to the detriment of personal autonomy (Thomasma, 1983).

The third point is this. Because the grid only *describes* most likely weights given to moral principles and rules in formulating an indicated course of action, one should not misconstrue the grid as claiming that physicians in tertiary care do not care about protection of autonomy, or that public health officials stress social responsibility to the exclusion of individual well-being. All the moral values should bear on a case. The grid only describes what values are most likely to take precedence in an indicated course of action.

The grid rests on a two-fold distinction: its coordinates. The first is the distinction between primary, secondary, and tertiary care, a standard distinction in medicine. Its importance for moral justification lies in the seriousness of the assault on personal wholeness represented by disease (Bergsma and Thomasma, 1982). Thus, a patient's wishes are more likely to be respected (protection of autonomy) in a primary care setting than in an emergency room after a heart attack, where a paternalistic response may be, and often is, more appropriate.

The second distinction or coordinate of the grid is that between the number of persons affected by the problem. The moral significance of this distinction is based on the increased complexity of moral values the more different persons are affected, and our increased tendency to protect the commonwealth rather than personal freedom as large numbers of persons are affected. Recall again that the purpose of the grid is to describe variable context rules, i.e., which moral principles and moral axioms will most likely be given more weight than others in formulating a moral policy or an indicated course of action.

Claims about the validity of the grid will be discussed in the final section of the paper (see Figure 1).

If the vertical axis of the grid be taken for the seriousness of the medical problem and the horizontal the number of persons affected, then:

1 quadrant 1A represents a single doctor-patient relationship in a primary care non- or mildly serious situation, 1B represents the same situation which also affects a family group and 1C the same situation which affect society in some way, or a health care team.

2 quadrant 2A represents a single doctor-patient relationship in a secondary-care setting, in which a serious medical problem is present. "B" and "C" describe larger involvement as above.

3 quadrant 3A represents a single doctor-patient relationship in a tertiary care setting, in which the patient has a very critical medical problem. "B" and "C" describe larger involvement as above.

Number of persons affected **FIGURE 1**

The Grid as a Moral Rule

Some points about moral rules can be made almost immediately. I shall organize these horizontally and vertically.

1 *Horizontal.* The further one moves to the right, the less the importance of individual rights and the axiom of individual beneficence, and the greater the principles of the common good and greatest happiness take precedence over the patient's individual rights. Bear in mind that the grid presents only a means by which to clarify the context and the most likely principles and rules in conflict. It does provide a means by which to resolve the conflicts, but not a normative guideline for a course of action. More about this point later. Secondly, the more one moves across the horizontal axis, the less personal responsibility of the physician and the more the entrance of social and community responsibility occurs.

2 *Vertical.* 1, 2, and 3 represent the three contexts of medical care, primary, secondary, and tertiary. Primary deals with front-line, non-invasive, preventive, and basic care for non-serious or mildly serious problems. In this context even considered horizontally, the patient and his or her values takes precedence over all other values, with corresponding horizontal diminishment. In secondary care settings, mostly hospitals and chronic disease centers, less of the patient's own values and more of the context's predominate. In tertiary care situations other individual values are sacrificed for the fundamental value of preserving the life of patients in critical situations.

Some descriptive examples will help clarify the grid. Take population ethics for an example:

1A An unmarried adult requests sterilization. The request is not medically indicated. The patient's right of self-determination is the primary value to be preserved (Graber, 1978).

1B A married adult requests sterilization. The request is not medically indicated. However, family obligations and economic factors demonstrate a reasonable cause. The patient's right of self-determination must be balanced with the physician's obligation to do no harm and the current situation and values of the family.

1C A married adult requests sterilization. The request is not medically indicated. Further, the married partner objects, or some member of the health care team objects, or hospital policy does not permit it. Since more social involvement occurs in this quadrant, social values and institutional values often predominate.

2A A married patient with a chronic illness requests sterilization, without which a pregnancy may threaten her life. It is medically indicated. Both the principle of self-determination and beneficence require the sterilization but the risks of the operation on the chronic illness must be weighed in the decision and alternative contraceptive methods explored.

2B A retarded adult, unmarried, is considered a candidate for sterilization, but objections from family members might override even a request from the retarded person.

2C A retarded child is sexually active and parents request sterilization. However, society values in eugenic laws, class interests of the retarded, or an absence of laws may override individual rights in this case.

3A A married, pregnant woman contracts leukemia, necessitating a therapeutic abortion because of radiotherapy and chemotherapy. Notice that while the individual rights of patients are horizontally preferred in quadrant 3, their values must be balanced against the factors of serious disease. A D and C after a rape, even though the victim may normally value children and be against abortion, I would place also in quadrant 3. Most often quadrant 3 cases are cases in the emergency room or intensive care ward in which the values of patients are hard to obtain and individual rights are protected only insofar as there are presumptions for a value of continued life.

3B A nuclear accident occurs in which five women and their fetuses are exposed to damaging amounts of radiation. Despite individual values in normal circumstances, the level 3 intensity of the danger to their lives and fetal damage might require terminating pregnancy.

3C In this quadrant the classic case of enforced sterilization of a population in a poor country without sufficient food can be placed. Individual rights are superseded here not only by the social crisis of overpopulation, but also by the common good of a decent economic development.

Before my final summary, I want to make an important point. This descriptive grid can be helpful for any number of broadly conceived ethical problems: prolongation of life, for example, is a totally different problem in quadrant 1 (a healthy patient has a seizure in a doctor's office) and quadrant 3 (a seriously ill patient has had four resuscitation attempts already). The obligation to preserve life is different in 2 (Hitler's physician was tempted to terminate Hitler's life after the bunker bomb blast by giving him an overdose of sedative) and 3C (the physician at a fire must act to preserve some lives rather than others due to the pressures of time and resources). Thus any attempt to discuss medical ethics problems (such as Hare's on abortion) without attention to these totally different quadrants or contexts at best provides only a polemic for one's moral principle or its refinement, and at worst demonstrates an insensitivity to concrete moral quandries which render the discussion fruitless.

CONCLUSION

The major features of this contextual grid, by way of summary, are as follows:

1 The grid presupposes that the aim of medical ethics is to propose resolutions to difficult medical dilemmas. Discussions of general principles might best be called ethics of medicine.

2 The grid presupposes the need to employ different moral principles which predominate in some quadrants more than in others. Medicine is too complex to admit a reductionistic ethical theory covering all its dilemmas.

3 A better developed grid can provide ethicists with ready access to the major medical values involved in each quadrant which must be respected in any moral policy developed. Advances in the limited axiom theory and revised professional codes can enhance the sophistication of the grid.

4 Finally, the grid does not provide immediate, computerized ethical solutions to medical dilemmas, principally because it is currently impossible to offer normative categories corresponding to the quadrants, not only because the bridge between the abstract and the concrete has not been completed, but also because we cannot foresee the patient values in each case. Thus, it is impossible to construct a normative calculus from this grid.

Having completed these qualifiers, one may again ask whether the contextual grid is merely *descriptive*. Does it just provide a description of the balances and priorities of principles and rules in suggesting either a policy or a course of action? Can it have any application in therapeutic and ethical decisions (i.e., medical decisions)? If one argued, as I have so far, that the grid were merely descriptive, then it would not address the problem of justification of indicated courses of action by appeal either to absolute moral principles, intermediate axioms, or moral policies. The grid should be seen as a suggestion of how one might rank conflicting values or rules in specific contexts.

A major problem in understanding how to justify particular ethical recommendations or an indicated course of action is that "intermediate principles" conflict in specific circumstances. Indeed, in some cases, moral principles also conflict. The task of medical ethics must, therefore, be to set priorities among these conflicts depending on the context. The context itself suggests how priorities should be made.

The validity of this argument can be tested by showing how resolution of conflicting principles, rules, and policies, without attention to contexts, condemns one to bald assertion or appeal to yet other principles or rules, and so on, *ad infinitum*. MacIntyre demonstrates the philosophical frustration in store for those who follow this approach (MacIntyre, 1979). The same medical problem would be treated differently in different circumstances and different rules would be weighted in these circumstances even when they involve the same patient. Justification for these different weights cannot be made by an appeal to a single moral principle because it is too "empty" of content to provide an indicated course of action. Other rules and values cannot justify the choice of precedence of one of their number over the others because they all, taken at face value, have equal force. Only the context itself, in conjunction with professional standards, can provide the reasons for ranking some values over others.

In different contexts we can state general claims concerning which rules take priority over others based on the context, as I have tried to show. In this way, the contextual grid could contribute to the identification of indicated courses of action in situations where moral rules conflict. Identification of priorities, however, differs from normative forces understood as the automatic direction for action in two important respects. First, the grid must be "filled out" or completed by medical work-up which may differ from case to case without the context. Second, the priority of one axiom over another, or of one principle over another, may still admit of several indicated courses of action, the justification for choosing one of which may require additional psychological, social, personal, or institutional values.

To summarize, then, the contextual grid for medical ethics supplies a descriptive bridge for relating abstract moral principle to concrete cases as well as intermediate classification of the priorities of one axiom over another depending on context. Indicated courses of action follow from this prioritization but not in normative fashion, because other therapeutic and social factors may intervene. The grid is less than normative but more than merely descriptive. I would suggest calling this intermediate position a "claim identification" standing because the grid does not identify claims for ranking values in conflict which rest less on social and cultural values (MacIntyre) than on the medical context. Obviously, to directly address Ingelfinger's challenge, one would have to develop a therapeutic standing on the grid, a complex feat beyond the scope of this paper but not beyond the realm of possibility.

If anything is valid in this paper, it has been the suggestion that medical ethics methodology must take the concrete, individual cases seriously, while providing a means to resolve medical problems which respects the case, medical context, patient and medical values, and general moral principles. At the stage of its current development, the grid cannot acquire any normative force in resolving medical ethics cases. But consensus about weights for moral principles and rules are at least more likely to occur than consensus about moral principles to govern a pluralistic society. I would suggest that intermediate axioms arguments would be more beneficial to the future of medical ethics than efforts to establish new abstract and universal moral principles. The contextual grid should be viewed as one means to achieve this end.

REFERENCES

Ackerman, T.F. What bioethics should be. *Journal of Medicine and Philosophy, 5,* 1980, 260–275.

Beauchamp, T., & Childress, J. *Principles of Biomedical Ethics.* New York: Oxford University Press, 1979.

Belmont Report of the National Commission for the Protection of Human Subjects. Washington, D.C.: U.S. Government Printing Office, 1978. DHEW (OS) 78-0012.

Bergsma, J. & Duff, R. A model for examining values and decision making in the patient-doctor relationship. *Pharos,* 1980, summer, 7–12.

Bergsma, J. & Thomasma, D. *Health Care: Its Psychosocial Dimensions.* Pittsburgh: Duquesne University Press, 1982.

Callahan, D. Shattuck lecture: contemporary biomedical ethics. *New England Journal of Medicine,* 1980, 22, 300–306.

Crane, D. Physician's attitudes toward the treatment of critically ill patients. In S. J. Reiser. A. Dyck, and W. Curran (Eds.). *Ethics In Medicine.* Cambridge, MA.: MIT Press, 1978, pp. 514–517.

Dyck, A. Ethics in medicine. In S.J. Reiser, A. Dyck, and W. Curran (Eds.). *Ethics In Medicine.* Cambridge, MA.: MIT Press, 1978, pp. 115–119.

Gorovitz, S. & MacIntyre, A. Toward a theory of medical fallibility. *Journal of Medicine and Philosophy,* 1976, *1,* 51–71.

Graber, G. On paternalism and health care. In J.W. Davis, B. Hoffmaster, and S. Shorten (Eds.). *Contemporary Issues in Biomedical Ethics.* Clifton, N.J.: The Humana Press, 1978, pp. 233–244.

Hare, R.M. Can the moral philosopher help? In H.T. Engelhardt, Jr. and S. Spicker (Eds.). *Philosophical Medical Ethics.* Dordrecht & Boston: D. Reidel, 1977, pp. 46–61.

Ingelfinger, F. Bedside ethics for the hopeless case. *New England Journal of Medicine,* 1973, *289,* 914.

MacIntyre, A. How virtues become vices: values, medicine and social context. In H.T. Engelhardt, Jr. and S. Spicker (Eds.). *Evaluation and Explanation in the Biomedical Sciences.* Dordrecht & Boston: D. Reidel, 1975, pp. 97–112.

MacIntyre, A. Patients as agents. In H.T. Engelhardt, Jr. and S. Spicker (Eds.). *Philosophical Medical Ethics*. Dordrecht & Boston: D. Reidel, 1977, pp. 197–212.

MacIntyre, A. Why is the search for the foundations of ethics so frustrating? *Hastings Center Report*, 1979, *9*, 16–22.

Mill, J.S. Dr. Whewell on moral philosophy. In J.B. Schnewind (Ed.). *Mill's Ethical Writings*, New York, Macmillan, 1965, p. 178.

Pellegrino, E.D. & Thomasma, D.C. *A Philosophical Basis of Medical Practice*. New York, Oxford University Press, 1981.

Pellegrino, E.D. Towards a reconstruction of medical morality, the primacy of the act of profession and the fact of illness. *Journal of Medicine and Philosophy*. 1979, *4*, 32–56.

Rachels, J. Medical ethics and the rule against killing: comments on professor Hare's paper. In H.T. Engelhardt, Jr. and S. Spicker (Eds.). *Philosophical Medical Ethics*. Dordrecht & Boston: D. Reidel, 1977, pp. 63–72.

Ramsey, P. The case of the curious exception. In G. Outka and P. Ramsey (Eds.). *Norm and Context in Christian Ethics*. New York: Charles Scribner's Sons, 1968, p. 78.

Ramsey, P. *The patient as person*. New Haven: Yale University Press, 1973.

Ruddick, W. Can doctors and philosophers work together? *Hastings Center Report*, 1981, *11*, 12–17.

Siegler, M. Cautionary advice for humanists. *Hastings Center Report*, 1981, *11*, 19–20.

Thomasma, D.C. & Pellegrino, E.D. The philosophy of medicine as source of medical ethics. *Metamedicine*, 1980, *2*, 5–11.

Thomasma, D.C. Beyond medical paternalism and patient autonomy: a model of physician's conscience for the doctor-patient relationship. *Annals of Internal Medicine*, 1983, *98*, 243–248.

Thomasma, D.C. The limitations of the autonomy model for the doctor-patient relationship. *The Pharos*, in press.

Thomasma, D.C. The possibility of a normative medical ethics. *Journal of Medicine and Philosophy*, 1980, *5*, 249–259.

Thomasma, D.C. Training in medical ethics and ethical workup. *Forum on Medicine*, 1978, *1*, Dec., 33–36.

Veatch, R. Professional medical ethics: the grounding of its principles. *Journal of Medicine and Philosophy*, 1979, *4*, 1–19.

ARE NURSES' MIND SETS COMPATIBLE WITH ETHICAL PRACTICE?

Mila Ann Aroskar

Ethical nursing practice often seems like a difficult and elusive goal. Why is this? The understanding and implementation of more ethical nursing practice are a challenge and an obligation for nurses as individuals and for the nursing profession collectively. The underlying assumption is that more ethical practice is a "good" to be sought in the delivery of nursing and health care. Understanding and implementation require processes of ethical inquiry, principled thinking, strategies for action and a spirit of compassion for one's self and for others. Nurses have support for more ethical practice in such documents as the ANA Code and ANA Standards for Nusing Practice. Yet one still hears arguments that ethical practice is too risky and requires a certain amount of heroism on the part of nurses.

THE "ETHICAL" IN NURSING PRACTICE

Ethics in nursing has to do with the critical examination of the moral dimensions of decision making at the daily practice level and the policy-making level. The concept of ethical nursing practice indicates practice that is based on and includes critical, reflective thinking about one's duties and obligations as an individual nurse in relation to clients and as a member of a profession fulfilling a social contract. Frequently, there is a lack of clarity as to what counts as the most

From *Topics in Clinical Nursing*, vol. 4, no. 1 (April 1982), pp. 22–32. © 1982. Reprinted with permission of Aspen Publishers, Inc.

"right" or "just" judgments, actions and attitudes in delivery of nursing care as a segment of the health care delivery system. A task of nurses and the nursing profession is to determine what is ethical practice in the context of the social contract between hospitals, other employing agencies, physicians and nurses and the larger social contract between a service profession and society. This task is not made easier by the shifting values evident in major social institutions such as families, economics, health, politics and education.

Marilyn Ferguson, author of *The Aquarian Conspiracy,* characterizes these personal and social shifts in society as paradigm shifts. Paradigm shifts have to do with new frameworks, perspectives and ways of thinking about old problems. In health care, changes such as the following are occurring: specialization is giving way to integration and concern for the whole person; emphasis on human values rather than efficiency is gaining; the patient is being viewed as autonomous rather than dependent; and the view of the professional as authority is shifting to one of the professional as therapeutic partner.[1] In these shifts, there are underlying tensions between the value of individual autonomy and the value of the common good in seeking a more just system.

NURSES AND DECISION-MAKING ENVIRONMENTS

Nurses as individual systems interact with other individual systems such as clients or colleagues in the environment. They also interact with larger and more complex social systems such as families and employing agencies which are generally bureaucratic and hierarchical in organization. Each of these systems has its own environments. The environments of nurses and nursing practice include two major dimensions. One dimension relates to the nurse's own internal environment, that is, the individual's own inner world. This world includes a mind set about the systems in which nursing and health care are delivered. The second dimension is the external environment. The external environment includes the mind sets of other individual systems such as providers and patients and the structures of the larger social systems within which these individuals interact.

The internal and external environments of individuals and the larger social systems including their formal and informal policies and norms are interacting and interdependent. They are often the context and source of actual and potential conflict for nurses who seek to achieve a more ethical level of practice.[2,3] See Figure 1 for a way of visualizing the dynamics of environments that impact on ethical practice in nursing.

INTERNAL ENVIRONMENTS AS MIND SETS

Internal as well as external environments affect if and how nurses deal with the ethical dimensions of practice. One aspect of the nurse's internal environment is the nurse's mind set or characterization of the health care system. The health

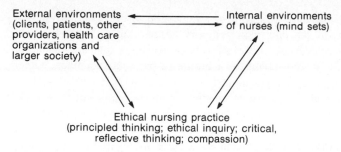

FIGURE 1.
Environments affecting ethical practice.

care system includes medicine, nursing and other types of services to care for the sick and to promote, restore or maintain health of individuals, groups and communities. Mind sets about health care can be characterized in at least four ways to include:

1 health care as medical cases or scientific projects with the cure of diseases as the single most important object;
2 health care as a commodity in the marketplace;
3 health care as the patient's right to relief from pain or a debilitating condition; and
4 health care as the promotion, maintenance and restoration of health within a cooperative community.

These views are adapted from an article by a philosopher, Lisa Newton.[4] They are used here to represent mind sets of nurses that influence efforts to achieve more ethical practice.

Health Care as Medical Cases

The first mind set—health care as medical cases or scientific projects with the cure of disease as the major goal—may predominate for nurses. It views the hospital or clinic as the "doctor's workshop." The physician may be viewed as the scientist who carries on projects with the hospital as the laboratory. Hospitals or clinics, including administrative activities, exist to facilitate these projects. Patients are the subject matter or case material. Nurses and other health care workers in the system carry on projects subsumed under those of the physician with nursing activities focused on meeting medical goals. Nurses are primarily accountable to physicians for their cases or projects. Medical values dominate the system in the decision-making processes related to patient care, services available and research conducted.

The legitimate focus of nursing activities for nurses who hold this as their predominant mind set about health care is the following of physician orders.

The nurse may feel that it is inappropriate to question or challenge physicians (still generally men) as the dominant authority figures under this view, even though the nurse may feel uncomfortable about decisions that are made for patients and families by physicians in a primarily paternalistic mode. Other consequences may include feeling blocked or frustrated with few or no options for personal, professional or institutional change. Or, nurses may unquestioningly equate ethical practice with following the wishes and orders of physicians. In some instances, this will be directly antithetical to the view that an appropriate activity of nursing is patient advocacy and to the current ANA Code which views the nurse as a competent professional with specific obligations to clients and society. Note that versions of the code as late as 1950 stated that the nurse's obligation was to carry out physician orders and to protect physicians' reputations. Nurse practice acts also contributed to the view of nurses as subservient to physicians. Efforts to change these practice acts in the past decade have not gone unchallenged.

Consider the power of this view in light of the following findings. Historically, the family was the institutional model for the operation of hospitals. This model still predominates in some hospitals and medical centers. The proper role of women, that is, nurses, was to care for this family and to keep it happy. Nurses were responsible for meeting the needs of all members of the hospital family—from patients to physicians. While nurses were capable of making decisions about patient care in the absence of physicians, they relinquished this role when the physicians returned. Nurses were also to be supportive and loyal to the institution and to preserve its reputation as well as that of the physicians.[5] This view of the appropriate role for nursing is radically different from that of the highly trained and appropriately remunerated professional envisioned by Nightingale more than a century ago.

Findings of a study done in the late 1970s of the moral reasoning of nurses including staff nurses and supervisors in hospitals and public health nursing agencies suggest that most of the participants were at a conventional level of reasoning. Participants at the conventional level stressed obedience to authority and the need for maintaining harmonious relationships with institutions and authority figures "even when patients' rights were being violated."[6] "Blame avoidance" behaviors of nurses are further evidence that they hold a mind set about health care as medical projects as exhibited in statements such as "the doctor ordered it" or "hospital rules require it."

One can still find arguments in the nursing literature in the 1980s for the subordinate role of nurses as functional in the contexts of medicine and hospitals where it is assumed that patients would be placed in jeopardy if health care providers other than physicians were making autonomous judgments about patient care. This assumes that physicians are always on the scene when the need for making clinical decisions does arise. Certainly, this is not a reflection of reality even in many intensive care units to say nothing of emergency rooms and other patient care units. Arguing for the maintenance of the nurse's subordinate role in the hospital environment, the author goes on to say that patients are comfortable with someone in such a role to whom they can ventilate safely. They can ventilate safely because the nurse can do nothing to change the patient's course of treatment. Nurses are seen, according to this author, as having no more control over the environment than patients.[7]

Speculations that nurse practitioners might demonstrate new patterns of behavior in relation to physicians are challenged by a report of in-depth interviews with 28 nurse practitioners. While these nurse practitioners saw themselves as providing a type of care that is currently lacking and desirable in the health care system, they still accommodate to the needs of physicians. They do this by submitting to the limits imposed by the medical profession. Nurse practitioners are legally accountable for their own practice, but the scope of their activities is generally established by physicians or the employing institution. It seems that they accept these restrictions for job security reasons and do so by remaining unobtrusive. Again, the nurse practitioners in this sample saw themselves as having little control over changes necessary to alter the nurse's traditional dependence on the medical community.[8]

The mind set of nursing as subordinate to medicine in health care delivery is still compelling for many nurses in the system. This mind set may well impede efforts to achieve more ethical practice which requires critical, reflective thinking and challenges to the decision-making structure of the present system.

Health Care as a Commodity

Under the mind set that views health care as a commodity to be sold in the marketplace, health care, that is, nursing and medical care, is offered for sale by hospitals and other health care agencies with the patient as a consumer or customer. The physician is an outside contractor and the nurse is an institutional employee. Under this view, the nurse's primary responsibility is to the administrative hierarchy of the institution. Institutional interests take precedence over the competing interests of traditional professional privileges such as those of the physician. They also take precedence over patient expectations and demands. Examples of this view as it relates more specifically to nursing may be seen in hospitals where packages of nursing services are offered to the patient/consumer or in agencies where competition for clients and the marketing of services become a major focus of nursing activities.

If this is the predominant view of health care held by nursing administrators and by staff, it follows that decisions would be based on a more utilitarian model. Using a utilitarian approach, one attempts to maximize utility or happiness for society and for the greatest number of people. One looks to consequences of alternative choices for the largest group. This approach is directly contradictory to the patient-centered ethic.

The patient-centered ethic is the traditional medical ethic which most nurses and health care providers are imbued with during their professional education. The patient-centered ethic commits nurses to meeting needs of individual patients, which, under this view of health care, often conflicts with the utilitarian goals of the institution. As an employee of the institution, the nurse then undoubtedly opts for primary accountability to the institution rather than to patients, thus upholding the goals of the institution. Or, nurses may feel the tremendous conflict which they have not had opportunities to learn to deal with constructively in many education or practice settings. This may be changing as institutions and the profession seek to deal with the stresses of nursing practice in complex social systems. Changes are occurring with development of new staffing patterns such as primary nursing and through such efforts as passage of the ANA resolution on teaching of ethics in continuing education and in basic nursing curriculums.

The point is that nurses who hold the view of health care as predominantly a commodity, whether or not it is consciously recognized, may not question openly what is right or wrong in terms of their own practice as long as it is congruent with institutional goals and policies. This may happen even if they feel personally uncomfortable. It was not too long ago that nurses were exhorted in nursing textbooks to follow the policies of the hospital in order to be ethical. Ethical concerns may not be raised at any system level if the bottom-line ethic in nursing administration is to view health care as a commodity like any other in the marketplace.

This view completely negates the viewpoint that claims there is something special about health care as a service to society. Energies will probably be focused on such issues as competition with other institutions and agencies and the marketing of services rather than the maintenance of standards and the troublesome and difficult ethical issues in delivery of nursing care where issues such as distributive justice constantly intrude. (Distributive justice has to do with who receives the benefits and who bears the burdens of decision making under some concept of need, equality of opportunity, equity or desert.) In reality, institutional interests related to survival are paramount with the current emphasis on cost containment and competition in the delivery of health care services. Yet sensitive nursing administrators and staff are often worried about issues such as justice in their decision making.

Health Care as the Patient's Right to Relief from Pain

Under the view of health care as the patient's right to relief from pain or a debilitating condition, hospitals and clinics exist in society to implement this right for clients who choose to come to these facilities. The nurse's primary obligation, along with that of other providers, is to meet needs and wants as identified by patients. Patient interests, rather than institutional or medical interests, would dictate what providers' roles would be appropriate in the system.

A major difficulty in implementing this view is that frequently patients identify different needs than those identified by nurses as providers. The patient (or family) might identify his or her need or preference for a private duty nurse while the nurse identifies a higher level of patient independence as more therapeutic. Or a new teenage mother's view of her needs may differ radically from that of the public health nurse who may see the mother's ideas as putting her infant in jeopardy. Under this view, the needs identified by the client based on his or her values would be decisive. This view of needs also raises the specter of health care delivery attempting to deal with a bottomless pit of identified needs or demands.

Some nurses have expressed opinions that this is a more desirable model from their points of view based on the promotion of a patient advocate role for nurses and meeting of patient needs as a primary goal of nursing care. However, this view logically puts the nurse then in the position of acting as an instrument to carry out what the patient wishes with patient values predominating. One wonders what happens to the integrity of nurses as persons and professionals under this view if it is accepted unquestioningly as ethical nursing practice.

Consumer movements, the Patients' Bill of Rights and some malpractice suits seem to point in the direction of more consumer control of the health care system. This model assumes that patients know what they need and how to use the system to satisfy their identified needs and wants related to health care. Educational efforts are being carried out by lawyers, physicians, nurses and others to assure more sophisticated consumers of health care.[9]

The above three views of the health care system make nurses primarily means to the ends of others. Nurses may be used by institutional administrators, physicians, researchers and patients to achieve goals based on values determined by individuals and groups other than nurses and the nursing community. These views, which may be held consciously or unconsciously by nurses as particular mind sets, have consequences for nurses as individuals and for the profession. Consequences may include patient care and damage to the nurses' personal and professional integrity. These mind sets may play a major role in the failure to develop more ethical nursing practice even though formal documents exist in support of more ethical practice. This is not to say that ethical practice is, or ever will be, easy.

These mind sets conflict directly or indirectly with the ANA Code which speaks to a broader vision of nursing's duties and obligations in society, with standards of practice developed by the nursing community, and with the development of nursing theories. These and other elements have influenced current nursing practice acts which point to a different view of nursing care within the health care delivery system in terms of responsibility and accountability. In this fourth view, nurses are not instruments of others such as institutions, other providers or patients.

One other possible implication of the above views (perhaps of even more serious import) is that nurses use other nurses to meet institutional, medical or client goals rather than questioning the appropriateness of these mind sets for nurses and nursing.

Health Care as Promotion of Well-being in a Cooperative Community

According to the view of health care as the promotion, maintenance and restoration of client well-being in a cooperative community, all participants' values are taken into account in decision-making processes at various system levels such as one-to-one interactions and policy making. This is a process that respects the values of the individuals involved in or affected by the decisions. The client is still the focus of care delivery, but the process implies that all participants are individually respected for their contribution to the goal of maximizing the individual's optimum level of health rather than simply means to the ends of others. Both providers and clients have rights and responsibilities under this view of health care delivery.

This view is not a panacea for all the problems in the system. For example, it could lead to a "blame-the-victim" syndrome in which clients would be considered responsible for their own conditions even though causes of the condition have not been identified (such as some types of cancer or alcoholism). This view could and does result in the asking of different questions and raises different concerns for nurses and others in regard to what constitutes more ethical nursing practice. Should, for example, nurses be responsible and accountable in the system for ensuring that clients have input into decisions affecting their futures?

IMPLICATIONS OF MIND SETS FOR ETHICAL PRACTICE

Each of the views discussed has implications for the ways in which nurses do, or do not, identify ethical issues and dilemmas in their practice. Each represents a mind set that has the potential for different nursing judgments, attitudes and actions in relation to how individual nurses and groups of nurses deal with ethical concerns and how they are interpreted. The added significance of these mind sets is that they are held not solely by nurses but also by the people with whom nurses interact such as other health providers, administrators, patients and families. These mind sets are then part of the nurse's internal *and* external environments.

Under the first three views of health care, one could say that the nurse whose practice is congruent with the goals of the employing institution, the medical community or clients is engaging in what could be considered to be at least morally correct if not ethical practice. Only the last view focuses on nurses as more individually and professionally responsible and accountable at a higher level than the legal minimum requirements of the other views. Under this last view, no persons are considered simply as means to the ends of others. Principled thinking, related to respect for individuals, would suggest that all individuals involved as providers and recipients of health care would be required to scrutinize their judgments, attitudes and actions in light of their impact on others' autonomy and values.

This is not meant to suggest that the first three views are necessarily immoral. Rather they are limited in terms of their requirements for the most fully ethical practice of nursing, if one views ethical practice on a continuum from less ethical to more ethical and considers requirements such as principled thinking, ethical inquiry and critical, reflective thinking. Thus the last view or "newer" view proposes a new paradigm for thinking about health care in which respect for all the individuals involved in or affected by major decisions to be made points to a different process and structure for the making of those decisions. The last view is implied in many current nursing documents and in professional and lay literature.

STRATEGIES AND SUPPORTS FOR NURSES WHO SEEK MORE ETHICAL PRACTICE

First, and perhaps most difficult, the acquisition of a new mind set requires that one acknowledge and give up the other mind sets where nurses are primarily means to the ends of others. This requires a change in one's own inner world, the internal environment. While it is evident that nursing and health care literature, significant nursing documents and many nurses in service, education and research are working to bring this new mind set to bear on delivery of care, it is also evident that many are comfortable with the old paradigms for decision making. While nurses may rail against the old paradigms as demeaning, they may also use them "to blame" others for what happens or does not happen in nursing care as long as nurses meet their legal responsibilities in practice. Reality is that legal responsibility establishes a bare minimum for practice whereas professional practice implies a higher order of obligations as promulgated by the profession through establishment of a code of ethics, standards of practice, educational requirements for entry into practice, and development of certification processes.

The other side of the coin is society's expectations of nursing. If society's expectations are that nurses simply follow physician orders and provide a safe sounding board, then some of the concerns raised here around a different paradigm or mind set for delivery of nursing and health care are moot. Evidence suggests other possibilities. Some nurses, physicians and consumers are concerned about how health care delivery and decision making are structured at present and how they should be structured in a more humane manner. In addition, alternative modes of health care delivery are being mandated by third party payers such as government and are developing from needs of consumers such as self-help groups that use professionals as consultants or in an educational capacity.

Our society and profession seem to value action and "busyness" per se. On the other hand, existing conditions of practice in many settings allow for little else. When do nurses on a busy hospital unit, in a crowded nursing home or in a community nursing agency with a heavy caseload have an opportunity to think through together the nursing care issues and challenges with which they are confronted at conscious or nonconscious levels?

Many of these issues and concerns have repercussions in judgments, actions and attitudes toward practice. Many have ethical dimensions related to distributive justice in the sense of the most "right" or "just" distribution of scarce nursing resources—a valuable and necessary social resource both locally and nationally. Or there are questions and worries about how decisions are made by and for patients or clients. One could argue that nursing administrators have an obligation to plan with their staff for staffing patterns that allow for such opportunities perhaps in an ethical rounds format where the purpose is to discuss the ethical dimensions of a patient care situation or a program change. It is appalling to discover how frequently nurses are unaware that they are involved in situations requiring consideration of ethical elements. An example is a nursing supervisor in a nursing home who said that she had no ethical dilemmas, yet there were elderly patients who were comatose and on respirators, and who were transported for renal dialysis. Nurses followed established medical protocols.

Hospital nursing administrators and staff nurses could look for support for the newer paradigm in the Nursing Services Section of the *JCAH Accreditation Manual for Hospitals* (1982 edition). Standards have been developed based on the principle that the nursing department "takes all reasonable steps to provide the optimal achievable quality of nursing care and to maintain the optimal professional conduct and practices of its members."[10]

Interpretations of standards include the requirement that a sufficient number of qualified RNs are available to give patients care that requires the judgment and specialized skills of RNs to achieve quality nursing care and a safe patient environment. Nursing care plans are individualized with goals set mutually with the patient and/or family whenever this is possible. While these standards are to be implemented consistent with the medical plan of care, they denote a more interdependent process of nursing responsibility and accountability that is more consistent with the view of a cooperative community of health care delivery.

The ANA document, *Nursing: A Social Policy Statement* (1980), is a formulation of nursing's social responsibility and is also more congruent with the cooperative community view of health care delivery. One might well ask where the professional and public arenas exist for discussion of this and other nursing documents which articulate nursing leaders' views of the profession. Basic consciousness-raising endeavors are needed within the profession and with other providers and the public that nursing serves.

Muyskens, a philosopher, argues that the notion of collective responsibility in nursing is "a weapon" to be used in seeking more ethical nursing practice by individuals and the profession through the development of organizational mechanisms for implementation of the ANA Code. While these mechanisms do exist in the profession nationally and in the professional nursing organizations in many states, they do not exist in all states or in all nursing service organizations. On the other hand, even if the mechanisms do exist, individuals may not know about them in order to use them.

Muyskens argues that while individuals may do all that is required of them, their responsibilities are still greater than someone who is not a member of the profession to work toward upgrading the group's conduct when it is below the professional standards that can reasonably be expected of that group.[11] Can the nursing profession claim that its standards are met in all practice settings? Or do the standards need to be changed? A critical example would be unsafe patient environments by virtue of a lack of adequate nursing staff in terms of numbers and necessary expertise.

The notion of invoking collective responsibility requires sensitive individuals within (or outside?) a profession who can articulate their concerns based on principles of "rightness" and the existence of a compatible mind set. Nurses who hold mind sets emphasizing health care as a commodity where institutional interests take precedence over other interests, health care as physician projects, or health care as implementation of patient rights where nurses are essentially means to the ends of others, may be paying a high price in terms of personal and professional integrity. There is conceivably a cost to the health care system in terms of their potential contributions as responsbile professionals. There is also a cost to the profession in terms of lack of progress on the journey toward more ethical nursing practice.

While there are no panaceas, there are assessment efforts that could be made in the nurse's inner world and in the nursing profession to deal as responsibly and effectively as possible with efforts to achieve more ethical nursing practice if individuals and the profession so determine. Have you identified your own current mind set on nursing within the health care delivery system? Perhaps this is a necessary step toward more ethical practice in nursing in complex social systems.

REFERENCES

1 Ferguson, M. *The Aquarian Conspiracy* (Los Angeles: J.P. Tarcher (1980) p. 246–248.
2 Davis, A.J. and Aroskar, M.A. *Ethical Dilemmas and Nursing Practice* (New York: Appleton-Century-Crofts 1978) p. 31–44.
3 Murphy, C.P. "The Moral Situation in Nursing" in Bandman, E.L. and Bandman, B., eds. *Bioethics and Human Rights* (Boston: Little, Brown 1978) p. 313–320.

4 Newton, L.H. "To Whom Is the Nurse Accountable? A Philosophical Perspective." *Connecticut Medicine* 43:10 (1979) p. 7–9.

5 Ashley, J.A. *Hospitals, Paternalism, and the Role of the Nurse* (New York: Teachers College Press 1976) p. 17.

6 Murphy. "The Moral Situation in Nursing." p. 315.

7 Newton, L.H. "In Defense of the Traditional Nurse." *Nursing Outlook* 29:6 (1981) p. 348–354.

8 Simmons, R.S. and Rosenthal, J. "The Women's Movement and the Nurse Practitioner's Sense of Role." *Nursing Outlook* 29:6 (1981) p. 371–375.

9 Gots, R. and Kaufman, A. *The People's Hospital Book* (New York: Avon Books 1981).

10 Joint Commission on Accreditation of Hospitals. *Accreditation Manual for Hospitals* 1982 ed. (Chicago: JCAH 1982) p. 115.

11 Muyskens, J.L. "Collective Responsibility and the Nursing Profession" in Mappes, T.A. and Zembaty, J.S., eds. *Biomedical Ethics* (New York: McGraw-Hill 1981) p. 102–108.

THE LEGAL AND PHILOSOPHICAL FOUNDATIONS OF THE RIGHT TO PRIVACY

Richard Wasserstrom

I

If there is one thing that is undeniably true of privacy, it is that there are several different phenomena that have been and that can be discussed under the heading of "privacy." Almost all of the discussion has been of comparatively recent vintage. In legal scholarship, the classic reference to a right of privacy is the article by Brandeis and Warren entitled, "The Right of Privacy," which appeared in *The Harvard Law Review* in 1890. The first enunciation by the United States Supreme Court of an explicit constitutional right of privacy occurred in 1965 in the case of *Griswold v. Connecticut*. And almost all philosophical and public policy examinations of privacy have appeared within the past fifteen years.

The topic of privacy is very much in the air and in the news today; it is the subject of appreciable discussion and legislation. As witness, for example, the 1973 Minnesota statute which enacted a patient's "bill of rights" and which included within those rights two that explicitly mentioned privacy: "Every patient and resident shall have the right to every consideration of his privacy and individuality as it relates to his social, religious, and psychological well-being" and "Every patient and resident shall have the right to respectfulness and privacy as it relates to his medical care program. Case discussion, consultation, examination, and treatment are confidential and should be conducted discretely."

Part of the problem in thinking about privacy, and in deciding, for instance, what this statute means, is, as I have said, that the same thing is not always meant at all by the term "privacy." In fact, there are, I believe, at least three distinct kinds of interests or claims that may be involved when commentators, the courts, legislatures, and ordinary citizens talk about privacy and its importance.

The kind of thing that Brandeis and Warren were concerned with was the unconsented use by an individual of another's identity in order to secure some special advantage. The central focus here is upon the improper use of a person's name or likeness for commercial purposes, as, for example, when a person's name and picture are included in the advertising for a product in order to enhance the sale of the product. But I include within this category cases in which true facts of a certain sort about an individual are made public, as for instance when there is an unconsented public showing of the films of a particular Caesarian birth.

The United States Supreme Court was concerned with a rather different sense of "privacy" in the Griswold case. That case involved primarily the constitutionality of a Connecticut statute which made it a crime for any person to use any drug, medicinal article or instrument for the purpose of preventing conception. One reason some of the members of the Court gave for holding the statute unconstitutional was that the statute intruded improperly into a constitutionally protected zone of privacy. That zone of privacy existed, apparently, in virtue of the fact that the behavior covered by the statute included that of married persons in respect to their own sexual relationship. This idea—that certain relationships and certain behavior occurring within the home were immune from governmental regulation—was also utilized by the Court in the abortion decision and in a case involving an individual's right to possess and read pornographic literature in his home.

The third sense of "privacy" is reflected in the contemporary concern over the wrong, if any, that was done by the members of the plumber's squad who broke into the office of Daniel Ellsberg's psychiatrist to see what they could learn about Ellsberg from the notes of his psychiatrist. It is reflected, as well, in the worry many persons have over the development and use of sophisticated spying devices which make it possible surreptitiously to overhear another's conversations or observe another's behavior. And it is reflected, too, in the concern over the large scale accumulation of data which now exists about each one of us and which is capable of being stored in and retrieved from large scale data banks. Here, it seems to me, the root issue captured by this idea of privacy is that of the control that an individual will be able to maintain over information about himself or herself.

It is this third sense of "privacy" that I propose to concentrate upon. I think it is the one that is centrally involved in that section of the patient's bill of rights that gives to every patient and resident the right ". . . to every consideration of his privacy and individuality as it relates to his social, religious, and psychological well being." But my interest is not legislative interpretation. What I am convinced of is that this sense of "privacy" is an important one and that it does figure in problems of medicine, as well as those of social existence generally. So that the issue I want to concentrate upon is that of the kind and degree of control a person ought to be able to exercise in respect to knowledge of or the disclosure of information about himself or herself. I want to consider primarily what this kind of privacy is all about and why persons might think it is of importance.

II

Information about oneself is not all of the same type; as a result control over some kinds may be much more important than control over others. For this reason, I want to start by trying to identify some of the different types of information about oneself over which persons might desire to retain control, and I want to describe the situations in which this information comes into being. To do this, I shall consider three situations and look at the ways they resemble each other and differ from one another.

There is first of all the fact that you can, if you wish to, look "inward" and become aware of the ideas that are running through your mind, the various emotions you are experiencing, and the variety of bodily sensations you are having—an itch on your scalp or a pain in your side. One thing that is significant about one's mental states—about one's dreams, conscious thought, hopes, fears, and desires is that the most direct, the best, and often the only evidence for another of what they are consists in my deliberately revealing them to you. To be sure, my nonverbal behavior may give an observer a clue as to what is going on in my mind. If, for example, I have a faraway look in my eyes you may infer that I am daydreaming about something and not paying very much attention to you. In addition, there is, no doubt, a more intimate and even conceptual connection between observable behavior and certain states of feeling. If I am blushing that may mean that I am embarrassed. If I am talking very fast that may lead you to infer correctly that I am excited or nervous. It is also sometimes the case that I will not know my own thoughts and feelings, etc., and that by saying what I think they are a skilled observer can, by listening to me and watching me as I talk, tell better than can I what is really going on inside my head.

But even taking all of these qualifications into account, it still remains the case, I believe, that the only way to obtain very detailed and accurate information about what I am thinking, fearing, imagining, desiring, or hating and how I am experiencing it is for me to tell you or show you. If I do not, the ideas and feeling remain within me and in some sense, at least, known only to me. Because people cannot read other people's minds, these things about me are known only to me in a way in which other things are not unless I decide to disclose them to you.

What about things that are going on in my body? In some respects the situation is similar to that of my thoughts and in some respects different. There are things that are going on in my body that are like my thoughts, fears and fantasies. If I have a slight twinge of pain in my left big toe, there is no way for anyone else to know that unless I choose to disclose it. Of course, if the toe is swollen and red, and if I grimace whenever I put any weight on it, an observer could doubtless infer correctly that I was experiencing pain there. But in many other cases the only evidence would be my verbal report.

There are other things about my body concerning which this privileged position does not obtain. Even though they are *my* ribs, I cannot tell very well what they look like; even though it is *my* blood, I cannot tell with any precision how much alcohol is there. A person looking through a fluoroscope at my ribs or at an X-ray of my ribs can tell far better than can I (just from having them as *my* ribs or from looking down at *my* chest) what my ribs look like. A trained technician looking at a sample of my blood in combination with certain chemicals can determine far better than I can (just from it being *my* blood) what the alcoholic content is or whether I am anemic.

So there are some facts about my body that I know in a way others logically cannot know them, that can be known to others only if I disclose them by telling what they are. There are other facts about my body that cannot be known by others in the way I know them but that can be inferred from observation of my body and my behavior. And there are still other kinds of facts about my body that I don't know and that can be learned, if at all, only by someone or something outside of myself.

In the second place, there is some information that is private only in virtue of the setting in which the information is disclosed or communicated. For example, suppose that I have broken my arm and that I am in a room with the door closed, alone with the doctor while he or she sets the break. Or suppose instead that I am in an enclosed telephone booth, calling a hospital to make an appointment to donate some blood. In both of these cases it is the setting that makes the behavior distinctive and relevant for our purposes. In both of these cases I believe I have a substantial degree of present control over the information about myself—that my arm is broken and is being set, or that I want to donate blood to the hospital—because of the situation in which the information is being conveyed or disclosed. If no one is in a position to see me and the doctor, then no one is in a position at that time to know about my arm. If no one is in a position to overhear (at my end) what I am saying to the person at the hospital, and if no one is tapping the telephone line, then no one is able at that time to hear what I am saying except for the person at the other phone. We can, I think, usefully describe cases of this kind as cases of things being done in private— meaning by that only that they are done in a setting in which there did not appear to be anyone other than the person to whom I was talking, etc., who was in a position to hear what was being said or to see what was being done. This is, of course, an extremely weak sense of privacy, and for at least two reasons. To begin with, the information is less within my control than is information about my mental states, not yet revealed to anyone, because the other person can if he or she chooses reveal what he or she has learned about me. And in addition, there is nothing about the character of the information which seems to make further revelation a source of concern.

It is this last point which leads to the third kind of case I want to discuss. Suppose that instead of having my broken arm set by a doctor, my wife and I are alone in a room engaged in sexual intercourse. Or suppose, that instead of calling the hospital to arrange to give blood, I have called my psychotherapist from a phone booth to tell her about some special problem I am having trouble dealing with right now. Both of these things are being done in private in the same sense in which the discussion with the hospital or the treatment of my broken arm were private, i.e., no one else could see or hear. But these also have an additional quality not possessed by the earlier two examples. When I call my therapist from a phone booth—or await her in her office—I certainly do expect that what I tell her is not being overheard by anyone else while I am telling her. In addition, though, I also reasonably expect that what I am telling her will be kept in confidence by her. Thus, it is private in the additional respect that the understanding between us is that it will not be subsequently disclosed to anyone— at least without my consent. It is what might be called a private kind of communication. And that is not the case with my phone call to the hospital. Absent special or unusual circumstances (like telling the hospital that I don't want anyone to know I am giving blood), I have no particular interest in retaining control over disclosure of this fact.

Similarly, engaging in sexual intercourse with my wife is private in the additional respect that it is the sort of intimate thing that is not appropriately observed by others or discussed with them—again, absent special or unusual circumstances, e.g., treatment at a Masters and Johnson clinic (and even here we would expect to be able to control quite specifically who would have access to this information, and under what circumstances). So, in addition to being done in private this act, too, is a private kind of thing. In this respect it seems unlike having my broken arm set by the doctor. For in that case there was no expectation on my part that what my arm looked like or how it was treated should not be made known to others. (This particular case is not a clear one and I will return to it later to say more about why it is not. For the present, though, let us suppose that it is private only in the sense of having been made so by the setting.)

The most obvious and the important connection between the idea of doing something in private and doing a private kind of thing is that we typically do private things only in situations where we reasonably believe that we are doing them in private. That we believe we are doing something in private is, often, a condition that has to be satisfied before we are willing to disclose an intimate fact about ourselves or to engage in the doing of an intimate act. I would probably have called the hospital to arrange to donate blood even if I were phoning from a crowded room where there were lots of people who could overhear what I was saying. The telephone was a convenient way to make the arrangements. But the fact that I was making them in a setting that appeared to be private was not important to me. It did not affect what I disclosed to the person at the other end. Thus, even if I had suspected that the telephone line was tapped so that an unknown person overheard my conversation, I would probably have called the hospital. In the case of my conversation with my therapist, however, it was the belief that the conversation was in a private setting that made me willing to reveal a private kind of thing. If someone tapped that telephone line and overheard what I said to my therapist they injured me in a way that is distinguishable on this basis alone from the injury, if any, done to me by tapping my conversation with the hospital. That is to say, at a minimum they would have gotten me to do or to reveal something that I would not have done or revealed if they had not hidden their presence from me.

It should be evident, too, that there are important similarities, as well as some differences, between the first and third cases—between my knowledge of my own mental states and my disclosure of intimate or otherwise confidential information to those to whom I choose to disclose it. What are they? Why might we believe that a special injury had been done to us if information of certain sorts became known, without our consent to others? Consider an extreme, somewhat fanciful case first.

III

Suppose existing technology made it possible for an outsider in some way to look into or monitor another's mind. What, if anything, would be especially disturbing or objectionable about that?

To begin with, there is a real sense in which we have far less control over when we shall have certain thoughts and what their content will be than we have over, for example, to whom we shall reveal them and to what degree. Because our inner thoughts, feelings, and bodily sensations are so largely beyond our control, we would, I think, feel appreciably more insecure in our social environment than we do at present were it possible for another to "look in" without our consent to see what was going on in our heads.

This is so at least in part because many, although by no means all, of our uncommunicated thoughts and feelings are about very intimate matters. Our fantasies and our fears often concern just those matters that in our culture we would least choose to reveal to anyone else. At a minimum we might suffer great anxiety and feelings of shame were the decisons as to where, when, and to whom to disclose, not to be wholly ours. Were access to our thoughts possible in this way we would see ourselves as creatures who are far more vulnerable than we are now.

In addition, there is always the more straightforward worry about accountability for our thoughts and feelings. As I mentioned, they are often not within our control. For all of the reasons that we ought not hold people accountable for behavior not within their control, we would not want the possibility of accountability to extend to uncommunicated thoughts and feelings.

Finally, one rather plausible conception of what it is to be a person carried with it, I believe, the idea of the existence of a core of thoughts and feelings that are the person's alone. If anyone else could know all that I am thinking or perceive all that I am feeling except in the form I choose to filter and reveal what I am and how I see myself—if anyone could, so to speak, be aware of all this at will I might cease to have as complete a sense of myself as a distinct and separate person as I have now. A significant, if not fundamental, part of what it is to be an individual person is to be an entity that is capable of being exclusively aware of its own thoughts and feelings.

Considerations such as these—and particularly the last one—help us to understand some of the puzzles concerning the privilege against self-incrimination, as well as some of the worries about coercive therapies. Because of the significance of exclusive control over our own thoughts and feelings, the privilege against self-incrimination can be seen to rest, ultimately, upon a concern that confessions never be coerced or required by the state. The point of the privilege is not primarily that the state must be induced not to torture individuals in order to extract information from them. Nor is the point even essentially that the topics of confession will necessarily (or even typically) be of the type that we are most unwilling to disclose because of the unfavorable nature of what this would reveal about us. Rather, the fundamental point is that required disclosure of one's thoughts by itself diminishes the concept of individual personhood within the society.

Similarly, non-consensual drug therapies which reduce if not destroy the patient's resistance to disclosing the things that he or she is thinking are subject to the same criticism. The objection to such therapies is not merely that the individuals involved will be led to say things which they would have not otherwise said, because they regarded such disclosures as shameful or otherwise reflecting badly on themselves (although this is certainly a substantial if not decisive consideration against ever doing this to individuals). The additional objection to such therapies is that they take away from the individual control over that one area which is for others exclusively within their control and by which they are helped to maintain a clear sense of their own selfhood and individuality.

The more prominent worry today does not, I think, concern intrusion into the domain of one's uncommunicated thoughts and feelings, but rather concerns the degree to which communications between persons about private things shall remain exclusively within their control. What, for example, would be the wrong that was done to me were someone to have tapped my phone conversation with my therapist, or if my therapist had told other persons what I had told her? Or what would have been the injury that would have been done to us if, unknown to my wife and me, one of the walls in our room had really been one-way glass and we had been observed engaged in intercourse by a class of prospective sex therapists and counselors?

The most obvious point, I guess, is that because of our social attitudes toward the disclosure of intimate facts and behavior, most of us would be extremely pained were we to learn that these had become known to persons other than those to whom we chose to disclose them. It is important to see that the pain can come about in several different ways. If I do something private with somebody and I believe that we are doing it in private, I may very well be hurt or embarrassed if I learn subsequently that we were observed but didn't know it. Thus if I learn after the fact that my wife and I were observed while we were having intercourse, the knowledge that we were observed will cause us distress both because our expectations of privacy were incorrect and because we do not like the idea that we were observed during this kind of intimate act. People have the right, I think, simply to have the world be what it appears to be precisely in those cases in which they regard privacy as essential to the diminution of their own vulnerability.

Reasoning such as this lies behind, I think, a case that arose some years ago in California. A department store had complained to the police that homosexuals were using its men's room as a meeting place. The police responded by drilling a small hole in the ceiling over the enclosed stalls. A policeman then stationed himself on the floor above and peered down through the hole observing the persons using the stall for eliminatory purposes. Eventually the policeman discovered and apprehended two homosexuals who used the stall as a place to engage in forbidden sexual behavior. The California Supreme Court held the observations of the policeman to have been the result of an illegal search and ordered the conviction reversed. What made the search objectionably illegal, I believe, was that it occurred in the course of this practice which deceived all of the persons who used the stall and who believed that they were doing in private something that was socially regarded as a private kind of thing. They were entitled, especially for this kind of activity, both to be free from observation and to have their expectations of privacy honored by the state.

There is an additional reason why the observation or disclosure of certain sorts of activity is objectionable. That is because the kind of spontaneity and openness that is essential to them disappears with the presence of an observer or the lack of a guarantee of confidentiality. To see that this is so, consider a different case. Suppose I know in advance that we will be observed during intercourse. Here there is no problem of defeated reasonable expectations. But there may be injury nonetheless. For one thing, I may be unwilling or unable to communicate an intimate fact or engage in intimate behavior in the presence of an observer. In this sense I will be quite directly prevented from going forward. For another thing, even if I do go ahead the character of the experience may very well be altered. Knowing that someone is watching or listening may render what would have been an enjoyable experience unenjoyable. Or, having someone watch or listen may so alter the character of the relationship that it is simply not the same kind of relationship it was before. The presence of the observer may make spontaneity impossible. Aware of the observer, I am engaged in part in viewing or imagining what is going on from his or her perspective. I thus cannot "lose" myself as completely in the activity.

Nor is this the only problem presented by a nondeceptive absence of privacy. Suppose that one is in a setting in which one can be certain that there will never be privacy, that virtually everything one does and virtually everything that happens to one will be recorded and known to others. Even if nothing particularly embarrassing, incriminating or intimate goes on (or is apt to go on) there is, I think, something else that is troublesome and objectionable about such an an-vironment. To begin with, it will be difficult for the individuals who are the objects of such scrutiny to continue to retain a sense of their own individuality and autonomy. Concomitantly, it will be difficult for the individuals who are conducting and maintaining the scrutiny to continue to retain a sense of the subjects as persons rather than objects.

This seems to me to be part of what is seriously wrong with the way medicine is often practiced, hospitals typically run, and patients almost always treated. Patients, and especially patients in hospitals, are observed, monitored, checked and the information obtained thereby routinely and regularly recorded in accordance with notions of institutional regularity, thoroughness and convenience. Much if not all of the observation and the collection of information may be for the patient's welfare. And I am certainly not suggesting that any of this is done maliciously. But I do think it likely that the absence of these malevolent features tends to disarm and thereby to make the practices even more dangerous . In an environment of the sort I have described, it will, as I have suggested, be difficult for a patient to preserve his or her sense of autonomy and individuality. In this environment it will be easy for those of the institution who are not patients to see themselves as different in important respects from the patients. They are not continually under scrutiny; the patients as objects are. In such a setting, medical personnel all too often become both manipulative and paternalistic in their relationship with their patients. A lack of privacy, in this sense, is not the only reason for the dominance of these modes of interaction between the medical personnel and the patients. But it, coupled with a lack of sensitivity toward the harm that can be caused, is certainly one of the significant causes.

IV

I want to say a word, finally, about the law's special concern for the relationship between medicine and intimate kinds of things as that concern is manifested in the evidentiary privileges.

There are two distinct evidentiary privileges that relate to medicine. These two privileges—the physician-patient privilege and the psychotherapist-patient privilege—establish the right that a patient has to have kept confidential most information acquired by the doctor or psychotherapist in the course of treating the patient, even though the communication would constitute otherwise relevant evidence at a trial.

The case for the psychotherapist-patient privilege is the easier one to make out. Because of the nature of the things typically discussed in psychotherapy persons very often see themselves as rendering themselves extremely vulnerable through their revelation to another. This comes about in two ways. First, psychotherapy typically deals with many things that the patient has never disclosed to another; things of which previously he or she alone has been aware. So psychotherapy often involves admission into what was previously the private self—the core of individuality. And second, the kinds of things revealed are often the sort that, individuals believe, would reflect badly upon them were these facts to become known to others. For psychotherapy almost always deals with the respects in which the person sees himself or herself as deficient. It is natural, therfore, that persons should want substantial guarantees of nondisclosure without which they would see themselves as having exposed themselves to unreasonable risk of injury from others. And it is appropriate that the law should provide those guarantees so that the processes of psychotherapy can go forward.

What is less clear and hence more instructive is why there should be a physician-patient privilege. Several alternative rationales present themselves. One is that the physician often plays the role of psychotherapist. Another is that diseases often *have* a "mental" or emotional component. Hence it is essential for the treatment of physical diseases that the physician be able to explore with the patient the related or underlying mental aspect. Both of these accounts fit comfortably into the kind of analysis already proposed, and if this were all there were to the physician-patient privilege it would not be much of a puzzle. But the privilege protects more than communications between the patient and physician about these sorts of intimate matters. It covers all of the things that the doctor discovers about the patient's body and all of the things the patient tells the doctor about his or her body. And this same concern is reflected in the sweeping language of that section of the patient's bill of rights which requires that "Case discussion, consultation, examination, and treatment are confidential and should be conducted discreetly." (The language is sweeping because it covers all case information and not just information about psychiatric or "intimate" details.)

What this reveals, I think, is that attitudes and beliefs concerning one's body, as well as one's diseases, are uncertain and varied in our culture. Much information about our bodies does not enjoy a privileged epistemic status. And much information about the physical condition of our bodies is not—it seems to me—the kind of information which is naturally seen as intimate and deserving of confidential status. Nevertheless, in our culture many persons do regard much, if not all, information about the state of their bodies as the kind of information which ought to be kept largely under their control.

I suspect that the reasons for this are varied and deep. Some have to do with the connection between the fact that it is *our* body and our sense of ourselves as distinct individuals. For there is a long and respectable philosophical tradition which takes the body to be the individuating element in existence. Some of the reasons have to do, instead, with a rather different philosophical-religious tradition; namely, that which regards the body as the least human and most corrupt feature of human life. The body *per se* is a source of shame and evil. Clearly, then, the less said and known about it the better. And finally, there is the sense in which a diseased body is seen by many as a kind of imperfection and one which somehow reflects badly upon them. It is easy, I think, to see how natural it is to want to keep hidden imperfections and blemishes of any sort. It is not even very hard to see how the move is made from that concern to a stronger desire to keep hidden deficiencies that are in some way or other one's fault. Whether rational or not, our attitudes toward beliefs about both physical and mental disease still contain many of these features within them.

What all of this shows, in addition, is how socially contingent much, if not all, that is deemed to be intimate and private is. What the patient's bill of rights protects, what the evidentiary privileges protect, what the concern for privacy protects is information which is deemed by the culture to render the individual unusually vulnerable and exposed. It is information which if known to others, except in special contexts, is unusually capable of causing injury to the person involved. It is, I think, an important and fascinating question—but one that is beyond the scope of this paper: to ask whether there is any information that is, so to speak, intrinsically private, rather than contingently so, or to ask whether it is even socially necessary that in every culture there be some information that functions in this fashion. I think there is much that can be said on both sides of these questions. For the purposes of our inquiry, however, it is I believe, sufficient to observe that for our culture at this time these concerns for and about privacy make very good moral sense.

ETHICS: NURSE, AM I GOING TO LIVE?

Diana G. French

One of the most compelling issues professional nurses always face concerns telling the truth to terminally-ill patients. Is it within the scope of nursing practice to disclose sensitive diagnostic or prognostic information? What is the effect of the illness experience on an individual? What factors influence the nurse's moral-ethical decisions in disclosing information?

Physicians, hospital administrators, patients' families, and patients themselves—all have differing expectations regarding the nurse's role which create serious ethical dilemmas for those attending the terminally ill. Particularly in such bureaucratic institutions as hospitals, can the nurse truly respond as the patient's advocate? The wisdom necessary to solve this particular ethical dilemma will not be found in technology. Rather, ethical solutions will evolve from the moral art of nursing: the humane and compassionate care of patients and clients.

"Terminal illness" is a categorical label applied to the condition of patients for whom medical technology can offer nothing more in curative treatment. Such patients are suffering from a sudden acute illness episode or traumatic injury, or from protracted and lingering forms of disease which may involve periods of exacerbation and remission. Even though the disease or injury may be intractable to curative or medical therapy, holistic care for the patient as a person should not decrease in importance or priority.

Reprinted with permission from *Nursing Management*, vol. 15, no. 11 (November 1984), pp. 43–46.

Although it is inescapable that living beings will at some time die, the human experience with dying and death is unique among all living creatures. Cortical awareness of the prospect of death is one element which separates us from all other forms of life and serves as a foundation for the concept of human dignity.

PATIENTS WITHOUT POWER . . .

Our society has become ever more vocal about individual rights and has increasingly asserted them. Patients, therefore, demand more autonomy in making decisions regarding their own health care.[1] Frequent denial of fundamental rights, including the right to information, has contributed to patient rebellion in the form of malpractice suits.[2]

Hospitalized individuals often feel impotent and helpless. Considering the events surrounding transformation to the patient role, this is not surprising. Traditionally, patients have had little, if any, control over even the most basic activities of daily living. Thrust into an alien environment, they have been surrounded by strange equipment and strange faces—including the one in the next bed. Meals, baths, medications, visitors, vital signs, and bedtime are all regimented to conform with the smooth operation of hospital routine. The hospital, as a health care delivery system, makes it extremely difficult for patients to retain their individuality and to have that individuality respected.

Even more than the unfamiliar, discomforting elements of the patient role, the very presence of disease itself impinges upon the person's sense of humanity.[3]

In the first place, the individual experiences a loss of independence as a human being. The illness infringes upon the person's autonomy by requiring that the individual petition another person to cure, or take care of, a deficiency or defect. This humiliation threatens one's self image and will affect interactions with others. Second, the illness may cause the patient to suffer a loss of freedom of action: whether verbal, locomotive, or intellectual, this further serves to diminish the self image. A third element deals with interferences with the patient's latitude in exercising the right of choice. The patient's ability as a decision maker is not at issue. Rather, this infringement should be examined in light of basic human rights: self determination, autonomy, and privacy.

. . . VS. PROFESSIONALS WITH AUTHORITY

A corollary of these three factors is the power ascribed to health care professionals. As the patient sees it, disease and the lack of controls over that disease severely threaten him. Fear of the unknown often compounds this anxiety. If we contrast the knowledge and information which the caregiver holds with that which the patient possesses, we can easily imagine the depth of the patient's sense of powerlessness and helplessness.

Many common examples in the care of the terminally ill illustrate infringements upon the patient's humanity, and hence, the patient's dignity as a person. Because of rigid time considerations, a nurse refuses a dying person's request for pain medication. Why? Need there be fear of the addictive effects of narcotic analgesia in such a case? A patient is cajoled and coerced into submitting his ecchymotic, frail arm for daily venipuncture and blood samples. Why? To provide empirical evidence to the dying process? A conspiracy of silence becomes the response to the patient's lucid, rational request for information. Why? To protect the patient from unpleasant news?

THE NURSE AND ETHICAL DECISIONS

Bioethicists as well as nurses are giving more and more attention to the variety of ethical problems to which the practice of professional nursing gives rise. Many conflicts are direct effects of the nurse's complex role within the health care delivery system. The nurse is in the incongruous position of undertaking considerable responsibility for managing patient care which requires her to have a high level of knowledge and skill while customarily holding little authority to make or execute decisions.

The medical establishment has long maintained a paternalistic attitude towards nursing.[4] In this relationship the question of the nurse's accountability—to physician or to patient—creates even further conflicts.

A nurse strongly committed to serving the interests of the patient may find herself an uncomfortable adversary to the physician on moral issues. Various authors have expressed concern for the moral problem of the nurse who, out of conscience, wishes to act as the patient's advocate.[5] In bureaucratic institutions other people make many of the key decisions which nurses ultimately must implement.

Particularly in a primary nursing system, daily intimate contact with the patient puts the nurse in a singular position among those in contact with hospitalized patients. It is the nurse who is present during the most elementary of human activities: bathing, eating, ambulating, and elimination. It is the nurse who performs specific care activities such as dressing changes, wound irrigations, and intravenous infusions. It is the nurse who psychologically and emotionally supports patients experiencing physical and mental pain, fear, anguish, sadness, joy and anger. From this constellation of caring activities, this special physical and emotional intimacy, the essential element for the therapeutic relationship is formed: trust. In the natural progression of this trusting relationship, questions will be asked of the nurse. Does the nurse have a moral duty to provide the answers?

ESTABLISHING A PERSONAL VALUE SYSTEM

Nursing decisions and actions are supposed to be based upon scientific or theoretical knowledge, clinical experience, and individual capabilities. However, the nurse's value system, beliefs, and particular stage of moral development, also play their part in clinical decision making.[6] Forming ethical decisions that the nurse can substantiate involves a rational, cognitive process which employs concepts of human rights and principles of justice.[7]

Lawrence Kohlberg's theory of moral development categorizes moral development of the individual into three levels: preconventional, conventional, and postconventional.[8] Each level proceeds in two stages. This cognitive developmental process is sequential in nature and progression through the stages varies greatly within society.

In the *preconventional level,* an individual's moral choices are primarily hedonistic; they may conform to the norm of right conduct only out of self-interest. In stage one, the punishment/obedience orientation, the individual obeys authority from fear of punishment rather than from respect for authority. Instrumental opportunism typifies stage two. The individual will reciprocate or retaliate within a relationship to achieve personal gain rather than to honor such abstract purposes as justice, duty, or honor.

At the *conventional level,* persons conform to societal norms and seek to maintain the social *status quo.* Individuals in stage three view conformity to social and peer pressure as a determinant of "good" or "right" behavior for the purpose of gaining social approval. Stage four is distinguished by a conformity to rules, either societal or institutional. This stage is the law and order orientation. For example, violation of hospital policy may be construed as "wrong" action irrespective of moral duty to the patient.

At the *postconventional level* of moral development, thinking becomes more autonomous and reasoning more complex. Stage five development recognizes the interfacing of duty, welfare of the majority, basic human rights, democracy and constitutionality on that which is determined "right" by conscience. The individual in stage six employs advanced reasoning in the application of universal ethical principles. This person may respond in conflict situations out of duty to abstract but ethical principles of justice, which may not conform with established regulations or laws.

A given nurse's level of moral development will strongly determine the direction of any ethical decision she undertakes.

MORAL FOUNDATIONS FOR DISCLOSURE

Curtin maintains that the nursing profession has evolved beyond an attempt to define the function of nursing in terms of tasks.[9] Rather, role definition should be based upon the philosophical foundation of nursing; the concept of advocacy, which determines the welfare of other human beings as the end purpose of nursing.

The advocate relationship with the patient supposes the underlying dignity of the human being and rights to freedom, respect, integrity, and self determination.[10] The relevance of these moral concepts to the health care delivery system involves the patient's right to: consent to treatment, information regarding care, confidentiality, informed consent, and privacy.

Denying the truth to a terminally ill patient or withholding essential information effectively denies that person the right to privacy, to consent to treatment, to choose the place of death, and to determine the disposition of his body after death.[11] It is unfair to expect a patient to provide informed consent to various plans to treat or withhold treatment from his condition, that is, to participate in the decisions regarding his care, unless he has sufficient information in terms he can understand.

The American Nurses Association Code of Ethics is very explicit regarding the nurse's responsibility in relation to the patient's right of self determination and information. "Each client has the moral right to determine what will be done with his/her person; to be given the information necessary for making informed judgments; to be told the possible effects of care; and to accept, refuse, or terminate treatment."[12]

According to Yarling, whether or not to disclose information to a terminal patient is a moral, not a medical, decison. Therefore, a physician's medical/scientific expertise does not give his opinion any extraordinary value.[13]

Consequently, exercising rights and obligations to the patient in disclosing information is not the singular province of any one member of the health care team. If relationships within the team were genuinely collegial, and if the team concentrated upon the patient per se in their deliberations concerning his care, the moral rights of the patient would be better served.

Based on the principles of self determination and autonomy, the patient who requests information about his condition or treatment has a moral right to that information. If an inquiry is addressed to her, the nurse has a reciprocal moral right and obligation to answer the inquiring patient according to her competence, in collaboration with others responsible for the patient, and out of respect to her rapport with the patient.[14]

A knowledge of the pathophysiology of the disease, with its possible treatments and consequences, and psychosocial skills in communication are indicative of competence. For example, a nurse with extensive clinical experience in and theoretical knowledge of oncologic nursing, would be considered competent.

Collaboration is established when the nurse consults with the physician and other nurses responsible for the patient's care regarding intent to disclose information and keeps the others informed of the action already taken. To plan care prudently, the nurse should develop appropriate responses to possible inquiries from the patient regarding his health status.

Rapport evolves from the trust formed in the therapeutic relationship. We delude ourselves if we think that a patient asks questions of such a serious nature of any person who happens to go into the room. The action of the patient in asking a particular person for specific diagnostic or prognostic information presupposes rapport. Therefore, the terminally ill patient's choice on questions of such a serious nature, whether physician, nurse, or clergyman, establishes a vital criterion for exercising the moral right to inform.

The Burn Care Team of the Los Angeles County-University of Southern California Medical Center is strongly convinced that to begin or withhold max imal therapeutic effort is more an ethical rather than medical judgment. Critically burned patients, for whom survival is unprecedented, are asked whether they desire a full therapeutic regimen or ordinary care. The patient is given sufficient information to make an informed decision while he is still lucid. This approach has not altered mortality rates for these patients but has increased the self determination that they exercise and the empathy they receive.[15]

The nurse's skills in assessing the whole situation and communicating appropriately are essential in making and carrying out the ethical decision whether to disclose or not to disclose information to the patient. We do not act as the patient's advocate if we give information which the patient did not seek and is not ready to hear—no matter how good the intent. The nurse must thoroughly assess the patient's behavior before responding to his question. In other words, exactly *what* is the patient asking? We all know the story of the youngster who asks his mother, "Where did I come from?" The mother replies with an attempt to answer the age-old bird and bees question. Puzzled, the child comments, "Gee, that's funny. Johnny comes from Toledo."

FACING THE CONSEQUENCES

Undoubtedly, the nurse takes risks in acting on the basis of moral right and obligation to the patient. In actual nursing practice, the nurse may have to face some unpleasant consequences. She may experience strained and uncomfortable working relationships. She may find herself sharply rebuked by the physician, hospital administration, the patient's family, and even her nursing colleagues.

When a patient asks a nurse for information which the physician has specifically told her not to divulge, a severe moral dilemma presents itself. How does the nurse honor the conflicting demands of physician and patient for her discretion and trust? Depending on several personal variables, including the nurse's level of moral development, the nurse may attempt to reduce or avoid the conflict.

Some nurses employ deception and distortion in unsuccessful efforts to represent the interests of both patient and physician.[16] Deception generally takes the form of gestures or omissions rather than more disquieting lies. Sharing only that information to which the patient will predictably respond is distortion. Good intentions notwithstanding, these tactics ultimately erode the trust relationship between patient and nurse.

TO TELL OR NOT TO TELL

Just because a person is hospitalized with a terminal illness, his basic human rights should not be alienated. Although health care providers do not intentionally or maliciously usurp patients' rights, the system lends itself to a layering effect which does circumscribe their meaningful exercise. Health care delivery in the modern hospital has become so technological and so complex that its processes becloud accountability to the patient. Increasing technology, medical and nursing specialization, malpractice suits, and costs, as well as the movement of industrial managers into hospital administration, are all factors which may contribute to depersonalizing health care.

Their duties of managing and coordinating care give registered nurses continuing access and close contact with patients. Thus, they are in the most favorable position to provide some measure of stability and some sense of security to patients within an environment which can easily appear confusing and threatening. Patients expect to rely upon their nurses to interpret that environment to them and to inform them of their status. As the most accessible representative of the health care delivery system, and as a professional person committed to preserve human dignity, the nurse must stand ready to respond to that basic human right of patients who, indeed, have the most "need to know"—the terminally ill. That obligation to respond becomes a moral responsibility from which no one can absolve her.

REFERENCES

1 Payton, R.J., "Information Control and Autonomy: Does the Nurse Have a Role?" *Nursing Clinics of North America,* March, 1979, 22–33.

2 Kelly, L.Y., "The Patient's Right to Know," *Nursing Outlook,* January, 1976, 26–32.

3 Curtin, L., "The Nurse as Advocate: A Philosophical Foundation for Nursing," *Advances in Nursing Science,* April, 1979, 1–10.

4 Payton, R., *loc. cit.,* and Yarling, R.R. "Ethical Analysis of a Nursing Problem: The Scope of Nursing Practice in Disclosing the Truth to Terminal Patients," Parts I and II, *Supervisor Nurse,* May, 1978, 40–50, and June, 1979, 28–34.

5 See, in *Hastings Center Report,* August, 1977, Aroskar, M. and Veatch. R.M., "Ethics Teaching in Nursing Schools," 23–26; Jameton, A., "The Nurse: When Roles and Rules Conflict," 22–23; Smith, J.M., "The Nurse and Orders Not to Resuscitate," p. 24; and Smith, S.J., and Davis, A.J., "Ethical dilemmas: Conflicts Among Rights, Duties, and Obligations," *American Journal of Nursing,* August, 1980, 1463–1466.

6 Mahon, K.A. and Fowler, M.D., "Moral Development and Clinical Decision Making," *Nursing Clinics of North America,* March, 1979, 3–12.

7 Sigman, P., "Ethical Choice in Nursing," *Advances in Nursing Science,* April, 1979, 37–51.
8 Mahon, K.A. and Fowler, M.D., *loc cit.*
9 Curtin, L., *loc. cit.*
10 Ibid.
11 Annas, G.J., "Rights of the Terminally Ill Patient," *Journal of Nursing Administration,* March–April, 1974, 40–44.
12 American Nurses Association, *Code for Nurses with Interpretive Statements,* Kansas City, 1976.
13 Yarling, *loc. cit.*
14 Ibid.
15 Imbus, S.H. and Zawacki, B.E., "Autonomy for Burned Patients When Survival is Unprecedented," *New England Journal of Medicine,* August 1, 1977, 308–311.
16 Payton, *loc. cit.*

DISCLOSURE OF INFORMATION TO ADULT CANCER PATIENTS: ISSUES AND UPDATE

Richard J. Goldberg

While problems involving disclosure of information are not unique to oncology patients, they somehow seem more dramatic and have attracted much attention in this specialty. This may be, in part, because of the assumption that the impact of hearing about cancer will be devastating to people. In deciding what information to provide patients during the course of the treatment, the provider routinely faces situations that seem to be dilemmas. Is it right always to insist that a patient be fully informed, and can it ever be in the interest of the patient to know less? Notwithstanding the burgeoning literature devoted to the ethical dimensions of these areas,[1-4] the clinician must frequently make decisions without the benefit of conferences or time for extensive reflection.

If one brings up the topic of disclosure of information among a group of experienced clinicians, one invariably hears a variety of anecdotal reports of an apparently contradictory nature. Some claim that withholding information at times turns out to be the humane approach; others tell of patients whose insistence on knowing detailed information seemed a model of the intelligent courageous patient. Other problems are commonly brought up: situations in which the patient seemed to want to know less than the physician wanted to tell; situations in which a family put the physician in a bind by not wanting the patient to know the truth; situations in which patients behaved as if they were unaware of what the physician communicated. Some providers publicly uphold their paternalistic

Reprinted with permission from *The Journal of Clinical Oncology*, vol. 2, no. 8 (August 1984), pp. 948–955.

approach to disclosure, in which they maintain that it is their professional duty to provide only as much information as makes sense for a particular patient at a particular time. Others maintain that it is the patient's right to know as much as possible. This apparent conflict between the presumed obligations both to inform and to protect can create an ongoing strain for the clinician. Decision making is further complicated by the prevailing context of social values that strongly influence the practice of individual clinicians and patients. Currently, the paternalistic style of medical practice is definitely being challenged by a more consumer-oriented and disclosure-oriented value system.[5]

CHANGING ATTITUDES TOWARDS DISCLOSURE

Attitudes towards disclosure have changed significantly over the past three decades. In 1953, a questionnaire of 442 Philadelphia physicians regarding the issue of disclosure of diagnosis found that 69% of physicians surveyed stated that they usually did not or never told their patients the details of diagnosis. Thirty-one percent said that they always or usually told the patients.[6] In 1960, a survey of 5,000 physicians found that the percentage stating that they never told the patient the diagnosis dropped to 22%, while 16% of the group stated that they always told the patient.[7] However, a survey one year later of 219 physicians in Chicago in 1961 found 90% stated that they generally did not inform patients of their diagnosis.[8] By 1970, another relatively small survey revealed that 25% of physicians said they always told the patient, and only 9% stated they never told the patient.[9] A more thorough population survey was conducted by Novack et al.[10] in Rochester. In this study which represented multiple specialists, 98% reported that it was general policy to tell the patients. Two thirds stated that they never or very rarely made exceptions to that rule. This data is in sharp contrast to the earlier studies. The most frequent factors that physicians reported as intervening in their decision to tell the patient were the patient's age, intelligence, the patient's (and relative's) expressed wish about information, and perception of the patient's emotional stability. Yet, how these factors actually related to decisions of imparting information about diagnosis remained largely unexplored and suggested that a priori personal judgments based on some attitudes and biases were the real determinants of policy. Eighteen percent of the sample reported they were less likely to tell a child and only 10% reported being inclined to tell a patient who was old or who had poor comprehension. Fourteen percent said that they would tell the patient less frequently or might delay telling if they thought the patient was prone to depression or suicide. Approximately 12% would tell the patient somewhat more frequently if personal business needed to be put in order. Hardy et al.[11] reported on a group of 185 physicians in Tennessee regarding their communications with cancer patients. Of the respondents (61% of sample), 97.7% reported "always" or "usually" informing the patient of the diagnosis. Factors reported to be important influences on decision making included: stage of disease (71%), age of physician (65%), treatment required (60%), family wishes (60%), and histopathology (58%). Unfortunately this report does not indicate the directionality of these factors such as how age of physicians or patients influenced decision making. A more recent study[12] of 98 Midwestern cancer clinicians indicated significant differences in attitudes towards communication with cancer patients. Only 25% indicated that they experienced any difficulty. About 40% thought patients really preferred not to know their condition, though 80% thought cancer patients should be told their history clearly and as soon as possible. Older physicians reported feeling greater communication difficulties than younger colleagues. Physicians with university appointments reported being more comfortable as were those whose practices included large numbers of patients with metastatic disease.

There are several possible interpretations that may account for the attitudinal changes reported in the review by Novack et al. (1979) of physicians' attitudes towards disclosure. Oken[8] suggested around 1960 that the diagnosis of cancer implied the expectation of death, depriving the patient of hope, and hence physicians were reluctant to tell cancer patients their diagnosis. (Paradoxically, 100% of the sample indicated a preference for being told if they themselves had cancer.) Yet, by the late 1970s physicians were telling the patients the diagnosis much more often. Part of this change could perhaps be accounted for by improved therapy that would allow physicians to be more optimistic about their patients. Another factor that may have contributed to (or coincided with) the trend to increased disclosure has been the upsurge of interest in death and dying, with a consequent opening up of previously taboo topics. Finally, the swing in the pendulum of social values towards consumerism and increasing public scrutiny of the medical profession have altered the physician-patient relationship. Whichever factors are actually possible, it appears that oncology providers cannot escape the clinical issues that emerge as a consequence of carrying out the ethical demands of informing patients.

PROBLEMS IN THE PROCESS OF DISCLOSURE

While the debate about disclosure is easily fueled and carried on, the actual determinants of clinical practice are difficult to analyze. Despite the documentable shift in physician attitude towards increased disclosure, what actually takes place in the office has not been adequately studied. There is probably a significant gap between espoused attitudes regarding talking to patients and actual behavior.[13] If indeed physician attitudes are widely divergent from their actual behavior, the importance of much of the surveyed literature is significantly attenuated. Furthermore, the nuances of the communication process make this a difficult area to untangle. The provider may communicate, by tone of voice or nonverbal expression, a message other than what the words themselves state. Disclosure may be masked by the use of words that are too technical or by the use of euphemisms. Information processing also will be inadequate when it occurs in a highly emotionally charged setting. The provider sometimes often assumes that a single communication will suffice and that once something is said, the topic has been addressed. Finally, even well-intentioned advocates of complete disclosure must make decisions about what to select from a relatively unlimited pool of possible information. It has been empirically demonstrated that variations in the way information is presented to patients can influence their choices between alternative therapies.[14] Disclosure is always selective and, therefore, dependent on the provider. The listener may be distracted by pain, anxiety, or information overload. Some patients may be limited by intelligence, vocabulary, or cultural orientation from taking advantage of generally available materials. Some may be afraid to ask questions or bother the physician by further inquiry. The patient's personality may affect the process: some will require more details, others will be confused by them; some may prefer an impersonal, scientific approach while others need the personal touch. Finally, the patient may consciously or unconsciously deny the information presented and behave as if it had not been presented.

How is the thoughtful and intelligent clinician to proceed given the societal pressure to disclose, the professional values to protect, and the inherent limitations of the communication process itself? All theoretical arguments in this area finally come down to particular events with particular patients. Decisions are always being made for better or worse. While in any single case it may be impossible to know the outcome of either telling something or withholding something, recognizing the strengths and limitations of each option is important. The basic ethical arguments that support the right of the patient to truthful disclosure have been summarized by Jonsen et al.[15] and also are reiterated in the President's Commission Report.[16] Telling the truth is a moral duty not easily overridden by speculation about possible harm. The patient has a need for truth to make decisions. Concealment can undermine trust in the physician and the profession. Further, concealment may be based on physicians' uneasiness rather than patients' inability to accept information. There are also arguments that provide justification for less than full disclosure.[17] There are several legal exceptions, such as those dictated by mandates of public health policy. Other exceptions include emergency treatment and incompetency of the patient to participate in decision making. The final justification for incomplete disclosure involves "therapeutic privilege," which permits professionals to refrain from making a disclosure that could so seriously upset the patient as to be countertherapeutic. The issue of therapeutic privilege has been seen by some in the broader context of paternalism. The essence of paternalism is the overriding of a person's freedom for their own good.[18,19] Physicians should be aware of the arguments that both support and oppose paternalism and of the clinical skills needed to carry out either policy of protection or disclosure. Supporters of full disclosure at all times should have an appreciation for the clinical impact on patients and the clinical skills that are necessary to deal with this. Supporters of full disclosure must also recognize the inherent limitations involved in the communication process. Whatever position one maintains, the clinician must develop skills in communicating, listening, and understanding patients as individuals. Many times, in fact, the apparent clinical ethical dilemma involving decisions about providing information is actually a misperception of an underlying clinical problem.[20]

Few, if any, studies have looked at exactly what or how physicians provide information to their patients in day-to-day practice. Despite evidence of changes in underlying attitudes, controversy over actual practice continues between those who are proponents for guarding individual rights and their opponents who claim that the attempt to achieve full disclosure is impossible due to limitations in patient understanding as well as the desires of patients not to be told.[21] Do people want to know the "truth?" How can the clinician determine how much a particular patient wants to know? Can truthfulness be harmful? Are there any available data that can shed some light on these questions?

Meisel and Roth[22] have recently reviewed the empirical studies in the area of informed consent, an area that has considerable overlap with the issue of disclosure. They found few, if any, studies that attempted to determine actual daily practice, though several studies have looked at some of the communication problems in this area.[23,24] Studies on whether patients want to be told appear contradictory. Some have found substantial numbers of patients who claim not to want to be informed.[25] In one study,[26] more than 75% of the patients surveyed recognized that they were dying of cancer and communicated that knowledge to staff members who displayed an attitude of openness. These patients indicated they preferred frank communication with their caregivers and were happier when such openness prevailed. In a review of nine other studies in the area, Veatch[27] found a significant majority of patients (60%–98%) indicated the wish to be told a diagnosis of a terminal illness. Kelly and Friesen[28] found that 98% of cancer patients indicated they preferred knowing their condition. McIntosh[29] reported observations on a Scottish cancer ward where many patients had incurable disease. He found that 88% of the patients knew or suspected they had cancer, over half wanted confirmations of their diagnosis, but only one patient wanted to know the prognosis, and none wanted to know whether the illness would be fatal. Henriques et al.[30] studied a large sample of Danish patients with abdominal diseases, asking if they wanted to be told their diagnosis if it were cancer. Fifty-four percent said definitely yes; 22% probably yes; 8% probably not; and 3% definitely not.

Unfortunately, there seem to be no studies that systematically examine whether disclosure causes "harm" to patients and what the nature of that harm might be. There has been some suggestion that informed consent can be "hazardous" to health[31] as a result of negative placebo effects. Yet, there is also evidence that the benefits from information can be considerable.[32] Generalization from many studies of disclosure is limited by failure to involve real patients with serious conditions, rather than healthy subjects responding to hypothetical situations. Possible "negative consequences" would also have to be carefully specified. Available studies on the negative consequences of disclosure have also been contradictory, with one demonstrating an increase in "apprehensiveness, anger, and anxiety,"[33] with another (about an impending surgical procedure) claiming to show a decrease in anxiety.[34] Cassem and Stewart[35] cite studies indicating patients' overwhelmingly positive attitudes in favor of being told their diagnosis and a lack of demonstrable negative effects. Overall, there is a paucity of studies in this area, and those currently available are of generally little help for the oncology provider. Despite the finding by Novack et al.[10] that 97% of physicians (in this sample) preferred to tell the patient their diagnosis, it is still not uncommon to find situations in which the patient behaves as if the physician has not done this, at least not in a way the patient has been able to process. For example, there may be a note in the record stating "a full and frank discussion about diagnosis took place today" only to find that the patient continues to behave as if unaware of important information. At times, this may be accounted for by low retention of information given to patients in stressful medical situations.[36-39] Since patients may not recall much information when the timing of it coincides with peak emotional stress, one wonders whether disclosure can usefully take place in a single frank discussion anyway, even when the clinician makes an effort to take into account the patient's intelligence, interest, etc.

Morrow et al.[40] demonstrated that providing patients with informed consent documents to take home before signing increased their demonstrable understanding of treatment. Reynolds et al.[41] studied the relative gains in information by using explicit categorization (a method that provides the patient with a list of possible questions to ask), and by providing tape recordings of the consultation. Tapes did not enhance recall beyond the method of explicit categorization alone, which resulted in patients recalling more information. Even so, patients without either intervention, though able to recall less, were just as satisfied with the amount of information they received. Clearly, how the patient is told is as important a factor as what the patient is told.

DISCLOSURE MUST BE A PROCESS

Disclosure of information is often not possible in a single or simple transmission event. It is a process that must take place over time and requires a clinician who can analyze and comprehend a variety of psychologic processes. Let us say that the physician accepts the premise that a single communication cannot, for many reasons, fulfill the intent of providing adequate information. This implies that the physician must continually monitor the "information status" of the patient and continutally reinfuse information as the capacity of the patient changes in terms of anxiety, physical status, receptivity, etc. This process places an increasing burden on the provider who, as a consequence, must face the difficulty of repetitively informing. The difficulties of providing unpleasant and often upsetting news become multiplied. Further, the provider continually faces a dilemma of whether it is wise to "insist" that the patient be and act "informed." The provider may be in a position of having to challenge the patient's denial and possibly undermine an important defense. It requires skill to approach a patient who is maintaining denial.

Informing the patient is not an "all-or-none" phenomenon, nor is the patient's awareness an all-or-none phenomenon. The patient may acknowledge one aspect of the illness while maintaining denial about the diagnosis itself. This has been referred to as "middle knowledge" by Weisman[42] in reference to a situation in which the patient verbally denies the medical condition but behaves as if he knows that it is present.

PATERNALISM AND DISCLOSURE

Does an ethically informed policy of full disclosure help the clinician confronted by the patient with terminal illness, who in the midst of some routine care, looks up and asks, "I'm going to make it, aren't I." Of course, there is no single answer correct for each time this question is raised. The comforting pat on the shoulder may be just the thing needed, while at other times it would be grossly inappropriate. Only the clinician can attempt to decide what the question means. Is it a request for reassurance, a plea for companionship, a way for the patient to break out of isolation, or a genuine request for information?

The clinical approach values aciton that is "in the patient's overall best interest." This position has been seen by some as excessively paternalistic. It has been pointed out that medical expertise is no guarantee of moral wisdom, and that the clinician's idea of the patient's "overall best interest" always involves some hidden evaluative components.[43] Physicians begin from a position of paternalism. The heritage of the profession creates this stance. Physicians felt, and possibly correctly perceived 50 years ago, that people came to them as God-like figures and said, "Take care of me. I have pain in my back; tell me how to make it go away. I don't want to understand what's causing it. I don't want to understand that I have options like this or that." Options were not offered. Even today one hears some physicians saying, "People pay me to take care of them, not to educate them. I'm to do the worrying for them." A lot of people in the public would disagree with this position now.

Many arguments have been raised against the paternalistic position.[44] One of the most detailed critiques of this position[45] has raised several areas that might trouble the thoughtful clinician. To begin, can the physician ever have knowledge sufficient to know what is really in the "best overall interest" of another person? However, if one argues that it is unlikely that one could ever know enough about a person to guarantee that a paternalistic approach is justified, then wouldn't the same argument apply to the act of providing information as well as withholding it? Underlying such debates, of course, is the position that the physician has some moral/professional obligation to play this role at all. If physicians become technicians and not healers, then it may be appropriate to abandon this role. Buchanan argues that no physician (or nurse) is in a position to make judgments about the quality of someone else's life. Hoffmaster has pointed out the catch-22 of such a stance. "The nature of the issue precludes participation of the person whose life it is." When a physician has diagnosed a terminal illness and is debating about whether to inform the patient about it, he cannot ask the patient, "If it were discovered that you had terminal illness, would you want to know about?" or "If it were discovered that you had a terminal illness, would you regard being informed about the terminal illness or not being informed about the terminal illness as leading to a more fitting completion in your life, when your life is viewed as a unified process of development?" Merely raising such a question would certainly be a tip-off to the patient about the severity of his disease.

Thus, the only person who, theoretically, is in a position to make such a judgment is, for practical reasons, excluded from making the judgment. Yet someone has to make the judgment. What skills might be important for making such a decision, and does the physician (or nurse) possess these skills? To begin with, paternalism requires a pater, a parent, someone who knows the patient in depth and detail. The physician's ignorance of the patient's values, culture, and life style can be as detrimental to good case as the patient's ignorance of medical factors.[46] It seems that a consultant or occasional contact is almost disqualified from paternalistic activity insofar as only the primary provider who has known the patient (and family) over time can at least make a claim for such knowledge. This is not to say that many specialists do not become involved with their patients to such an extent that they are not in a position to do the same. In depth knowledge of the patient, then, seems a prerequisite for a paternalistic position. The clinician should not assume anything. Instead, through a series of questions, patients should gradually be led to reveal their experience of the illness and treatment process. The patient is allowed to maintain denial if necessary but is also invited to open up areas for more discussion. It is the obligation of the clinician to provide such an opportunity and to listen carefully in order to spot clues that the patient wants to continue. The clinician would contend that it is important to first understand the patient's experience before following through on any general intervention policy regarding methods or details of disclosure. The individual bias of the clinician must be supplemented as much as possible by the unique life data of the particular patient. How has the person dealt with similar situations in the past? What is the family style of dealing with such situations, etc.? Such knowledge requires an ongoing relationship, exploration of the patient's subjective values, and knowledge of the patient's psychologic resources. Even when the physician or nurse possess the skills to elicit such information about a patient over time, how certainly can future responses be predicted? While the warnings to the paternalistic position are clearly sounded, there remain strong proponents that such behavior can be a morally valued aspect of the physician's effectiveness[47] and that most patients, no matter how well informed, need the physician to choose for them at times.[48]

CONCLUSIONS

The strain created by lack of information unnecessarily isolates patients and can create an atmosphere of mistrust and perplexing communication. The perceptions of children and old people are generally underestimated, and those groups are at special risk for not receiving appropriate information, despite extensive literature investigating the child's perception of their diagnosis.[49,50] The lack of information may also deprive patients of coming to terms with their own existence and may also paradoxically increase stress through the torment of fantasies conjured up to fill the void.

Physicians' attitudes toward disclosure have changed considerably over the past several decades. However, exactly what they actually say, how they actually say it, and the impact of such decisions have not been adequately addressed. Disclosure cannot take place in a single "telegram" form. The process of assimilation of information must be recognized by the clinician who intends to provide information in an assimilable form. The assumption that there is a simple answer to the question of disclosure should be questioned and replaced by the intent to create an ongoing dialogue with the patient. Maintenance of such a dialogue challenges the clinician to develop skills such as how to identify psychologic defenses, a respect for moral ambiguity, as well as awareness of one's own feelings, as for example, concerns about being the bearer of bad tidings.

The ethical principle that upholds the obligation to disclose information to the patient is currently in the ascendancy. Perhaps this position is an appropriate corrective measure for excessively arbitrary withholding in the past. However, even when the clinician recognizes the need to have this ethical position guide behavior, informing the patient is a complex clinical process and no simple matter of information transmission. The standards that guide medical behavior cannot displace the requirement for the provider to know the patient and understand the meaning of an event or a procedure for a particular patient.[51] Changing attitudes that lead to more disclosure must be accompanied by a recognition of the need for appropriate psychologic and emotional support that a patient's knowledge may demand. The more that patients are told, the more they respond either in words or actions that require improved observational and listening skills on the part of both the physician[52] and nurse. It has been suggested that disclosure of information is analogous to giving a blood transfusion: "like a transfusion of blood, the dispensing of certain information must be distinctly indicated, the amount given consonant with the needs of the recipient, and the type chosen with a view of avoiding unfavorable reactions."[53]

REFERENCES

1 Beauchamp TL, Childress JF: Principles of Biomedical Ethics. New York, Oxford University Press, 1979.
2 Jonsen AR, Cassel C, Lo B, et al: The ethics of medicine: An annotated bibliography of recent literature. Ann Intern Med 92:136–141, 1980.
3 Reich WT (ed): Encyclopedia of Bioethics. New York, The Free Press, 1978.
4 Walters L (ed): Bibliography of Bioethics, vol 7. New York, The Free Press, 1981.
5 Taub S: Cancer and the law of informed consent. Law, Medicine & Health Care 10:61–66, 1982.
6 Fitts WT, Ravdin IS: What Philadelphia physicians tell patients with cancer. JAMA 153:901–904, 1953.
7 Rennick D (ed): What should physicians tell cancer patients? N Med Materia 2:41–53, 1960.
8 Oken D: What to tell cancer patients: A study of medical attitudes. 175:1120–1128, 1961.
9 Friedman HS: Physician management of dying patients: An exploration. Psychiatry Medicine 1:295–305, 1970.
10 Novack DH, Plumer R, Smith RL, et al: Changes in physician's attitudes toward telling the cancer patient. JAMA 241:897–900, 1979.
11 Hardy RE, Green DR, Jordan HW, et al: Communication between cancer patients and physicians. South Med J 73:755–757, 1980.
12 Greenwald HP, Nevitt MC: Physician attitudes toward communication with cancer patients. Soc Sci Med 16:591–594, 1982.
13 Blanchard CG, Ruckdeschel JC, Blanchard EG, et al: Do attitudes predict behavior: Correlation of oncologists' attitudes with their observed behavior toward cancer patients. 16th Annual Meeting of American Association of Cancer Education. 1982 (Abstr 49A).
14 McNeil BJ, Pauker SG, Soc HC, et al: On the elicitation of preferences for alternative therapies. N Engl J Med 306:1259–1262, 1983.
15 Jonsen AR, Siegler M, Winslade WJ: Clinical Ethics. New York, Macmillan, 1982.
16 Commission for the Study of Ethical Problems in Medicine and Biomedical and Behavioral Research: Making Health Care Decisions, vol 1. US Government Printing Office, Washington DC, October, 1982.
17 The Values Underlying Informed Consent, in Commission for the Study of Ethical Problems in Medicine and Biomedical and Behavioral Research: Making Health Care Decisions, vol 1. US Government Printing Office, Washington, DC, October, 1982.
18 Dworkin G: Paternalism. The Monist 56:64, 1972.
19 Gert B, Culver CM: Paternalistic Behavior. Philosophy and Public Affairs 6:45–57, 1976.
20 Lo B, Jonsen AR: Ethical decisions in the care of a patient terminally ill with metastatic cancer. Ann Intern Med 92:107–111, 1980.

21 Meisel A: The exceptions to informed consent. Conn Med 45:27–32, 1981.

22 Meisel A, Roth LH: What we do and do not know about informed consent. JAMA 246:2473–2477, 1981.

23 Golden JS, Johnston GD: Problems of distortion in doctor-patient communications. Psychiatry Medicine 1:127–149. 1970.

24 Boreham P, Gibson D: The informative process in private medical consultations: A preliminary investigation. Soc Sci Med 12(5A):409–416, 1978.

25 Alfidi RJ: Controversy, alternatives, and decisions in complying with the legal doctrine of informed consent. Radiology 114:231–234, 1975.

26 Hinton J: Whom do dying patients tell? Br Med J 281:1328–1330, 1980.

27 Veatch RM: Truth-telling. I: Attitudes, in, Reich WT (ed): Encyclopedia of Bioethics, Ne York, Macmillan, 1978.

28 Kelly WD, Friesen SR: Do cancer patients want to be told? Surgery 27:822–826, 1950.

29 McIntosh J: Patients' awareness and desire for information about diagnosed but undisclosed malignant disease. Lancet 2:300–303, 1976.

30 Henriques B, Stadil F, Baden H: Patient information about cancer. Acta Chir Scand 146:309–311, 1980.

31 Loftus EE, Fries JF: Informed consent may be hazardous to health. Science 204:4388, 1979.

32 Brody D: The patient's role in clinical decision-making. Ann Intern Med 93:718–722, 1980.

33 Lankton JW. Bachelder BM, Ominsky AJ: Emotional responses to detailed risk disclosure for anesthesia: A prospective, randomized study. Anesthesiology 46:294–296, 1977.

34 Denney MK, Williamson D, Penn R: Informed consent—emotional responses of patients. Postgrad Med J 60:205–209, 1975.

35 Cassem NH, Stewart RS: Management and care of the dying patient. Int J Psychiatry Med 1:295–305, 1970.

36 Robinson G, Merav A: Informed consent: Recall by patients tested postoperatively. Ann Thoracic Surg 22:209–212, 1976.

37 Leonard CO, Chase GA, Childs B: Genetic counseling: A consumer's view. N Engl J Med 287:433–439, 1972.

38 McCollum AT, Schwartz AH; Pediatric research hospitalization: Its meaning to parents. Pediatr Res 3:199–204, 1969.

39 Reading AD: Psychological preparation for surgery: Patient recall of information. J Psychosom Res 25:57–62, 1981.

40 Morrow G, Gootnick J, Schmale A: A simple technique for increasing cancer patients' knowledge of informed consent to treatment. Cancer 42:793–799, 1978.

41 Reynolds PM, Sanson-Fisher RW, Desmond Poole A, et al: Cancer and communication: Information-giving in an oncology clinic. Br Med J 282:1449–1451, 1981.

42 Weisman AD: Coping with Cancer. New York, McGraw Hill, 1979.

43 Veatch RM: Models for ethical medicine in a revolutionary age. Hastings Center Report 2 3:5–7, 1972.

44 Hoffmaster B: Physicians, patients and paternalism. Man and Medicine 5:189–202, 1980.

45 Buchanan A: Medical paternalism: Philosophy and Public Affairs, 7:370–391, 1978.
46 Kleinman A, Eisenberg L, Good B, et al: Culture, illness and care: Clinical lessons from anthropological and cross-culture research. Ann Intern Med 88:251–258, 1978.
47 Cross AW, Churchill LR: Ethical and cultural dimensions of informed consent. Ann Intern Med 96:110–113, 1982.
48 Ingelfinger FJ: Arrogance. N Engl J Med 303:1507–1511, 1980.
49 Kellerman J, Rigler D, Siegel SE, et al: Disease related communication and depression in pediatric cancer patients. J Pediatr Psychol 2:52–53, 1977.
50 Spinetta JJ, Maloney LJ: The child with cancer: Patterns of communication and denial. J Consult Clin Psychol 46:1540–1541, 1978.
51 Katz J: Informed consent in the therapeutic relationship: Legal and ethical aspects, in Reich W (ed): Encyclopedia of Bioethics, Vol 2. New York, The Free Press, 1978, p 771–778.
52 Saunders C: The moment of truth: Care of the dying person, in Pearson L (ed): Death and Dying, Cleveland, Case Western Reserve University Press, 1969, p 49–78.
53 Meyer BC: Truth and the physician, in Torrey FF (ed): Ethical Issues in Medicine: The Role of the Physician in Today's Society. New York, Little, Brown, 1968, p 166–177.

INFORMED (BUT UNEDUCATED) CONSENT

F. J. Ingelfinger

The trouble with informed consent is that it is not educated consent. Let us assume that the experimental subject, whether a patient, a volunteer, or otherwise enlisted, is exposed to a completely honest array of factual detail. He is told of the medical uncertainty that exists and that must be resolved by research endeavors, of the time and discomfort involved, and of the tiny percentage risk of some serious consequences of the test procedure. He is also reassured of his rights and given a formal, quasi-legal statement to read. No exculpatory language is used. With his written signature, the subject then caps the transaction, and whether he sees himself as a heroic martyr for the sake of mankind, or as a reluctant guinea pig dragooned for the benefit of science, or whether, perhaps, he is merely bewildered, he obviously has given his "informed consent." Because established routines have been scrupulously observed, the doctor, the lawyer, and the ethicist are content.

But the chances are remote that the subject really understands what he has consented to—in the sense that the responsible medical investigator understands the goals, nature, and hazards of his study. How can the layman comprehend the importance of his perhaps not receiving, as determined by luck of the draw, the highly touted new treatment that his roommate will get? How can he appreciate the sensation of living for days with a multi-lumen intestinal tube passing through his mouth and pharynx? How can he interpret the information that an

Reprinted by permission from *The New England Journal of Medicine* 287, 9 (August 31, 1972): 465–466. © 1972 Massachusetts Medical Society.

intravascular catheter and radiopaque dye injection have an 0.01 per cent probability of leading to a dangerous thrombosis or cardiac arrhythmia? It is moreover quite unlikely that any patient-subject can see himself accurately within the broad context of the situation, to weigh the inconveniences and hazards that he will have to undergo against the improvements that the research project may bring to the management of his disease in general and to his own case in particular. The difficulty that the public has in understanding information that is both medical and stressful is exemplified by [a report that] only half the families given genetic counseling grasped its impact.[1]

Nor can the information given to the experimental subject be in any sense totally complete. It would be impractical and probably unethical for the investigator to present the nearly endless list of all possible contingencies; in fact, he may not himself be aware of every untoward thing that might happen. Extensive detail, moreover, usually enhances the subject's confusion. Epstein and Lasagna showed that comprehension of medical information given to untutored subjects is inversely correlated with the elaborateness of the material presented.[2] The inconsiderate investigator, indeed, conceivably could exploit his authority and knowledge and extract "informed consent" by overwhelming the candidate-subject with information.

Ideally, the subject should give his consent freely, under no duress whatsoever. The facts are that some element of coercion is instrumental in any investigator-subject transaction. Volunteers for experiments will usually be influenced by hopes of obtaining better grades, earlier parole, more substantial egos, or just mundane cash. These pressures, however, are but fractional shadows of those enclosing the patient-subject. Incapacitated and hospitalized because of illness, frightened by strange and impersonal routines, and fearful for his health and perhaps life, he is far from exercising a free power of choice when the person to whom he anchors all his hopes asks, "Say, you wouldn't mind, would you, if you joined some of the other patients on this floor and helped us to carry out some very important research we are doing?" When "informed consent" is obtained, it is not the student, the destitute bum, or the prisoner to whom, by virtue of his condition, the thumb screws of coercion are most relentlessly applied; it is the most used and useful of all experimental subjects, the patient with disease.

When a man or woman agrees to act as an experimental subject, therefore, his or her consent is marked by neither adequate understanding nor total freedom of choice. The conditions of the agreement are a far cry from those visualized as ideal. Jonas would have the subject identify with the investigative endeavor so that he and the researcher would be seeking a common cause: "Ultimately, the appeal for volunteers should seek . . . free and generous endorsement, the appropriation of the research purpose into the person's [i.e., the subject's] own scheme of ends."[3] For Ramsey, "informed consent" should represent a "convenantal bond between consenting man and consenting man [that] makes them . . . joint adventurers in medical care and progress."[4] Clearly, to achieve motivations and attitudes of this lofty type, an educated and understanding, rather than merely informed, consent is necessary.

Although it is unlikely that the goals of Jonas and of Ramsey will ever be achieved, and that human research subjects will spontaneously volunteer rather than be "conscripted,"[3] efforts to promote educated consent are in order. In view of the current emphasis on involving "the community" in such activities as regional planning, operation of clinics, and assignment of priorities, the general public and its political leaders are showing an increased awareness and understanding of medical affairs. But the orientation of this public interest in medicine is chiefly socioeconomic. Little has been done to give the public a basic understanding of medical research and its requirements not only for the people's money but also for their participation. The public, to be sure, is being subjected to a bombardment of sensation-mongering news stories and books that feature "breakthroughs," or that reveal real or alleged exploitations—horror stories of Nazitype experimentation on abused human minds and bodies. Muckraking is essential to expose malpractices, but unless accompanied by efforts to promote a broader appreciation of medical research and its methods, it merely compounds the difficulties for both the investigator and the subject when "informed consent" is solicited.

The procedure currently approved in the United States for enlisting human experimental subjects has one great virtue: patient-subjects are put on notice that their management is in part at least an experiment. The deceptions of the past are no longer tolerated. Beyond this accomplishment, however, the process of obtaining "informed consent," with all its regulations and conditions, is no more than an elaborate ritual, a device that, when the subject is uneducated and uncomprehending, confers no more than the semblance of propriety on human experimentation. The subject's only real protection, the public as well as the medical profession must recognize, depends on the conscience and compassion of the investigator and his peers.

NOTES

1 Leonard, Claire O., et al. Genetic counseling: a consumer's view. N Engl J Med 287:433–449, 1972.
2 Epstein, L. C., Lasagna, L. Obtaining informed consent: form or substance. Arch Intern Med 123:682–688, 1969.
3 Jonas, H. Philosophical reflections on experimenting with human subjects. Daedalus 98:219–247, Spring, 1969.
4 Ramsey, P. The ethics of a cottage industry in an age of community and research medicine. N Engl J Med 284:700–706, 1971.

PARENTALISM[1]

M. Benjamin and J. Curtis

In its most general sense, parentalism means that an adult is being treated as if he or she were a child by persons acting as if they had the authority and concern of a parent.[2] Just as a parent may force an unwilling child to go to bed at a certain hour or take bitter medicine, so too, it is argued, a nurse may sometimes force an unwilling patient to get rest or receive treatment. Like the parent, the nurse will claim to be acting *on the behalf*, although *not at the behest*, of the patient; for, like the child, the patient is presumed unable to appreciate the connection between the nurse's behavior and his or her own welfare.[3]

Where a parent forces or manipulates a child into doing something for his or her own good, the assumption is that the child lacks the capacity to understand, endorse, and act in accord with the parent's benevolent aims. When a child is, in fact, able to understand and appreciate the parent's reasoning, but nonetheless disagrees with it, parental force or manipulation may no longer be justified. Thus, it is one thing for a parent to force a four-year-old to brush his or her teeth; it is quite an other for a parent to prevent a fourteen-year-old from going to any but "G"-rated movies. Parents are justified in coercing or manipulating children into doing things "for their own good" when: (1) it is reasonably clear that the result will be in the child's interests; (2) the child is unable to understand or resists rational appeals to the connection between the act in question and his

From *Ethics in Nursing*, Second Edition, by Martin Benjamin and Joy Curtis. Copyright © 1986 by Oxford University Press, Inc. Reprinted by permission.

or her own (long-term) interests; and (3) it is reasonable to assume that, in the absence of special "brainwashing " or indoctrination, the child will endorse or ratify the parents' behavior at a later date when he or she can understand and appreciate the parents' aims and reasoning. It is because forcing four-year-olds to brush their teeth clearly meets all of these conditions, while preventing four-teen-year-olds from going to any "PG" movies does not, that we are inclined to think the former more justifiable than the latter.

Insofar as parentalistic coercion or manipulation of an adult involves a refusal to accept at face value the choices, wishes, or action of an individual who is presumed to be autonomous and self-determining, it bears an even heavier burden of justification. Parentalistic behavior, regardless of benevolent motives or the magnitude of the benefit to be secured or the harm to be avoided, overrides the right of an adult to be treated as a person. To be a person, as the term is used here, is to regard oneself as having the ability and right to formulate various projects and make various commitments, and then to attempt to fulfill them. A human being is identified as a particular person by the values and life plan that guide his or her conduct. To respect another as a person, then, is to take full account of his or her values and life plan and to give them as much consideration in determining the effects of one's conduct as one wants given to one's own values and life plan. Conversely, to disregard or give only perfunctory consid-eration to the values and life plans of others is to show contempt for them as persons. It is to regard them as mere objects or things rather than one's equals as persons, *even if one's aim is to benefit them or protect them from harm*. In Kant's terms, it is to treat them as mere means to an end, and not as ends-in-themselves.[4] And nothing is more demeaning to a person, more damaging to self-respect, than to be so treated. To deal with a sick individual as a person, then, is to place his or her values and plans, as far as possible, in the center of the picture and to attempt to preserve his or her sense of capacity for reflective choice.[5]

Nonetheless, as the following case illustrates, there may be times when an adult's capacity for reflective choice is seriously impaired.

PARENTALISTIC RESTRAINT

Sixty-seven-year-old Henry Young had suffered a stroke and was being kept under continual restraint in the hospital at the direction of Kirsten Bennett, the supervising nurse. A locking waistbelt was used, whether Mr. Young was in bed or in a chair. The belt was of a "humane" design, permitting him as much freedom as possible while assuring that he could not fall out of the bed or chair.

Mr. Young had had a fall earlier in this hospital stay, having attempted to walk while unattended. He was only slightly injured in this episode, but because of the possibility of serious injury that such a fall presents, Kirsten required him to be restrained in the waistbelt whenever he was left unattended, even for a very short period. Mr. Young vigorously protested that he was being deprived of his dignity, that he felt as if he were in prison, that he was afraid of being unable to escape in the event of a fire, and that he was perfectly competent to be left free and responsible for his own safety. In response, Kirsten repeatedly told him that the restraint was a "standard procedure" for patients in his condition and that he had no choice in the matter as long as he remained in the hospital and his condition remained unchanged.

Underlying her decision was the fact that, as is not uncommon in such cases, Mr. Young's mental capacities seemed to swing back and forth so that sometimes he was undoubtedly competent to move about at liberty, but at other times he became confused and lost some degree of motor control. It had, in fact, been during such a confused period that he had suffered his earlier fall. Another important consideration was the fact that the nursing staff did not have time to keep continual watch over him. Thus, as Kirsten explained to Mr. Young's family, the restraint was "for his own good" even though contrary to his wishes. All things considered, she maintained, it was best for him to be kept in the waistbelt, even during periods of mental clarity, in order to insure that he would not, when unattended, lapse into mental confusion and seriously hurt himself. Mr. Young's family agreed with the supervising nurse and fully supported her decision.[6]

If we assume that Kirsten's appeal to Mr. Young's best interests is not a rationalization for a more basic concern with the hospital's legal liability, the convenience of the nursing staff, or an authoritarian desire to exercise complete control over all patients, her reasons for keeping him in restraints are purely parentalistic. She believes that Mr. Young's capacity to decide for himself on this question has been seriously impaired and that because he runs a significant risk of harm from being left unrestrained while unattended, he must, for his own good, be kept in the waistbelt even if he resists and protests. The question now is whether this parentalistic intervention is justifiable.

Parentalistic behavior requires justification because it refuses to accept at face value the choices, wishes, or actions of an individual who is presumed to be autonomous and self-determining. Thus, in justifying a particular parentalistic intervention, one must show that the presumption of autonomy or self-determination no longer holds—that the choices, wishes, or actions of the individual are not genuinely autonomous or authentically self-determined.[7] Even John Stuart Mill, whose defense of individual liberty is often considered to be antiparentalistic in the extreme,[8] allowed that we may interfere with a person's acting on his or her expressed desires when we can be certain that they are not his actual desires.

If either a public officer or anyone else saw a person attempting to cross a bridge which had been ascertained to be unsafe, and there were not time to warn him of this danger, they might seize him and turn him back without any real infringement of his liberty; for liberty consists of doing what one desires, and he does not desire to fall into the river.[9]

Similarly, we might conclude that Mr. Young does not desire to injure himself while walking around unattended. Thus, insofar as he is prevented from doing so, the nursing staff no more violates his right as a person to do what he (genuinely) wants to do than the intervener in Mill's example violates the rights of the person crossing the bridge.

In both Mill's example and the case of Mr. Young, the defense of the intervention rests on two conditions: (1) the ignorance or impaired capacity for rational reflection of the agent; and (2) the magnitude and probability of harm that would result without parentalistic intervention. Although some would argue that only the first of these conditions is *necessary* to justify parentalistic interference, and others would maintain that the second is by itself *sufficient* to justify such interference, we believe that both are necessary.[10] If a person meets condition (1), but does not thereby run an increased risk of significant harm, one cannot say that the "lesser evil" (the deprivation of liberty or choice) is justified by appeal to the avoidance of a "greater evil" (harm to the person whose liberty or choice is restricted); hence, the intervention is not clearly in the person's best interests. And if a person meets condition (2), but is mentally competent and fully aware of the magnitude and probability of harm that may result from his or her action, interference cannot be justified on parentalistic grounds unless one is willing to say that people should not be free to drive racing cars, smoke cigarettes, or refuse certain forms of medical treatment.

Although a parent may be justified in making a child do things judged to *benefit* the child as well as to protect him or her from harm, we believe that generally a health professional can override an adult client's right to self-determination *only to prevent harm*. Although the difference between preventing harm and providing a benefit is not always clear, often it is both clear and useful. The main difference between the promotion of benefit and the prevention of harm, for our purposes, is that it is much easier to obtain agreement on what constitutes a harm than on what constitutes a benefit. People may, for example, differ widely about whether public funds should be used to promote the arts, athletics, ethnic festivals, libraries, or parks, but there is usually significant agreement among the same people that such funds should be used to prevent foreign invasions, crime, and disease. The latter are regarded as harms of great magnitude by most any set of values, while whether one or another of the former is regarded as a vital benefit will vary widely from one set of values to another. Thus, unless one has a more or less explicit prior consent for interventions conceived mainly as providing a benefit rather than preventing a harm, the *presumed* benefit (which may simply reduce to the imposition of one's own values on a vulnerable patient) cannot override the *certain* infringement of a person's right to self-determination.

Underlying this emphasis on harm as opposed to benefit is an assumption that parentalistic behavior is justifiable only if the subject of the intervention in some sense consents to it. For example, a parent's forcing the child to brush his or her teeth is justified, in part, by the reasonable assumption that the child at a later date when the parent's aims and reasoning can be understood and appreciated, will endorse or ratify the parent's behavior. As Gerald Dworkin puts it, "Parental paternalism may be thought of as a wager by the parent on the subsequent recognition of the wisdom of the restrictions. There is an emphasis on what could be called future-oriented consent—on what the child will come to welcome, rather than on what he does welcome."[11] Similarly, just as Mr. Young, the stroke victim, . . . does not want to injure himself, and the person about to walk over the bridge in Mill's example does not want to fall into the river, those who parentalistically interfere can reasonably assume that their interventions will later be ratified by the subjects of the interference.[12] Thus, we may now add a future consent condition to the two we have already provided for the justification of an act of parentalism. An act of parentalism will now be said to be justified if and only if:

1 the subject is, under the circumstances, irretrievably ignorant of relevant information, or his or her capacity for rational reflection is significantly impaired (the *autonomy* condition);
2 the subject is likely to be significantly harmed unless interfered with (the *harm* condition); and
3 it is reasonable to assume that the subject will, at a later time, with greater knowledge or the recovery of his or her capacity for rational reflection, ratify the decision to interfere by consenting to it (the *ratification* condition).[13]

Recent discussions of the justification of parentalism often distinguish two forms: "strong" and "weak." Strong parentalism emphasizes doing what is ostensibly for the patient's own good or welfare regardless of his or her capacity to consent. Weak parentalism, on the other hand, involves acting to benefit a person or limit harm when, due to irretrievable ignorance or mental impairment, the patient is substantially unable to make the decision for him- or herself. Our emphasis on the autonomy and ratification conditions indicates that we are endorsing a "weak" and not a strong" form of parentalism. Our restriction of condition (2) to harm, and excluding benefit or welfare, indicates that ours is also among the weaker versions of "weak" parentalism. Our main reason for rejecting stronger versions of parentalism is that they are usually too quick to override that patient's autonomy in the name of a conception of the good that cannot be shown by cogent argument to be superior to the patient's own conception of the good. On the other hand, the form of weak parentalism outlined here can, in many instances, be justified in the context of health care.

Let us now become more thoroughly acquainted with our three conditions for justifiable (weak) parentalism by applying them to three more cases.

CONVINCING THE PATIENT

"The job of a primary nurse," in Debbie Rokken's words, *"is to provide care to the patients; and that includes basic assessment, basic nursing care, bathing, and different kinds of nursing duties; also more sophisticated care, such as giving chemotherapy, blood components, IVs, and medications. If I personally cannot give the care directly, then I have an LPN or an orderly who will work along with me to see that the care gets done. I work the three to eleven shift, and another RN from the day shift is my associate. Between the two of us, we organize the care and provide it to the same group of patients."* In the primary care system the primary nurse, being ultimately responsible for the patient's nursing needs, exercises considerable influence over the patient.[14]

Debbie and her associate cared for Mrs. Cotton, who was thought to have metastasis to the pelvic area and for whom a total pelvic examination was recommended. Both nurses agreed to help Mrs. Cotton decide about having surgery, which "might be radical." Mrs. Cotton was apprehensive about surgery, afraid of losing control with the anesthesia, and afraid that the procedure would be too radical. According to Debbie, Mrs. Cotton "had very little support from her husband or her children; no one talked about surgery, much less helped her decide whether or not to have it done." Debbie had seen two women recently "do very well with similar extremely radical procedures." She also thought that the other alternatives, no treatment at all or a less radical treatment, would lead to a much more rapid demise and certainly a lowered quality of life with dependence on narcotics for pain. Therefore, she attempted to convince Mrs. Cotton that such surgery might be a good idea. Debbie spent time talking about why Mrs. Cotton needed the surgery and what could happen as a result of her not having it. She spent time with Mrs. Cotton and carefully chose interpersonal relations skills that might enhance feelings of trust. She sat close to Mrs. Cotton, occasionally held her hand, and once put her arm around her shoulders to comfort her. After several days Mrs. Cotton decided to undergo the surgery.

Months later Debbie reconsidered her actions, not because of Mrs. Cotton, whose pelvic mass was not malignant, but because in her words, "After more experience I saw a lot of women not do so well, and suffer more from that kind of treatment. It certainly makes you ask yourself whether you're doing them a service or not." Debbie's parentalistic intervention in this case seems to meet none of the conditions we have suggested as necessary to justify such an intervention. It does not meet the first condition because there is no evidence that Mrs. Cotton's capacity for rational reflection is impaired (her fears seem to be those that most people would have about major surgery), and her ignorance of the risks of the procedure could be remedied simply by providing her with information. Debbie's intervention does not meet the second condition because, as she later learns, her belief that Mrs. Cotton is likely to be significantly harmed by not having the operation is based on insufficient evidence. Debbie's initial assessment of the risks and benefits of the surgery were based on a sample of only two cases. Finally, for the same reason, Debbie could not reasonably assume that Mrs. Cotton would later consent to her interference and hence ratify it; thus the third condition was not met. We may, therefore, conclude that Debbie's parentalistic intervention in this case was not justified.

The question of justified parentalism also arises in the following case.

BREAKING THE CIGARETTE HABIT

Twenty-three-year-old Fred Winston had attempted suicide by shooting himself in the head. He was hospitalized with permanent brain damage, which left him largely helpless and his body deformed by muscular contractions. He required assistance for almost every activity. He was usually incontinent, though this was attributed more to a lack of concern than to physical incapacity. In addition, his speech was barely audible, and the combination of brain damage and emotional difficulties resulted in stammering, repetitive speech patterns.

Fred failed to eat well, and his primary pleasures seemed to be watching television and smoking cigarettes. After his initial period of hospitalization, those responsible for his nursing care decided to try to limit his smoking "for his own good." Thus, he was often falsely informed that his cigarettes were all gone, or that there were only one or two left and he ought to save them for later, or that no one was available to supervise him while he smoked (a safety requirement necessary because of his limited fine motor control). The nursing staff reasoned that since he did not appear to care about what was in his own best interest, they would have to take measures to limit his smoking even if he protested.

When he sensed what was happening, Fred protested as strongly as his limitations would allow. In response to the nurses' explanation that what they were doing was for his own good, he insisted that since there was little hope that his condition would improve, he was entitled to whatever gave him pleasure at the present moment. Given his condition, he maintained, smoking was "for his own good." But inasmuch as his physical debilities and difficulties with speech limited his capacity to resist or vociferously protest the nurses' behavior, their will prevailed.[15]

Before determining whether the nursing staff's conduct meets our three conditions for *justifiable* parentalism, we may want to ask whether their actions are, at bottom, parentalistically motivated. Parentalistic reasons for forcing or manipulating people to do certain things often function as rather high-minded rationalizations for conduct that is actually motivated by anger or a concern for one's own advantage or convenience. In such cases parentalistic reasoning, which we may characterize as primarily other-regarding, simply acts to conceal reasoning that is basically self-regarding, though we may be reluctant to admit this—even to ourselves. In the case before us, for example, it would not be surprising if the nursing staff's behavior were motivated by an underlying, un-articulated anger with Fred. After all, patients like Fred are not likely to make the nurse's already difficult job any easier. He requires a great deal of care and shows a lack of respect and consideration for the nurses by his apparently willful incontinence. His failure to eat well is also likely to frustrate the nurses and, like most people, they are probably threatened to some degree by Fred's self-destructive repudiation of society and all they hold dear, regardless of what drove him to attempt suicide. Thus, it is important in this case for the nursing staff to determine whether their conduct is actually, or only apparently, parentalistic.

Even if their plan to help Fred cut down on his smoking is intended for his own good, and not simply a rationalized expression of anger, it does not meet the conditions we have set out for justified parentalism. It does not meet the first condition because, as far as we can tell from the case description, Fred is neither ignorant of the dangers of smoking nor is his capacity to reason about his decision less impaired than that of other smokers. (It should be noted that other patients in the same part of the hospital were, subject to safety rules, allowed to smoke as they wished). The staff's parentalistic behavior fails to meet the second condition, not because cigarette smoking is not harmful, but rather because it has not been regarded by the society as a whole to be *so* harmful that adults, after being duly warned, are not free to decide for themselves whether the benefits outweigh the risks. Consistency demands, then, that we regard the probability and magnitude of harm to Fred from smoking at this point no greater than that to Fred before his hospitalization or to other people in or out of the hospital. Finally, the nurses cannot reasonably assume that Fred will, at some later date, ratify their decision by consenting to it. As he himself suggests, given his limitations, the pleasure derived from smoking has taken on a greater significance than it had before his hospitalization. As these limitations are apparently permanent, it is unlikely that he will ever be able to replace the pleasures of smoking with anything else.

If the nurses' conduct is not an instance of justified parentalism, it must be regarded as an attempt to take advantage of Fred's dependence and vulnerability to impose their values on him. Surely if he were strong enough to smoke without supervision or to protest vociferously, the nursing staff would be forced to change their treatment of Fred. Insofar as their force prevails, so too does their will. This, of course, is not the first time that professional dominance has violated the rights of patients to be treated as persons. But here as elsewhere, a precedent for the violation of someone's personhood ought never to be confused with an ethical justification for it.

The recent emphasis in nursing on health promotion and teaching constantly raises questions about justifiable parentalism. How far may a nurse go in trying to alter a client's way of living in the name of better health? Can one be parentalistic when the situation is very complex and the likelihood of harm cannot be reliably gauged? And if so, what form should the parentalistic interference take? Are exaggerated threats and lies acceptable if nothing else appears likely to be effective? Consider, in this connection, the following all too typical case.

PROMOTING A HEALTHY LIFESTYLE

Donna Boyd, staff nurse, faces the task of interpreting Alan Spencer's current health risk appraisal form to him. The appraisal, a computer printout sheet, indicates the risks he faces from various health, problems, given his age and physical condition. In Donna's professional judgment, Mr. Spencer's health risk appraisal shows that he should reduce his smoking and intake of food and alcohol, exercise more, and take his medicine with greater regularity. Although Mr. Spencer, who is fifty years old, reports that he watches his diet, has cut down on his smoking, and regularly takes his medicine, he has nevertheless gained fifteen pounds during the past year; he came into the hospital with a blood pressure of 220/140, cholesterol level of 500 mg/dl, and triglycerides level of 450 mg/dl. Donna knows that during other hospitalizations and clinic visits other nurses have tried to persuade Mr. Spencer to change his lifestyle, but he has become irritated by such efforts and what he has termed, "preachy nurses." He has indicated that he wants no further discussion of his personal behavior. Donna, however, is strongly inclined to make another effort to get him to change his ways, for his own good.

Since previous discussions to this end seem to have been unsuccessful, what should Donna do? Should she simply hand Mr. Spencer the assessment with no further comment? Should she try to overcome his reluctance to change by using subtle or open threats, or even lies, about the likelihood of a painful and early death? Or is there a more plausible course of action that lies between these two extremes?[16]

We leave it to the reader, at this point, to answer these questions for him- or herself. The answers, we believe, are not obvious. A good way to begin is to determine whether parentalism might be justified in this case; and, if so, whether threats or deception about the likelihood of a painful and early death can in this case be parentalistically justified. Other relevant considerations include the possibility that further efforts to alter the client's lifestyle might only increase his antagonism to medicine and nursing and thus be counterproductive, and whether or not the nurse can reasonably expect the high value she, quite understandably, places on health to be shared by the patient.

NOTES

1 By "parentalism" we mean what is conventionally referred to in the literature as "paternalism." But since women are no less capable than men of occupying the "paternal" or "father knows best" role in their dealings with others, we prefer the sexually neutral term.

2 An important distinction can be drawn between "parentalism" *as a social practice* having certain roles and expectations governing the behavior of patients and health

professionals in the total health care system and parentalism *as a justification for particular acts* of manipulation or coercion on the part of health professionals. Unless otherwise indicated, we use the term "parentalism" in the second sense.

3 James Childress, "Paternalism and Health Care," in Wade L. Robison and Michael S. Pritchard, eds., *Medical Responsibility* (Clifton, N.J.: Humana Press, 1979), p. 18.

4 As Charles Fried puts it, "even if the ends are the patient's own ends, to treat him as a means to them is to undermine his humanity insofar as humanity consists in choosing and being able to judge one's own ends, rather than being a machine which is used to serve ends, even one's own ends." Charles Fried, *Medical Experimentation: Personal Integrity and Social Policy* (Amsterdam: North Holland, 1974), p. 101.

5 *Ibid.*, p. 95.

6 This case has been provided by Bruce Walters, student in the College of Human Medicine at Michigan State University.

7 See Bruce Miller, "Autonomy and the Refusal of Lifesaving Treatment," *Hastings Center Report*, 11 (in press, 1981).

8 H.L.A. Hart, *Law, Liberty, and Morality* (New York: Vintage, 1966), p. 32–34.

9 John Stuart Mill, *On Liberty* (New York: Library of Liberal Arts, 1956), p. 117.

10 Childress, p. 24.

11 Gerald Dworkin, "Paternalism," *Monist*, 56 (January, 1972), p. 76f.

12 Kirsten Bennett in Case 3.2 might thus be criticized for not having worked harder at obtaining consent from Mr. Henry, during his lucid periods, to his being restrained, if necessary, in the future. The case, as presented, suggests that she may have been more concerned with securing his family's consent than his own.

13 Ultimately this condition must be modified to account for subjects who will never recover their capacity for rational reflection.

14 See Chapter 5, Section 1, Part B, for a further account of the role of the primary nurse.

15 This case has been provided by Bruce Walters.

16 This case was provided by Dorothea Milbrandt, Vice-President for Nursing, Ingham Medical Center, Lansing, Michigan, and Marilyn Rothert, Director for Lifelong Education, College of Nursing, Michigan State University.

AUTONOMY AND PATERNALISM: TWO GOALS IN CONFLICT

Elias S. Cohen

The development of concepts of autonomy and paternalism, as applied to children, women, the mentally ill and mentally retarded, and the elderly, has been a remarkable journey for philosophers, lawyers, physicians, caregivers, and politicians. Autonomy and paternalism have moved together in uneasy company to new definitions and applications derived in an extended dialectical process that has not only refined the definitions but also moved them away from the extreme ends of the gamut. To the extent that autonomy is equated with independence of action and paternalism is equated with coercive actions contrary to an individual's wishes or desires in order to achieve a beneficent end, we have exercised some of the most extreme and benighted paternalism while permitting in some sectors of our lives great independence on grounds of classical autonomy. Refinements of these concepts have moved us to new levels of sophistication and have made us aware of new issues and problems with which we have yet to wrestle.

In 1908, Justice Brewer of the United States Supreme Court mustered an array of paternalistic arguments in *Muller v. Oregon,*[1] a case testing the validity of a statute that limited the work hours of women in a laundry to 10 hours a day. In a classic statement, he argued for individual paternalism, social paternalism, and hard, direct, and active paternalism when he wrote:

That woman's physical structure and the performance of maternal functions place her at a disadvantage in the struggle for subsistence is obvious. . . . By abundant testimony of the medical fraternity continuance for a long time on her feet at work, repeating this from day to day, tends to have injurious effects upon the body, and as healthy mothers are essential to vigorous offspring, the physical well-being of woman becomes an object of public interest and care in order to preserve the strength and vigor of the race. Still again history discloses the fact that woman has always been dependent upon man. He established his control at the outset by superior physical strength, and this control in various forms with diminishing intensity has continued to the present. As minors, though not to the same extent, she has been looked upon in the courts as needing special care, that her rights may be preserved. . . . It is still true that in the struggle for subsistence, she is not an equal competitor with her brother. Though limitations upon personal and contractual rights may be removed by legislation, there is that in her disposition and habits of life which will operate against a full assertion of those rights. She will still be where some legislation to protect her seems necessary to secure a real equality of right.[2]

At the same time as Justice Brewer's paternalistic reasoning, some peculiar notion of autonomy had stilled the birth of products liability. Courts were secure in the belief that rational, deliberate consumers acting in their own self-interests could protect themselves against the risk of harm from negligently made products by the exercise of free choice in purchasing.[3] Similarly, juvenile courts dealt willy-nilly with children, placing and "protecting" them, although society's reluctance to enact child labor laws permitted the horrendous industrial employment of children.

Our notion of autonomy as independence was reflected in the way that economic relief for the poverty-stricken was provided. What little economic relief there was consisted of workhouses, almshouses, and restricted food, coal and rent chits, but every man was free to sleep under the bridge. That the United States waited until 1935 to take the first steps toward a policy of national economic relief was a testament to the power and persistence not only of the belief in individual responsibility, but also of the belief that autonomy reasonably and rationally exercised would necessarily produce desired results both for individuals and for society. One must note, however, that when the United States did move away from that position in 1935 it did so with one of the most remarkable legislative embodiments of the principle of respect for persons: the act granted an unprecedented degree of autonomy to poor persons by prohibiting federal participation in any economic relief that was not provided in the form of an unrestricted cash grant.[4] This provision stands alongside the civil rights acts[5] and the great constitutional amendments[6] when measured on any autonomy/paternalism scale.

Our early history of paternalism, which persists in many instances today, is reflected in the exercise of police powers under a sweeping *parens patriae* doctrine.[7] Applied to children, idiots, imbeciles, lunatics, drunkards, and old people, all in some respect legally disabled, the doctrine was used to incarcerate hundreds of thousands, to deny them education, treatment, even protection against fellow residents in institutions or their keepers, and to strip them of personhood, all in the questionable name of beneficence and against their wishes. That due process was not honored is simply another part of the rough and ready way that paternalism was meted out. For all of these individuals, it was clear that they were no longer persons, and therefore respect for persons was never an issue.

Until recently, it was appropriate to speak and write of autonomy and paternalism as two goals in conflict. The Justice Brewers of our courts held firm views about paternalism as protection. Those who argued on behalf of individuals resisting the state held relatively unsophisticated, albeit quite correct, views about autonomy and independence. As society has developed, and as we have explored the meaning of respect for persons, the ways in which we define autonomy and protect the objects of our beneficent concerns have become complex. Nevertheless, the dichotomies that the law loves so well do persevere to a large extent: guilt or innocence, sanity or insanity, and contract or no contract. Increasingly, however, the shades of gray intrude upon the blacks and whites: examples are the new California probate code,[8] which eschews sweeping findings of incompetency, or the blurring of the rights of children (still far from resolved), represented by *In re Gault,*[9] which gives children due process rights. *Gault,* however, is offset by more recent Supreme Court decisions, such as *Parbam v. J.R.,*[10] which permits parents to commit their children to mental hospitals under a "voluntary admission" without any representation of the child's interest independent of his parents.

Writers in the field have made enormous contributions to our thinking about the nature of autonomy and paternalism, providing refinements which ultimately will be reflected in law and practice. Childress's analysis has led him, with others, to the development of a concept of limited paternalism.[11] Just as John Locke's view of independent man and John Stuart Mill's views on liberty of action no longer suffice, just so early views of paternalism as coercive action interfering with liberty of action by reason of the welfare, good, happiness, needs, interests, or values of the person being coerced are insufficient for today's more complex understanding of paternalism.

In health care of the elderly, issues of autonomy and paternalism, even in their most recent evolutions, are not entirely sufficient to guide us in the formulation of legal limits or an articulation of rights, duties, and obligatons. Even current notions of autonomy and paternalism perseverate with the law's demand for neat boundaries and its dichotomous approach that places persons or events on this or that side of a legal line.

This article first examines the formal structure of autonomy, the interrelationship that has developed between autonomy and independence, the assumptions this has imposed upon society, and the impact this may have had upon the elderly. Second, the article explores paternalism and its applications. Third, some goals for new syntheses in the ongoing dialectical process that explores and redefines autonomy and paternalism are discussed.

Autonomy is that quality which describes the degree of mastery an individual exercises over his or her life. It has to do with the exercise of choices—choices of a life plan and choices of the intermediate steps one takes to carry out that plan or a freely and rationally arrived at modification of the plan. To be autonomous is not necessarily to be original. It is rather to assert "ownership" over the life plan and its intermediate steps. Autonomy is not limited to the impact on oneself, for surely autonomy and its exercise clearly have an impact on others.

Autonomy, it is said, may be measured along four axes; these may be said to be four concurrent "tests" of autonomy, all of which have found their way into law in varying degrees.[12] First is the axis of free action, i.e., action by an individual free of internal or external constraints or coercions. Second is action grounded in rational deliberation, i.e., action that is based upon consideraton of pros and cons, long- and short-range consequences, consideration of known facts, and application of logical thinking. This is not to say that rational deliberation always yields the right results. Right results are not an essential concomitant of autonomous action. Third is authentic action, i.e., action that is consistent with the attitudes, values, dispositions, and life plans known to be characteristic of the individual. Thus, to act "out of character" may be to raise questions about the autonomy of the action. Finally, autonomy as moral reflection is a measure of the degree to which one may have considered complete sets of values, attitudes, and life plans. It is distinguished from rational deliberaton by the depth of its analysis. It is more than a "buy-in" to a particular set of religious or moral values which, for example, permit or prohibit the termination of life, withholding of treatment, or blood transfusions.

Autonomy is not the same as liberty, although notions of autonomy inform notions of liberty rights. Both conceptions of liberty, as license and as independence, provide for the curtailment of liberty. Curtailment of liberty as license requires justification on the grounds of protection or prevention of harm to others or to society at large. Curtailment of liberty as independence requires a finding that one is not competent to have a reasonable conception of good and evil, is ignorant, or has "wrong" values. Such curtailments demean the individual and are affronts to dignity and independence. As such, they require narrow definitions that are extreme in the sense that a free society requires high degrees of freedom in setting the standard of what is competent action, good action, and informed action.

Autonomy is not the same as independence in the image of the lone American, making choices and taking responsibility, as articulated in the John Wayne paradigm. Yet, it is that paradigm that has been transported into law, culture, and economic behavior. This conception of autonomy has set the patterns for asserting rights and making claims, and has been built into our social, commercial, and legal structures. Much conservative economic theory (and current law) suggests that autonomous behavior driven by rational self-interest will yield the greatest good for the greatest number.[13] Competition engendered by the pursuit of self-interest constrains the exercise of excessive self-interest, and in fact beneficent self-interest leads to both the social good and good social results.[14]

A benevolent Congress, politically responsive federal, state, and local officials, and a relatively affluent society have conferred a wide array of benefits upon an elderly population. A panoply of programs is available to assist the elderly in varying degrees depending upon where they live, what their income is, what their work experience was, the state of their housing, the state of their health, and so on. What is important in the context of autonomy and paternalism is the way in which the elderly gain access to such benefits and entitlements.

Benefits and entitlements in America are not self executing. Whatever economic benefits have been conferred upon us, they have been conferred in a way which typically requires the assertion of a claim to secure it. Whether one speaks of public benefits or private benefits, of a Social Security entitlement or an automobile warranty, to take advantage of the entitlement one must file a claim. Tax refunds, food stamps, nutrition programs, housing assistance, and health care must be affirmatively asserted regardless of whether they are constrained by specific eligibility requirements. Outside the criminal courtroom, entitlements are unlikely to be conferred *sua sponte*.

The claim-based approach to rights is founded on the mythical American: independent and assertive, who stakes out his claim on the prairie, protecting it from marauders and contributing to the public good by pursuing self-interest. Such an approach presumes that individuals have vigor, independence, knowledge, and the resources to pursue those claims to a successful conclusion. It also assumes that society is beneficent and responsive to asserted claims. This approach also assumes that claims not asserted reflect rational affirmative decisions not to do so.

Operationalizing autonomy in this fashion overlooks the constraints on freedom of choice which too often are the lot of elderly people—constraints imposed by frailty, poverty, lack of personal resources, sensory deficits, intellectual deficits, emotional changes, and a coercive living environment. These constraints, even taken together, may not be sufficient to determine incompetency and to permit the assertion thereafter of police powers related to guardianship, conservatorship, and the repeal of personhood in whole or in part.

Furthermore, these constraints on freedom of choice, which are not an infrequent accompaniment of old age, have been reduced to shorthand phrases or terms which substitute for pathological conditions and incorporate negative prejudices and stereotypes into law, rules, and regulations. Negative stereotyping, i.e., the attribution of negative characteristics to older people as a whole, are found frequently in statutes which set forth the standards for determination of incompetency. For example, the Arizona statute states that " 'Incapacited person' means any person who is impaired by reason of . . . advanced age . . . to the extent that he lacks sufficient understanding or capacity to make or communicate responsible decisions concerning his person. . . ."[15] The Indiana code states that an " 'incompetent'. . . is a person who is . . . incapable by reason of . . . senility . . . old age . . . or other incapacity, of either managing his property or caring for himself or both."[16] Old age in these states is equated with mental illness, insanity, imbecility, idiocy, chronic alcoholism, mental deficiency, drug addiction, inebriety, and other similar pathologies.

Still other statutes have had the further effect of excluding the elderly from treatment facilities or programs on the grounds of chronic brain syndrome, often referred to in statutes or regulations as "senility," a pejorative term that connotes weakness of mind, forgetfulness, childishness, and similar characteristics.[17] Legislators seem to have reasoned that the psychic pain and distress brought on by the dementias of late life are unworthy of the attentions of psychiatrists, psychiatric nurses, social workers, or other psychiatric personnel. For example, in Pennsylvania, the Mental Health Procedures Act provides that "senile" persons shall receive mental health treatment "only if they are also diagnosed as mentally ill,"[18] leaving those who suffer from senile dementia of whatever type to shoulder the burden of proving that their psychic pain is the product of a mental disease unrelated to multiple infarcts or Alzheimer's Disease. In other words, those who are old and whose psychological problems stem from a physiological disorder are constrained in their choice and opportunity for mental health treatment, whereas the nonelderly who may suffer from physiologically induced mental disorders (such as psychomotor epilepsy or other pathology of the brain which discloses itself in bizarre behavior) do not need to prove or qualify the etiology of their illness. That this statute was conceived in benevolence to spare those suffering from mild cerebral arteriosclerosis from the horrors of mental hospital back wards does not alter the result. The simple and sad fact is that the law has been used effectively to exclude hundreds of thousands of elderly from both in-patient and out-patient mental health services.

The 1950s and 1960s brought the United States to an unusual point in the development of its notions of autonomy. Occurring at the same time were moral outrage over the disgrace of America's mental hospital back wards, the evolution of legal doctrine culminating in *O'Connor v. Donaldson*.[19] the growth of such medical technologies as the new ataractic drugs, and the development or rediscovery of medico/social technologies concerned with day hospital, out-patient, and community service techniques. These events resulted in radically revised notions about how and where America's mentally ill were to be cared for. These notions were benevolent in their origin, simplistic in their application, and less than fully successful in the achievement of their desired goals and objectives. The deinstitutionalization and transinstitutionalization of America's mentally impaired elderly from its mental hospitals to boarding homes, nursing homes, and streets and alleys of America were grounded in, among other things, our black-and-white notions about competency and incompetency, dependence and independence, and autonomy. Policy makers apparently believed that those who were not incompetent were fully competent and sufficiently powerful to be able to assert their claims.

I do not argue for a return to the monstrous state hospitals of a generation ago—hospitals like Pilgrim State Hospital on Long Island with 13,000 beds, or Manteno State Hospital where 8,000 mentally ill patients were confined on any given day. Rather, it is to suggest that there are no sharp lines between competence and incompetence or, for that matter, autonomous or non-autonomous behavior. What exists is a set of behaviors more common in the late stages of life than in the early ones, that requires interventions to empower the individual and to assist him or her in the assertion of claims and rights. Entitlements ought to be made available *without* being claimed and without being imposed against the will of the individual; instead, they ought to extend and maintain the individuals' ability to act free of internal and external constraints, to deliberate rationally, to act in ways consistent with past behaviors and sedimented values (to use Neveloff-Dubler's happy term),[20] and to act on the basis of moral reflection.

Recognizing the realities of biological, psychological, and social and economic decrement, much of which is inevitable in old age, does not require a conclusion that old age is inevitably accompanied by incompetence. What old age is accompanied by, more often than not, is a diminution of power or a diminution in autonomy. The proper response to diminution of power, however, may not be paternalism, as conventionally conceived.

Paternalism has been defined in terms of two elements: (1) a beneficent (or non-maleficent) motive and intent, and (2) action or non-action to achieve an end contrary to an individual's wishes or desires.[21] Although coercion can be a component in the paternalistic act, it is not essential (as, for example, in cases of withholding information under a therapeutic privilege). In some ways, this definition maintains the myth of the assertive, self-determining person. It does not admit to the problem of the acquiescent, fearful, defeated, apathetic individual caught in the web of circumstance, unwilling or unable to assert himself against a harsh world despite his reasonable orientation to time, place, or person.

In contrast, doctrinaire proponents of autonomy (or critics of paternalism) may, as James Childress points out, "stand back [and] frequently deny . . . any responsibility for what happens to others, sometimes remaining unmoved by the needs of others."[22] Grounded in the notion that rational man prefers life to death, pleasure to pain, knowledge to ignorance, and mastery to slavery, the narrow proponent of autonomy regards the selection of a road taken as the road affirmatively desired.

Winter in Philadelphia confronts us sharply with the dilemma of choosing between conventional paternalism and autonomy. There are in Philadelphia, on any given night, an estimated 2,100 homeless street people, many of whom are old.[23] In cold weather they sleep on grates or prop themselves in doorways or in the entranceways of buildings not far from the federal courthouses and parts of the old city. In early 1985, when the temperature dropped to zero, Mayor Wilson Goode ordered the police in this district to pick up people who seemed to be spending the night outside and to take them to a shelter.[24] If there were protests or if it appeared that the individual was disoriented, he or she was to be brought in, and a proper emergency commitment paper was to be filed. Civil libertarians were understandably nervous about the sweep, but did not intervene. The issue was not that the shelters were inaccessible to the street people nor that the street people did not want to go to the shelters. Rather, the issue was the government's attempt to reach middle ground between autonomy, i.e., the exercise of choice, and paternalism, an action born of beneficent motives and contrary to an individual's wishes or desires. This middle ground needs to be explored but is fraught with ambiguities. For the elderly it is an important one.

Childress's analysis of paternalism in *Who Should Decide* is instructive, and his arguments for limited paternalism deserve our attention. He argues that the principle of respect for persons requires that we adopt a concept of limited paternalism. First, Childress argues that limited paternalism overrides the individual's wishes, preferences, and desires for the good of the patient and because the patient is in some way impaired and cannot act rationally and independently, or cannot articulate an authentic course of action. Therefore, the exercise of limited paternalism requires the rebuttal of the presumption of competence. In addition, limited paternalism requires the probability of harm unless the intervention occurs. It also requires proportionality; that is, the probable benefit to be achieved by the intervention should outweigh the probable harm which would arise as a result of non-intervention. Childress notes that the principle of limited paternalism would require an assessment of the mode of intervention—effectiveness is not enough. In general, the intervention must be the least restrictive, least humiliating, and least insulting to the individual. Finally, Childress argues that limited paternalism would recognize the importance of procedural fairness.[25]

Application of this approach would alter considerably the results that have been reached in protective service cases affecting thousands of elderly persons. For example, in *Vecchione v. Wohlgemuth*,[26] a federal district court decreed that the state could not automatically take Social Security funds from patients, who were institutionalized in mental hospitals and schools for the retarded and who had not been declared incompetent, in order to pay for the cost of their care. The court required that each patient receive a due process hearing before the funds were taken away.[27] Although the state showed careful obedience to the court's order, the Public Interest Law Center of Philadelphia, which was a major objector in the settlement proceedings, has received no reports that alleged incompetents were found competent. To be sure, they *were* found to be incompetent. However, no palpable benefit to the individuals was demonstrated, nor was any consideration given to the nature of the harm that would befall the patients in the event the intervention was not undertaken. This "protective" service, like that provided by the state of New York in the 400–500 cases studied by Alexander and Lewin in their landmark study, *The Aged and Need for Surrogate Management*,[28] provided no benefits to the individuals themselves but did furnish benefits to the Commonwealth and, presumably, its taxpayers. Furthermore, the court considered, but rejected as too novel, a less restrictive, less humiliating, and less insulting alternative, i.e., an effort to provide bona fide agents to the patients to manage funds at their direction and give effect to their desires, wishes and preferences.[29]

Paternalism, when applied to the elderly, is the harshest widespread application of paternalism in our society. For example, in the arena of protective services, the current law relating to incompetency and protective services (the new California Probate Code[30] notwithstanding) continues to be, in John Regan's words, "antiquated . . . repressive . . . [and] basically unchanged. . . ."[30] Properly and eloquently, he scores the failures of those who followed a due process approach toward improvement and failed, as well as the abolitionists who would never intervene against the will or wishes of an individual. Regan suggests a middle-ground approach between the due process advocates whom he characterizes as adopting a " 'minimal intervention' approach to guardianship and adult protective services."[32] He develops a seven-point agenda:

1 The criteria for determining incompetency must be narrowed. . . .

2 Determination of incompetency should be based on client behavior which threatens vital personal interests. Statutory requirements that the source of the disability be identified (such as mental illness or mental defect) should be reconsidered. . . .

3 Determinations of incompetency should be situation-oriented and therefore total guardianship should be abolished and only limited ones permitted. . . .

4 Public guardianship, as an ongoing fiduciary relationship between a public agency and an individual client, should be abolished. Instead, public agencies should be limited to providing services willingly accepted by clients and to seeking court authorization for providing specific services to individual clients in emergencies and high risk situations, but not in the role of a guardian. . . .

5 Basic procedural safeguards for the client must be provided as an essential part of any protective services program. . . .

6 The ethical responsibilities of the social worker toward protective services clients must be better defined. . . .

7 Steps should be taken both by state legislatures and by state and local service agencies to emphasize and promote client control of intervention.[33]

The news from the protective services front is not all bad, however. The widespread adoption of Durable Power of Attorney statutes is a major step forward in the extension of autonomy to periods of incapacity;[34] nevertheless, the probate and surrogate courts have not been sufficient to protect the elderly against protective services.

The second example of the harshness of paternalism applied to the elderly is drawn from the practice of consigning elderly persons to nursing homes. Tonight, approximately 1.2 million elderly persons will go to sleep in America's nursing homes.[35] A conservative estimate is that at least half of them suffer from a seriously dementing illness.[36] There is a wide range of estimates of the numbers of nursing home patients who could reasonably manage in a less restrictive environment. Whether demented or not, few patients entering the nursing home do so under a court order of commitment. In the author's experience, however, for only a tiny proportion does the entry into a nursing home represent an affirmative act comporting with desires, wishes, or preferences, and it is only recently that some jurisdictions have begun to explore less restrictive alternatives.

The consequence of this sort of paternalism, resulting from a near conspiracy of physicians, social workers, the legal profession, medical assistance workers, and mental health professionals to take advantage of the aquiescence of elderly, disabled, and ill individuals in need of long-term care, is the widespread application of a new doctrine, the least *resistive* alternative.

Solutions are not simple. Neither procedural reform providing adversarial due process hearings nor new definitions of eligibility will suffice. What is required is a sweeping approach and methodology grounded in a theory of limited paternalism as expressed by Childress and implemented by Regan's agenda, supplemented by a service system that potentiates and enhances the autonomy of those who may be acquiescent and defeated. Such a system must be consumer-oriented rather than agency-oriented. That is, the system should respect the consumer's values, lifestyle, and, where appropriate, follies. Its motto should be "the ultimate test of liberty is the right to folly." The system must also have the ability to assess disability with some precision and arrive at limited interventions which, wherever possible, should be furnished under the law of agency rather than guardianship, and should be directed by the object of the beneficence. Finally, the system must have available an array of limited interventions, as well as a cadre of agents, who can serve at the direction of their principal and who assist in the assertion of claims.

To achieve this, however, requires careful consideration of the nature of our acts and our behavior in relation to diminished individuals, still competent by any definition and not subject to coercive paternalism, but who, nevertheless, have been subjected to and have acquiesced in substantial reductions in their personhood.

REFERENCES

1 208 U.S. 412 (1908).

2 *Id.* at 421–22.

3 This was the prevailing judicial view until the case of Henningsen v. Bloomfield Motors, 161 A.2d 69 (N.J. 1960).

4 Pub. Res. 11, 74th Cong., 1st Sess., 49 Stat. 115 (1935).

5 18 U.S.C. §§241 *et seq.* 372, 2384 (1976); 28 U.S.C. §§1343. 1443, 1446 (1976); 42 U.S.C. §§1981 *et seq.*, (1976).

6 U.S. Const. amend. I–V. XIII–XV, XIX, XXI (repeal of prohibition). XXIV, XXVI (lowered voting age).

7 Horstman, P., *Protective Services for the Elderly: The Limits of Parens Patriae,* Missouri Law Review 40(2): 215 (Spring 1975); Regan, J., *Protecting the Elderly: The New Paternalism,* Hastings Law Journal 32(5): IIII (May 1981).

8 Cal. Probate Code §§1801, 1827.5, 1828.5 (1984).

9 387 U.S. 1 (1966).

10 442 U.S. 584 (1979).

11 J.F. Childress, Who Should Decide? Paternalism in Health Care (Oxford University Press, New York, N.Y.) (1982).

12 *Id.* at 61–66.

13 *See* M. Friedman, R. Friedman, Free to Choose (Harcourt Brace Jovanovich, New York, N.Y.) (1980).

14 I am inclined to agree with Frederick Jackson Turner, who suggested that much of the American character and our political and social styles were created by our historical proximity to a frontier which offered free land and apparent unbounded opportunity up until the end of the last century. Turner, F.J., *The Significance of the American Frontier in American History,* in Proceedings of the Historical Society of Wisconsin (Madison, Wis.) (1894). *See also* F.J. Turner, The Frontier in American Society (H. Holt and Co., New York, N.Y.) (1920).

15 Ariz. Rev. Stat. Ann. §4-5101 (1975).

16 Ind. Code Ann. §29-1-18-1(C) (2) (West 1979).

17 *See, e.g.,* S.C. Code §43-29-10(4) (definitions). *But see* Md. Ann. Code, Health Gen. §10-609(d), which requires for all persons 65 and over subjected to involuntary commitment proceedings a special evaluation by a geriatric evaluation team to identify the least restrictive alternative available, *and* Mont. Code Ann. §53-21-102(14) which incorporates for commitments of elderly people the standard of "danger to self or others."

18 Pa. Stat. Ann., tit. 50, §7101 (Purdon 1985).

19 422 U.S. 563 (1975).

20 Neveloff-Dubler, N., Outline distributed at conference, Legal & Ethical Aspects of Health Care for the Elderly (sponsored by the American Society of Law & Medicine, Washington, D.C.) (1983).

21 Childress, *supra* note 10, at 12–13.

22 *Id.* at ix.

23 Report of the Mayor's Public-Private Task Force on Homelessness—1984–85, Philadelphia, Pennsylvania, at 7.

24 *Police Transport the Homeless in Freezing Weather,* Adult Protective Services Network News, iss. 13, p. 1 (Spring 1985).

25 *See* Childress, *supra* note 1, at 102–23.

26 377 F. Supp. 1361 (E.D. Pa. 1974), *cert. denied,* 434 U.S. 943 (1977).

27 377 F. Supp. at 1370.

28 G. Alexander. T. Lewin, The Aged and the Need for Surrogate Management (Syracuse University Press, Syracuse, N.Y.) (1972).

29 *See* Vecchione v. Wohlgemuth, slip opinion at 23 (E.D.Pa June 30, 1978) (Becker, J.) (unpublished opinion given after settlement hearing).

30 Cal. Probate Code §§1801-1911 (1984).

31 Regan, J., *Adult Protective Services: An Appraisal and a Prospectus*, in National Law and Social Work Seminar: Proceedings and Prospects (University of Southern Maine, Portland, Me.) (1982).

32 *Id.* at 14.

33 *Id.* at 15–18.

34 *State Statutory References that Recognize the Durable Power of Attorney*, in E. Cohen, Durable Power of Attorney: an Important Alternative to Guardianship, Conservatorship, or Trusteeship (Temple University Long Term Care Gerontology Center, Philadelphi, Pa.) (1984) at app. B.

35 U.S. Senate Special Committee on Aging, Developments in Aging: 1983 (U.S. Gov't Printing Office, Washington, D.C.) (1984).

36 Office of Technology Assessment, Congress of the U.S. *Selected Chronic Conditions Technology and Biomedical Research*, in Technology and Aging in America (U.S. Gov't Printing Office, Washington, D.C.) (1985).

THE "RIGHT" NOT TO KNOW

David E. Ost

ABSTRACT. There is a common view in medical ethics that the patient's right to be informed entails, as well, a correlative right not to be informed, i.e., to waive one's right to information. This paper argues, from a consideration of the concept of autonomy as the foundation for rights, that there can be no such 'right' to refuse relevant information, and that the claims for such a right are inconsistent with both deontological and utilitarian ethics. Further, the right to be informed is shown to be a mandatory right (though not a welfare right); persons are thus seen to have both a right and a duty to be informed. Finally, the consequences of this view are addressed: since the way in which we conceptualize our problems tends to determine the actions we take to resolve them, it is important properly to conceptualize patients' requests not to be informed. There may be many reasons for acting in accord with such a request, but it is a mistake to conceptualize one's act as 'respecting a right possessed by persons.'

There is a widely-held view in medical ethics that the right of the patient to give informed consent to treatment carries with it at least two important corollaries: the first is the right to refuse treatment, since, without this right, consent would be meaningless; the second is the right to refuse information, inasmuch as the patient's right to be informed would seem to entail the possibility of his waiving that right. Thus, in their book, Tom L. Beauchamp and James F. Childress

From *The Journal of Medicine and Philosophy*, vol. 9, no. 3 (August 1984), pp. 301–312. © 1984 by D. Reidel Publishing Company, Dondrect, Holland. Reprinted by permission.

consider the question of information-waivers and offer the following hypothetical case:

> For example, if a deeply committed Jehovah's Witness were to inform a doctor that he wishes to have everything possible done for him, but does not want to know if transfusions or similar procedures would be employed, it is hard to imagine a moral argument to the conclusion that he must be told. (Beauchamp and Childress, 1979, p. 79).[1]

The suggestion seems to be that, inasmuch as the right to be informed flows from the individual's status as an autonomous moral agent, so, too, does a right *not* to be informed. Since the health professional is obliged, in virtue of the 'contractual relationship' between them, to respect the patient's autonomy, pressing unwanted information upon that patient constitutes a prima facie violation of that patient's autonomy.

Interestingly, Robert M. Veatch (1972), who is a strong advocate of the contractual conception of the physician/patient relationship, holds a view which seems to deny the patient a right not to be informed:

> It is possible to grant that the principle of patient freedom would be sufficient to restrain a physician from imposing unwanted bad news upon such a patient and yet hold that human dignity requires responsible decision making by individuals especially about matters of such ultimate significance as life and death . . . there may still be a moral duty to know one's self and one's fate (Veatch, 1976, p. 247).[2]

The apparent opposition between these views, however, is complicated, for Veatch has elsewhere maintained that, where a research subject declines further information, such information ought not to be imposed (Veatch, 1978). And Beauchamp and Childress, in the same work in which they seem to accept the patient's right to waive information, also argue that

> when a patient's or subject's autonomy is clearly limited by his own ignorance, as in the case of false belief, it may be legitimate to promote autonomy by attempting to impose the information (Beauchamp and Childress, p. 80).

Thus, Veatch seems to hold that, while a patient does not have a right to refuse information—and may even have a *duty* to accept it—a physician would be unjustified in attempting to impose that information on the patient. Beauchamp and Childress seem to hold that the patient has the right (at least a prima facie one) to refuse information, but that physicians are sometimes justified in violating that right in order to 'promote' patient autonomy. The implications ingredient in these positions are at least odd: for Veatch, the physician is obliged to respect an autonomous patient's assertion of a right, where no such right exists; for Beauchamp and Childress, the physician is not obliged to respect an autonomous patient's assertion of a right, where that right does exist, in order to enhance that patient's autonomy.[3]

I shall, in this paper, argue that Veatch is fundamentally correct: that there is not, nor can there be, a *right* not to be informed; that the recognition of such a right is seriously damaging to a coherent theory of ethical agency; and further, I shall suggest why I think that patients have an obligation to be informed. Finally, I shall assess the impact of such a view on the physician/patient relationship.

AUTONOMY, RIGHTS, AND RATIONALITY

The fundamental question addressed in the issue of refusal of information is whether or not the autonomy of the individual is violated by acting against his expressed desire not to be informed. Resolving this question requires a closer look at our concept of autonomy.

In purely formal terms, autonomy is that quality of entities which establishes them as *persons* (Kant, 1785, p. 45), i.e., bearers of rights and duties. Historically, the kind of content given to this formal characterization has been based on the traditional theological formulation of the concept of a soul: an entity possessed of intellect (*ratio*) and will (*voluntas*). Kant, for example, describes such a *person* as a *rational, free* agent; only such an agent can bear the burden of responsibility that morality requires. Similarly, in considering the question "Whether there is anything voluntary in irrational animals?" Thomas Aquinas notes:

> [I]t is essential to the voluntary act that its principle be within the agent, together with some knowledge of the end. . . . Perfect knowledge of the end consists not only in apprehending the thing which is the end, but also in knowing it under the aspect of end, and the relationship of the means to that end. And such knowledge belongs only to the rational nature (Aquinas, p. 646).

Thomas's observation is an articulation of two basic components in the concept of autonomy: rationality and freedom of the will. The act of an individual whose will is constrained or unfree is not, on this description, autonomous, insofar as the principle of the act is not internal to the agent; and the act of an individual who is irrational is not autonomous insofar as he knows not what he does.

There is, however, a tension between rationality and freedom, a tension which becomes evident when each of these principles is taken to its ultimate level. The common view among medieval theologians, for example, with respect to God's freedom of will was that God can do anything that can be done. He could not, then, will to create a being greater than Himself, or to square a circle, etc. In other words, God's freedom of will was constrained by the laws of reason, insofar as He could will only what was logically possible to be willed. Some late medieval and Reformation theologians, rebelling against any a priori constraint against God's freedom, gave His freedom ultimate primacy and made the laws of reason contingent upon it. The laws of logical possibility are themselves, on this view, dictated by such a supreme being, and thus they could have been otherwise, although, as subject to a universe in which they apply, man may be unable to conceive of a universe in which they do not apply, or in which a different set of such laws applies.[4] In the first case, God's will is rational, but not ultimately free; in the second, it is free, but not ultimately rational (i.e., it has no ground of determination).

What is true at the ultimate level is also true at the finite, human level; we sometimes emphasize one dimension of autonomy over against the other. Thus, libertarians like J. S. Mill emphasize liberty, freedom from external constraint, as autonomy in the primary sense, while others, like Kant, emphasize freedom from internal constraint (i.e., freedom *to be* rational) and minimize the factor of external constraint—though there is in each, to be sure, a strain of the other.

These differing emphases show up in the contrasting views presented in the first section of this paper. The following similarity between them should be noted: both positions agree that the freedom condition of autonomy prevents the physicians from imposing unwanted information on the patient, externally coercing him to accept it—we shall return to this point later. Our question, however, is not yet about the physician, but rather about the patient himself: does he have the *right* to refuse information?

If we can show that refusal of information is irrational, we will have shown that there is no such right. For if such refusal is irrational, and irrationality is an autonomy-defeating condition, and autonomy is the basis of rights, then to refuse information is *ipso facto* to claim that one is not autonomous, i.e., not a *bearer* of rights.

Before going any further, I should note the limits of this argument, lest the next poor individual who asserts that he has a "right not to know" be summarily treated as if he were irrational and non-autonomous. Human beings do many irrational, even self-contradictory things, and we would feel uncomfortable— not to mention threatened—if we advocated denying them their moral or political freedom on these grounds. It is the *recognition* of the right which is incoherent, not the assertion of it (which may be misguided rhetoric), nor action in accord with the assertion (which may have many motives other than obligation to respect a right). Rights-talk here—as in many other contexts in which it is promiscuously used—is inappropriate. To recognize a *right* not to know is to assert that a right is borne by a non-right holder. This argument holds, as I've said, if we can establish that refusal of relevant information is indeed irrational.

THE IRRATIONALITY OF INFORMATION WAIVERS

In a famous passage in his essay 'On liberty,' John Stuart Mill presents us with a case of what has come to be known as 'justified paternalism'—a legitimate interference with the liberty of another individual in his own best interest. Suppose we were to come upon a man who was about to cross a bridge which we knew to be structurally unsound, so that, in our best estimation, his attempt to cross it could place his life in jeopardy. We are justified, Mill thinks, in infringing upon his liberty—but only for as long as it takes to provide a warning to him. Once he has been warned, we may not legitimately interfere further, for "no one but the person himself can judge of the sufficiency of the motive which may prompt him to incur the risk" (Mill, 1859, p.1025).

There are some things we need to notice about Mill's example. First, we should notice that we are justified—surprisingly, for Mill—in violating the liberty of another in order to assure *ourselves* that he is, in fact, acting autonomously. If we were to extend Mill's example, we might note that, should the man involved prove to be deaf, or otherwise incapable of comprehending our warning (or of giving a response which satisfies us), we would presumably be justified in a fairly lengthy restraint of his liberty. It is not the autonomy of the man's act which is genuinely in question, but rather our assurance that it is in fact autonomous which figures in this justification.

Second, we should observe that our infringement of the bridge-walker's liberty has the purpose of (1) ascertaining whether or not he possesses certain relevant information: and (2) to impart that information if it is unknown to him. The implication is that our interference is warranted because the sort of information we possess is the sort of information which would be relevant to a rational appraisal of the act of walking across the bridge.

It is, I think, clear that what counts as relevant information is determined by what counts as 'rational appraisal.' In part, medical ethicists—and lawyers— have addressed this issue by means of a conception of a 'reasonable man'—that is, the relevant information is the sort of information that a reasonable man would require in order to make a sound decision. But the information that a 'reasonable man' would require is heavily a culturally-dependent standard; dependent upon the conceptual framework of the society and the amount of information available to be imparted. Perhaps we would do best to leave this problem alone; and we may do so, I think, inasmuch as our topic is the *refusal* of information, not dispute as to its relevance.

Suppose, then, our bridge-walker were to stop us short with a statement such as: "I don't want to hear your information; no information you could possibly impart to me would be relevant to my decision to cross this bridge." Such a statement is, I think, equivalent to that of the patient who refuses information about his diagnosis and treatment alternatives and puts himself, wholly and ignorantly, into the hands of his physician.

Now, I submit that there are only two grounds for a statement of this sort— and *both* of them are irrational. First, the individual's intentions may be so fixed and unalterable that no information would, in fact, be relevant to them. But this is almost a textbook definition of an obsession. If *no* information is relevant, then the decision can have no rational grounds of determination, i.e., it is irrational. Second, the individual may be claiming to know what he *cannot* know prior to your disclosure of the information; namely, his evaluation of its relevance to his decision. But to claim to know what you cannot know is contradictory, i.e., irrational.

One need not have a full-blown and comprehensive definition of rationality to conclude that a decision which refuses to admit any information as relevant is a decision which has no rational grounds of determination. Thus, the refusal of information is irrational, and this, as we noted earlier, is sufficient to show that there can be no *right* to refuse information. The further question remains: is there a *duty* to receive information?

THE DUTY TO BE INFORMED

Clearly, if there is, as Veatch suggests, a *duty* to receive information, then a right to refuse it is incoherent. One might argue that receiving such information is not an absolute duty; as is the case with other duties, we may admit excusing conditions as justifications relieving one of one's duty. But excusing conditions do not establish *rights*. The point that I wish to establish is that the right to be informed, in the doctrine of informed consent, is a mandatory right—i.e., it is not an option right which one may or may not exercise; rather, it is a right which we are *obliged* to exercise.

The concept of mandatory rights is often assimilated to that of positive welfare rights. As Joel Feinberg has noted,

> the performance of the duty is presumed to be so beneficial to the person whose duty it is that he can *claim* the necessary means from the state and noninterference from others as *his* due. Its character as claim is precisely what his half-liberty shares with the more usual (discretionary) rights and what warrants his use of the word 'right' in demanding it (Feinberg, 1978, p. 34).

I want to argue that the right to be informed is a mandatory right, but not that it is a welfare right; rather, its mandatory quality is bound up with the concept of an autonomous agent itself.

The problematic feature of the claim that receiving information is a duty is that it runs squarely against the question: If there is a duty to accept relevant information, to whom would such a duty be owed? The hypothetical case presented by Veatch stipulates that the patient is a bachelor with no family ties; the welfare of others is not at issue; and no one will benefit by the patient's being informed, not even the patient himself. There would seem to be only two possible candidates to whom such a duty could be owed: to humanity at large, or to the patient himself. Given John Stuart Mill's arguments against the restriction of liberty in the case of self-regarding conduct, and given the serious questions which can be raised against Kant's claim that there is a 'duty to oneself,' Veatch's suggestion—it is hardly an argument—seems, on its face, implausible at best. I hope to make it rather more plausible.

Where the patients involved are not autonomous agents, capable of making their own decisions, the doctrine of informed consent requires that proxy consent must be given in any treatment decision. Take the case of children, for example: children are not regarded as rational, insofar as their wills are conceived to be constrained by an inability to control their own desires and subordinate them to rational ends. It thus becomes appropriate for proxy decision makers to evaluate the relevant information and to decide what course to pursue on behalf of these children.

Normally, the task of proxy decision making falls to the child's parents, who may then be said to have both a right and a duty to give informed consent to treatment of their child. Parents who simply refused information that was relevant to assessing the possible risks and benefits of alternative courses of treatment are parents who would be violating their obligations as proxy decision makers. We need to consider the following set of possible actions:

1 Parents might refuse relevant information, yet make the decision, in which case they would be failing in their obligation to act in the best interest of their charge.

2 Parents might refuse relevant information *and* refuse to make the decision, leaving it in the hands of the physician, in which case they violate their obligation to *be* proxy decision makers.

3 Parents might accept relevant information, and leave the decision in the hands of the physician. To do this is not to avoid a decision, but to make one—namely, that given the relevant information, the best decision is to delegate decision making authority. That is, they have decided not to rule out any alternative courses of action.

This example illustrates the possibility that receiving information may be both a right *and* a duty. But the case we have been discussing is not a case of proxy consent, in which it might be argued that the obligation in question is owed to one's child, and is actually a welfare right. Rather, ours is a case of what Mill would call self-regarding conduct. By stipulation, no obligation of care is owed to another, and thus no obligation of this sort is violated by a refusal of information.

But self-regarding conduct, even for Mill, has limits. He argues quite straightforwardly that one's liberty, even in self-regarding matters, cannot include the liberty to sell oneself into slavery. Mill has a good deal to say—most of it unconvincing, as his commentators have noted—about why this particular instance of self-regarding conduct should not be permissible: "It is not freedom," Mill contends, "to be allowed to alienate his freedom" (Mill, 1859, p. 1031). Part of Mill's problem in making this argument stick is the conceptual emphasis he adopts in viewing liberty primarily as an autonomous agent's freedom from external coercion.

This problem is a direct result of the systematic ambiguity and internal tension, noted earlier, of the concept of autonomy as it is customarily deployed. On the one hand, we use it to refer to the exercise or expression of autonomy: we're inclined to say that X is autonomous if he is free from external coercion, and we seek to guarantee this sense of 'autonomy' by legislation. Hence, in the doctrine of informed consent, we have a right not to be coerced into a course of action which we have not autonomously chosen.

On the other hand, we use the concept of autonomy to designate a moral status which justifies the predication of rights and duties. This *status* is unaffected by any number of external constraints placed upon a person's *actions*. A person gagged and rendered immobile does not, in virtue of that fact, lose his *status* as an autonomous agent. Further, we would not regard a person's avowed 'surrender' of his status as a moral agent as sufficient cause for releasing him from his moral obligations; he retains these obligations insofar as he retains their foundation: his status as a rational, free agent. Similarly, however many of his rights a person may waive, he cannot waive the foundation of those rights, which is, again, his status as a rational, free agent. We may surrender our rights to many autonomous *actions*, but we can never surrender our status as autonomous agents. It is this sort of consideration, I suspect, which underlies Mill's prohibition against selling oneself into slavery.

Autonomy as an inalienable status, then, would seem to entail an obligation to *be* autonomous, inasmuch as one may be held morally 'to account' despite one's efforts to be non-autonomous. One does not have a 'right' to be autonomous, which one may then waive; rather one simply *is* autonomous, inescapably, and efforts to escape one's autonomous status are foredoomed to conceptual failure. Being autonomous is, in this sense, *mandatory*.

If autonomy includes rationality, then one's efforts to act irrationally are violations of one's autonomy. If one's refusal of information is irrational, then this refusal is a violation of the mandatory character of autonomy, even where that refusal is self-regarding. Thus, we can say that the right of informed consent is a mandatory right, and that receiving information about one's diagnosis, alternative treatments, etc., is both a right *and* a duty.

CONCLUSION

What, concretely, does all this mean? Does it mean that when a patient refuses information about his diagnosis and treatment options, we ought to grab him by the front of his hospital gown, hoist him half off his bed, and say something like: "Listen, fellow, you've got an obligation to be informed, whether you like it or not?" Clearly not.

The question of refusal of information is an important one in medical ethics because it brings into direct confrontation two value-orientations which are often conflated in ordinary experience: the humane and the humanistic. When we act humanely, we act in such a way as to minimize the pain, harm, or discomfort which inheres in a particular situation as a result of the human condition which we all share. Thus, for example, we act humanely when we accede to a patient's request for a stronger tranquilizer when he is having trouble coping with his levels of anxiety and stress. Humanistic values, by contrast, are demanding ones, for they project for us an ideal of what human actions and choices ought to be: free, self-determining, responsible. Thus, we act humanistically when we accede to a patient's request to step down his tranquilizer dosages in order to learn to cope better, without medication, with his anxiety levels, even though we know the price he will initially pay in terms of increased anxiety and tension. Humane acts have compassion as their underlying motive; humanistic ones, respect.

I do not mean to suggest that these two value-orientations are diametrically opposed, but only that they are different. Nor do I mean to say that one cannot reconcile conflicts between them, for we do that every day. I do mean, however, that we ought not to confuse one with the other.

A physician who does not tell his patient of a diagnosis of terminal cancer because he does not want to inflict the pain of that information acts humanely, but not humanistically. A physician who recognizes his patient's right to know, but who imparts that information bluntly and callously acts humanistically, but not humanely.

One of the foundational principles of medicine is, of course, *"primum non nocere,"* a principle which adumbrates an ethic of humaneness. In the case of refusal of information, one might be led on humane grounds, knowing the kinds of internal conflict and suffering the patient faces, simply to honor that request. If one conceptualizes this act as a case of respecting a patient's right not to be informed, one may be inclined to honor this request, and do no more. But if the aim of medicine is, as I think it is (though I will not try to defend this view here), to assist patients to achieve the optimal level of autonomy possible to them, then simply 'doing no more' is insufficient. Underlying medicine is another, humanistic value-orientation which calls upon the physician to do what he can to help the patient make autonomous decisions. What the physician does will be tempered by the principle of humaneness, but its ultimate aim is humanistic. It is an insight of this sort, I suspect, that leads Beauchamp and Childress to the conclusion that it is sometimes permissible to violate the patient's autonomy (in the sense of freedom from external coercion) in order to promote autonomy.

NOTES

1 On the contrary, one can easily imagine such a moral argument, since Jehovah's Witnesses hold that acquiescence to treatment which may include transfusion constitutes acquiescence to the transfusion, and that intentional ignorance of whether or not transfusion is to be used does not relieve one of moral guilt. In short, a minister might well point out that claiming the status of "committed Jehovah's Witness" is inconsistent with claiming a right not to know if transfusion is to be used, and that Witnesses are thus obliged to be informed if possible.

2 It is worth noting, here, that Veatch (1976) is *not* claiming that patients have both a duty to know and a right not to know about themselves and their fate, which would be an incoherent claim. Rather, the physician is restrained from imposing information by the principle of patient freedom, an operational principle of medical practice, *not* by a moral obligation to respect a patient's 'right' not to know.

3 It might be objected that Beauchamp and Childress stipulate that the patient's autonomy is already limited by ignorance, and thus that they are not discussing an autonomous patient's right not to know. But this begs the question. To assert that a patient has a right not to know is to assert that the patient has a *right* to his ignorance, a right which would be violated by the attempt to impose information. Ignorance, then, could not be a defeating condition for autonomous choice. One cannot, it should be noted, have it both ways: in their earlier Jehovah's Witness example, Beauchamp and Childress present us with a patient whose autonomy is "clearly limited by his own ignorance, as in the case of false belief" concerning the requirements of the religious doctrine to which he subscribes. On this view, this alone should constitute a moral argument to the conclusion that he must be told.

4 See, for example, Martin Luther (1500).

REFERENCES

Aquinas, T.: 1265–1273, *Summa Theologica* II–I, Q. 6, A. 2, *Respondeo*, trans. Fathers of the English Dominican Province, Encyclopedia Britannica, Inc., Chicago, 1952.

Beauchamp, T. L. and J. F. Childress: 1979, *Principles of Biomedical Ethics*, Oxford University Press, Oxford.

Feinberg, J.: 1978, 'A postscript to the nature and value of rights,' in Elsie L. Bandman and Bertram Bandman (eds.), *Bioethics and Human Rights*, Little, Brown and Co., Boston, 32–34.

Kant, I.: 1785, *Fundamental Principles of the Metaphysic of Morals*, trans. Thomas K. Abbott, Bobbs-Merrill, Indianapolis, 1949.

Luther, M.: 1500, 'The bondage of the will,' in J. Dillenberger (ed.), *Martin Luther*, Anchor Books, Garden City, New York (1961), 166–203.

Mill, J. S.: 1859, 'On liberty,' in Edwin A. Burtt (ed.), *The English Philosophers from Bacon to Mill*, Modern Library, New York, Modern Library, New York, 1939, 949–1041.

Veatch, R. M.: 1972, 'Models for ethical medicine in a revolutionary age,' *Hastings Center Report* 2 (June, 1972), 5–7.

Veatch, R. M.: 1976, *Death, Dying, and the Biological Revolution: Our Last Quest for Responsibility*, Yale University Press, New Haven.

Veatch, R. M.: 1978. 'Three theories of informed consent: philosophical foundations and policy implications,' in the National Commission for the Protection of Human Subjects of Biomedical and Behavioral Research, *The Belmont Report*, Appendix, Vol. 2, (DHEW Publication No. 78-0014), Washington, D.C., 26–33.

ALLOCATING AUTONOMY: CAN PATIENTS AND PRACTITIONERS SHARE?

Sally Gadow

On the surface, conflicts between professional authority and patient autonomy seem almost obsolete. After great expenditure of federal funds and local time, health care is becoming so humanized and patients so educated that—instead of meeting each other halfway—they have all but exchanged places. As professionals become increasingly human and patients increasingly professional, little turf remains that belongs exclusively to one or the other. Health care would seem to be well on its way to a situation of "shared autonomy."

A closer look, however, suggests othewise. Neither consumers nor providers are well on the way to sharing autonomy, in spite of appearances. At the policy level, physicians retain exclusive control, for example, of patients' use of prescription drugs, while patients, from their side of the fence, litigate increasing control over physicians. At the clinical level, practitioners anguish over patient's noncompliance, while patients study texts such as *How to Manage Your Doctor*. The very concept of noncompliance betrays the professional's concern about patient autonomy, and the growing movement in patient assertiveness suggests the patient's view of professional autonomy.

It is my premise that the issue of who should control whom in health care is a function of a specific philosophy, namely, that in which the autonomy of one party is assumed; that of the other suspended. However, since this familiar view

Reprinted with permission from Nora K. Bell, ed., *Who Decides? Conflicts of Rights in Health Care*, pp. 95–106. © 1982 by Humana Press, Inc.

of medicine, fondly termed paternalism, already has been soundly thrashed by its critics, I shall direct my discussion to an alternative philosophy.[1]

A radical reconceptualization of health care is called for if we are to extricate ourselves from the assert-and-counterassert struggle. Wresting power from the provider and transferring it to the consumer may achieve cooperation, but, as every child on the playground learns, cooperation that is achieved by force will always depend upon who happens at the moment to be stronger, not who is "in the right." For pragmatic reasons, then, if not for ethical ones, professional autonomy ought not be "taken by force," stormed like a citadel in order that the consumer's flag finally be raised over the smoking ruins. What is called for instead (unfortunately, for those interested in a quick coup, is a complete philosophical reorientation of the health professions.

SELF-CARE PHILOSOPHY

Nothing less than a new philosophy of health care is required. The view that I shall develop and defend here is a view that can be called the self-care philosophy of health care.

First, a word of caution against a possible confusion. "Self-care" is a term usually met in the context of the lay revolt against professional care. Viewed in that way, it is no more than a guerilla tactic in the attempted overthrow of medicine. It is billed as an *alternative to* professional care *rather than a philosophy of* professional health care.[2]

What is meant by self-care as a *philosophy* of health care? Specifically, how does such a philosophy advance us beyond the struggle for control between patients and practitioners?

The view of self-care I am proposing is this: that professional health care have as its purpose a positive assistance to individuals in the development and exercise of their autonomy in health matters. Self-care, as I am using the term, refers to actions personally selected and initiated, and thus freely performed by an individual in the interest of promoting that person's health as he or she construes it.

Two assumptions are crucial here. The first, which I shall not elaborate, is that self-care is an essential expression of individual freedom. Consequently, it is an aspect of human existence that, ethically speaking, ought to be enhanced. The second assumption is that self-care must express the individual's uncoerced self-determination if it be care that is, in truth, personally initiated and freely performed.

Clearly, "self-care" in this sense means much more than is usually meant by the term. On this view, self-care does not make the patient a "physician extender." That is, self-care is not carrying out the doctor's orders at home. But neither does it make the clinician irrelevant. That is, self-care is not a form of "alternative health care" that uses the professional—if at all—strictly as a consumer's guide.

What then *is* the place of the professional on this view? The concept of self-care that I am proposing involves two dimensions, and in both of these the professional provides a necessary assistance. These dimensions we can distinguish as *action* and *agency*. Self-care *action* is the health behavior that is performed. Self-care *agency* is the process of self-determination, the decision making with respect to the choice of behaviors and, more fundamental still, the determination of an individual's own values and concept of health upon which to base health care decisions. For all health behavior that has not become automatic, conscious choice necessarily is involved, a decision must be made. That decision is not "Can I do it?" but "Shall I choose to do it? Does the behavior represent a value for me? Does it facilitate my health as I understand it?" The conscious addressing and answering of that basic question about personal health and values is the exercise of self care *agency*, the process of self-determination.

Health practitioners have long been familiar with patients' needs involving self-care action, for example, in chronic illness and rehabilitation. Needs involving agency are not as familiar, especially since many professionals assume that agency is so impaired in illness that heroic measures are always indicated, namely, the substitution of professional authority for patient decisions. Within the self-care framework, however, self-determination is central. Coerced, enforced, or directed health behaviors may be conducive to health (professionally defined), but they *are not self-care actions* because they *do not originate in self-care agency*, that is, in the patient's own free decision.

Two forms of agency can be distinguished in self-care: one, the exercise of moral autonomy; the other, the formulation of clinical judgment. I shall argue that they are finally inseparable in self-care.

SELF-CARE AGENCY: MORAL AUTONOMY

The philosophy I am describing involves the obligation that professionals assist patients with agency as well as action. This means that, while practitioners are obligated to act in their patients' best interest (as they are in any philosophy of health care), here it is the patient and not the professional who decides what "best interest" shall mean. This is not only morally entailed by the self-care philosophy. It is also required by the fact that "best interest" for a patient—that is, patient self-interest—cannot be professionally defined. A definition of self-interest, or patient's best interest, that is determined by anyone other than the patient is not only unethical on this view, but in fact impossible.

Exactly what is the difficulty in ascertaining for a patient the course of action that is in that person's best interest? Is not that very determination the essence of health care?

Some of the difficulties in determining "best interest" for patients are by now familiar. The difficulty of defining "health" has been widely discussed.[3] As a result, although we have not yet reached the point of complete relativism, we at least acknowledge multiple levels on which to meaningfully define health and illness, from the molecular to the political. But that diversity among concepts of health is only part of the difficulty in determining the self-interest of patients. The other difficulty is that the concept of "self" is as elusive as that of health. To illustrate, there are at least three dimensions that must be examined in determining one's own best interest and thereby (subjectively) defining the self. These dimensions are the inner complexity, the outer boundaries, and the uniqueness of the self.

Complexity

For what *part* of the self should one care? The psychological? Intellectual? Physical? Spiritual? Seen from the outside, the self may seem to be a simple unit. In reality, it can be dismayingly complex, in spite of personal and professional efforts to subdue dissident elements. Consequently, certain aspects of the self may receive care at the expense of other parts. A decision that seems to ignore health needs may be a reasoned choice to care for the part of the self that the individual values most. A woman may sustain an "unhealthy" drug dependence in order to have available all of her energy for dealing with an overwhelming grief. She chooses to care for the part of the self that is suffering and in effect may be using the drug as a responsible form of self-care. The objection will arise that this is not true self-care, but is, at best, misguided; at worst, irresponsible or abusive. But a health care philosophy cannot have it both ways. Either a decision is valid because it is based upon self-determination and represents the individual's own definition of self and self-care, even if that definition conflicts with objectively established standards. Or, objective norms are imposed as the appropriate standard of care, in which case, health care is based not upon a philosophy of self-care, but upon the tradition of normative care.

Boundaries

A second difficulty in defining self-interest, in addition to the inner complexity of the self, is the extensiveness of the self. Is a human being essentially a free-standing, atomic entity, a self-contained unit? Or, does the individual exist primarily in relation to others? If the latter is the case—as it is whenever we choose to define ourselves through our relationships—then self-care would be an attending to the union rather than the individual, the "we" rather than the "I." Thus, a father might choose to give up a valued position in order to spend the first years of his child's life developing a close relationship with the child. He chooses to live essentially in a union with another person rather than as an independent entity, at least for a time. He has not chosen to sacrifice his own interests to those of the child. Instead, he regards the child and himself not as two self-contained individuals (who would in that case indeed have competing interests), but as a union.

Uniqueness

A third difficulty with any objective definition of self and self-care is that not only is the self complex and at times wider than a solitary individual, but it is unique. The fundamental health needs that self-care addresses may be universal, but they are perceived and understood in (often vastly) different ways by individuals. Therefore, no universal standard of self-care is applicable. Any generalization compromises uniqueness, since it assumes that individuals are more alike than different, that is, that uniqueness is not a central, but a peripheral feature of human experience. That assumption has merit, of course, if we are concerned with establishing general norms of health conduct and achieving compliance by imposing those norms upon persons. But the adoption of health behaviors by an individual in compliance with standards governing *persons in general* does not constitute *self*-care. The basis of self-care is self-determination, freely exercised choice expressing the individual understanding and values of the patient rather than the normative expectations of health authorities. Paternalism, the coercing or forcing of persons to act in their (externally and generally defined) best interest, is therefore—to repeat an earlier point—not only morally, but logically impossible on this view. Because each self is unique, a decision about the best interest of an individual cannot be made by anyone except that individual.

The uniqueness of the self is especially significant in relation to persons who, we readily admit, differ from the "normal", but who—for that very reason—are allowed *less* self-determination than other persons. I alluded to this issue when I observed above that many practitioners feel that the need for assistance in one's health care is tantamount to the need for professional decision-making. According to that belief, the greater the health need, as in severe injury or life-threatening illness, the greater the justification for substituting professional judgment for patient self-determination. In extreme situations, of course, patient decision-making is often impossible because of uncontrolled pain, unconsciousness, disorientation, lack of information, or other reasons. But in non-acute situations the reasons are not as clear, that is, in cases of chronic physical, psychological, or intellectual handicap, early childhood, advanced age, and so on. Persons in all of these situations deviate so far from "normal" self-care capacity that we have even developed clinical specialities to address their needs. Yet, for persons in these very groups, we seem to know less rather than more about their distinctive self-care needs, in particular, their need for assistance with self-care *agency*. It does not seem an exaggeration to say that the more unmistakably unique and nongeneralizable a situation is, such as the self-care of a multiply handicapped child, the more likely we are to tailor our assistance to general standards rather than to decisions arising out of the uniqueness of the individual.

It must be acknowledged that for many reasons, including limited resources, self-determination cannot be fostered in certain complicated situations. There, the external approach must be taken if health in any sense is to be maintained. However, it should be clear that in those cases, and even in cases in which patients willingly practice the behaviors prescribed, self-care has not yet been achieved. Patients who have been taught only to observe *standard* health care practices have not yet been helped to practice self-care, that is, care based upon *individual agency*.

The question now must be addressed, how does the professional assist patients in the exercise of self-care agency? That assistance involves the professional in helping individuals become clear about what they want to do, by helping them clarify their values and beliefs in the situation and, on the basis of that clarification, to reach *decisions that express their understanding* of themselves and the situation. That assistance is needed because clarification can be the most difficult exactly when it is the most urgent, when a situation arises that calls into question beliefs and values that are often the most deeply embedded in the person's life, and thus perhaps are the least defined or developed.

The role of the professional in self-care then is not merely to *protect* patients' freedom of self-determination against institutional encroachments, inadequate information, or professional prejudices. It is far more than that. It is *active assistance* to individuals in their exercise of self-determination. It entails participating with patients in discussion that has as its mutually agreed upon purpose the discernment of the patient's view and values and the examination of health care options in the light of those.

In the self-care framework, a practitioner is not relieved of ethical deliberation simply because it has been ascertained that the patient "owns the problem." On the contrary, the professional participates in the deliberations as fully as if he or she "owned the problem." The crucial difference is that that participation serves to assist the patient rather than the practitioner. Thus, as much preparation and proficiency in ethical reflection is required of the professional on this view as on the paternalism model where the professional shoulders all of the decision-making. More, in fact, is required, since the practitioner is concerned with a problem involving not his or her own values, but the patient's, which at the beginning may be undefined with regard to health.[4]

SELF-CARE AGENCY: CLINICAL JUDGMENT

The discussion of agency thus far has centered around freedom, self-determination, and values—all of them moral concepts. I have attempted to establish the *moral autonomy* of individuals in the self-care framework.

Now, a further issue arises in connection with agency. Even if we grant the *moral* agency of patients in regard to decisions about values, can we possibly suppose that patients should exercise autonomy in essentially clinical matters such as the formulation of diagnosis, the determination of etiology, or the selection of treatment? To phrase the problem differently, even if patients ideally ought to have as much autonomy as practitioners, can they possibly have as much knowledge?

The self-care philosophy of the patient as agent means that the professional incorporates the patient's personal, unique perspective on the situation as not only ethically, but clinically, primary. The patient's view must be valued as being as credible and as crucial as the clinician's approach. The reason for this is not the imperfect state of medical science. The reason for the validity of the patient's perspective is the phenomenological difference between viewing an experience as the subject or agent of that experience (as the patient views his or her illness) and viewing an experience objectively (as an object that is not largely constituted by the viewer, the clinician). Philosophical phenomenology has shown that the subjective activity of giving sense and meaning to one's complexity is at least as important as the application of objective categories in trying to understand a situation.[5] Inevitably, the patient brings his or her own perspective to bear on the problem at hand, and within a philosophy of patient agency, that perspective becomes an essential, not an optional, corollary to the professional's view in their combined clinical judgment.

It is not intended that the patient become an amateur clinician. Instead, it is proposed that the patient-practitioner relationship combine and make mutually enhancing the two different perspectives represented; either one alone must be seen as inadequate, one-sided.

To accept the validity of the patient's input into the formulation of a clinical judgment, we only need to accept the essential complexities in the experience of illness. Earlier I suggested some of these complexities in relation to the definition of "self." To compound the difficulty—or to add to the richness, depending upon one's view—there may be as great a complexity attending "the body." We can distinguish at least three modes of experiencing one's body, and a brief description of these may illustrate my point. Two of these modes phenomenologists refer to as the lived body and the object body: the third, I shall call the body as subject. They can be understood as different levels of the relation between self and body.[6]

Lived Body

At this level no distinction is experienced between self and body. The body is not that with which I act; it *is* my acting. Conversely, it is also my immediate vulnerability to the world acting upon me, my direct relation with the world, unmediated by any awareness of the body "over against me."

Object Body

When pain or incapacity disrupt the immediacy of the lived body, a distinction emerges between self and body. The body is then an encumbrance, an impediment that the self must take into account. The body is that which the self must either learn to control or be controlled by it. In contrast to the *lived* body unity, the body is now *object*.

"Object" refers here, not to the abstract theoretical body that the anatomist studies, but to the existential otherness, the concrete "thinghood," of the self. In this sense, the person who understands nothing about the body as neuroanatomical object experiences the existential object body in using the arms to lift a paralyzed leg.

Subject Body

In illness, the body is not only object, but enemy. The body mutinies, the self is overthrown. However, if we suspend the object body framework, a different phenomenon is possible; in illness the body insists, not that the aims of the self be surrendered, but that the body's own reality, complexity, and values be acknowledged. The acceptance of that reality as valid is the experiencing of the *body as subject*. That is, when the body is experienced as subject, it is considered to be part of the self with the same intrinsically valid claims as any other part of the self.

The contrast between object body and subject body can be illustrated by the difference, for example, between experiencing a phenomenon such as shortness of breath as limitation upon activity that might be alleviated with proper conditioning, or as an expression—a symbol—of the body's own perspective on the value of activity, speed, endurance. The slowing of the aging body thus can have either negative or positive meaning, as either the inability to move as quickly as the object body was once conditioned to do, or as the new capacity for "opening time," that is, for exploring experiences "not in their linear pattern of succeeding one another, but in their possibility of opening entire worlds in each situation."[7] By positive meaning, then, is meant a consideration of the particular phenomenon, such as slowing, as the body's expression or symbol of its own meaning.

The terms in which the subject body is perceived and understood cannot be the language of physioanatomy with which the clinician approaches the body. The classifications of science presuppose a body whose reality already is fully established or is developing along a typifiable course. But that is not the kind of reality that characterizes a subject, a self. Thus, categories that comprehend only a fixed, predeterminable object are inadequate for perceiving and interpreting the development of the body as subject.

In effect, scientific language is inadequate for describing the subject body because it is designed to express only a finite reality and meaning. However, *as self*—that which develops its own reality and meanings—the body is infinite. It is not of course infinite as *object,* able to transcend space and time. Its infinity is the infinity of self, that which transcends fixed determinations.

With this brief excursion into the phenomenology of the body, I am suggesting that even one of the body's realities, namely, the patient's own experience of the body, is not a simple affair. Now add to this complexity other perspectives toward the patient's body—notably, the clinician's view of the body as scientific object—and it should be apparent how elaborate the process of clinical judgment must be, to do justice to all of the realities present in a single determination about care. This does not mean that clinical judgment in the self-care framework is an unhappily mixed marriage of competing views. On the contrary, my point is that only within self-care practice *as a collaborative enterprise* between patient and professional *can either one* exercise clinical judgment, that is, informed decision-making about diagnosis and treatment. Thus, it is as important that the clinician's perspective be incorporated into the judgment as it is that the patient's view of the problem be respected and incorporated as phenomenologically valid. Finally, however, in the task of their together creating as comprehensive an understanding of "the whole person" as possible, it will be the patient who determines which findings are to count as thematic for the clinical judgment.

CONCLUSION

The discussion has indicated one way in which a complete reconceptualization of health care might proceed. In suggesting a fundamentally new philosophy of health care, I have not proposed self-care as an alternative to professional care, nor as a means of subverting the medical establishment. In both of those cases nothing substantive can be accomplished as long as the consumer-provider antagonism persists. Giving the power "to the people" may put the consumer in control. But my point is that any health care philosophy in which considerations of control and power are pivotal *cannot* in principle provide a framework for sharing autonomy, and—for reasons both ethical and medical—the sharing of autonomy as I have described it in terms of self-care is the preferred alternative to both of the two power extremes, consumerism as well as paternalism.

In the philosophy I have proposed, the professional actually contributes more than in a paternalistic framework. At the same time the patient exercises even greater self-determination than on the consumer model.

First, the professional contributes more than on the paternalist model because the clinician is not concerned with reaching a unilateral clinical judgment *about* a patient, but instead engages *with* the patient in an endeavor to reach a joint understanding of the situation—an understanding that expresses the patient's values and concepts of the body, the self, and health, as well as the practitioner's own perspective on these same issues. This unquestionably is an endeavor far more involving intellectually and ethically than simple decision-making *on behalf of patients*.

Second, patients exercise greater self-determination on the self-care model I have described than on the consumerism model. They are frankly supported instead of challenged by the clinician in their exercise of autonomy. In fact, patients who claim to want professionals to make all of the decisions may find themselves gently drawn by the practitioner into the clinical deliberations in order that their freedom of self-determination not be waived for trivial reasons, that is, out of habit or deference. In short, the aim of the health professional on this view is to actively assist patient self-determination. Given the difficulties inherent in clarifying one's view of the self, one's relationship to the body, and one's concept of health, that assistance from the health professional cannot fail to enhance the degree of self-determination that is exercised by patients.

NOTES AND REFERENCES

1 The usual arguments against paternalism are grounded in the principle of individual autonomy. Ivan Illich and Thomas Szasz are probably the most vociferous defenders of that principle in the health care context. A different approach is developed by Allen Buchanan ("Medical Paternalism," *Philosophy and Public Affairs,* (No. 4), 1978), who develops an antipaternalist critique that meets the paternalist "on his own ground" without recourse to rights-based arguments.

2 For a discussion of the potential role of the layperson as self-provider of primary care, see: Levin, Lowell S., Katz, Alfred H., and Holst, Erik. *Self-Care: Lay Initiatives in Health:* New York, Prodist, 1976. The authors, though suggesting that "a new lay-professional partnership may emerge," do not commit themselves philosophically to such a partnership.

3 See, for example, Englehardt, H. Tristram, Jr. "The Concepts of Health and Disease," *Evaluation and Explanation in the Biomedical Sciences.* Englehardt, H. Tristram, Jr., and Spicker, Stuart F., eds. Dordrecht, Holland, Reidel, 1975; Callahan, Daniel. "The WHO Definition of 'Health'," *The Hastings Center Studies,* Vol. 1, No. 3 (1973); and Boorse, Christopher. "On The Distinction Between Disease and Illness," *Philosophy and Public Affairs* **5** No. 1 1975.

4 In "An Ethical Model for Advocacy: Assisting Patients with Treatment Decisions," I propose guidelines for professional assistance to patients in their deliberations about values and treatment opinions (in *Dilemmas of Dying: Policies and Procedures for Decisions not to Treat,* Wong, Cynthia B., and Swazey, Judith P., eds. G. K. Hall, Boston, 1981).

5 See especially Merleau-Ponty's discussion of the body in *Phenomenology of Perception* (Colin Smith, trans.), New York, Humanities Press, 1962.

6 For a more detailed discussion of these levels, see my "Body and Self: A Dialectic," *The Journal of Medicine and Philosophy,* **5,** No. 3, September 1980. For an analysis

of the lived-body in particular, see: Schag, Calvin O. "The Lived-Body as a Phenomenological Datum," *The Modern Schoolman* **39** (1961–62), 203–218.

7 Berg, Geri, and Gadow, Sally, "Toward More Human Meanings of Aging: Ideals adn Images from Philosophy and Art," in *Aging and the Elderly: Humanistic Perspectives in Gerontology*, Spicker, Stuart F., et al. (eds.). Humanities Press, New York, 1978, 83–92.

TWO PHILOSOPHIES
OF CARING

D. Gary Benfield

Twentieth century America can be characterized as an era in which relationships between people in various walks of life have become increasingly impersonal and dehumanized. Just as mass production and computerization seem to influence our lives at every turn, the hospital practice of medicine has come to resemble an assembly line where people are perceived as "things" and patients as "pathologies."[1]

From my personal observation and the writing of others,[2,3] two philosophies of caring in medicine seem to exist. One is predominantly oriented to the disease in the body (disease-oriented) and the other, though primarily concerned with disease in the body, focuses more upon the needs of the individual patient (person-oriented). At the risk of oversimplification, let us explore how each of these two philosophies influence the care of critically or teminally ill patients and their families.

DISEASE-ORIENTED CARE

The disease-oriented philosophy is common in medicine. Actions based on this philosophy, in concert with advances in technology, have brought great benefits to people throughout the world; many diseases have been prevented or cured, and disability has been reduced. Using the latest in medical technology, this

Reprinted with permission from *The Ohio State Medical Journal*, (August 1979) pp. 508–511.

philosophy demands that health care personnel aggressively treat "the disease in the body in the bed." Though most people would agree that medical technology should continue to advance, one difficulty with this philosophy is that caretakers may think that death must be avoided for now and postponed to the future and the patient's views in the matter ignored. Thus a disease-oriented philosophy of caring can create painful problems for those terminally ill patients who wish to die, as illustrated in the following story adapted from an article by N. L. Caroline.[4]

A 78-year-old man was admitted to a midwestern teaching hospital for treatment of a bowel obstruction. He believed that he was dying, but no one would listen. When his elderly roommate, suffering from cancer of the colon, was unsuccessfully resuscitated while naked and lying in a pool of excretions, the patient frantically implored the doctor: "Please don't ever do that to me. Promise you won't ever do that to me."

Three days later, the patient developed congestive heart failure and was intubated, placed on a ventilator, and monitored with electrodes on the chest and arms, all against his will. During the first night of ventilator care, the patient was found dead in bed. He had awakened, reached over, and switched off his ventilator. On the bedside table, the doctor found a scribbled note: "Death is not the enemy, doctor, inhumanity is."

The author of "Dying in Academe" describes the 20th century as the "Age of Arrogance." In the tertiary-care hospital setting, all indiscretions are tolerated except death. To die is an unforgivable breech of faith with the staff and an outrage against physicians, nurses, technicians, orderlies, aides, and others. In the Age of Arrogance, man does not have to die—at least not at the conventional time. If his kidneys fail, he can be sustained by dialysis; if his lungs tire, a ventilator can help him to breathe. Even man's heart can be bypassed or maintained mechanically. Man's appointment with death must be rescheduled whether or not he agrees. For the disease oriented physician, death is the enemy.

Because the physician often is considered to "know best," patients and families may relent to the disease-oriented point of view though unaware that all options for caring have not been explored. In this way, patients and families may experience dehumanizing indignities, economic hardship, and emotional upheaval. For little or no gain, patients, families, and nursing personnel may suffer a great deal, as illustrated in the following story.

Immediately following an automobile accident, a 40-year-old man was admitted to the hospital in a comatose condition. Emergency CAT scan showed massive intracranial hemorrhage. He was intubated, placed on a respirator, and transferred to the intensive care unit (ICU). The family was informed of a "very poor prognosis" at that time.

Although an electroencephalogram (EEG) was isoelectric on both the second and fourth hospital days, the family had no communication from the attending physician except to be told that the outlook was "very poor." The patient continued to receive respirator care in the ICU until the 12th hospital day, when a crisis developed: the ICU was filled to capacity. A decision was made to transfer the patient to a general medical floor, an area where the nursing staff had never cared for a respirator patient before.

Following a 24-hour period, during which the nurses on the general medical floor received a "crash course" in respirator care, the patient was transferred out of the ICU. Two days later, he died.

Comments from two of the general medical nurses who cared for the patient highlight the suffering and sense of frustration felt by individual nurses and the patient's wife.

Nurse 1: I was so scared because I didn't know that much about respirators and I feared doing something wrong that might cause his death. His wife sat beside him, cried a lot, and looked so pathetic. Her questions upset me and I never knew what to say to her. I felt like I wanted to go somewhere and have a good cry. How do you talk to his wife? How far can we go? Where were the doctors? They would visit for maybe ten minutes in a day. We were involved 24 hours each day. It's easier for them—they can leave and see someone else—we can't.

Nurse 2: When the physicians made rounds, they would check the respirator, listen to his heart and lungs, write new IV orders, and leave. They never said anything to us or the family. If he had brain death why did they continue with everything?

You know how some doctors are—they don't want nurses to tell the patient or the family anything. They say that they will tell them. But they don't tell the family anything other than: 'It doesn't look good' or 'His condition is critical.' Where does this leave the nurses when the family says: 'Is he dying?' or 'How long will it be?' It happens all the time and makes me mad! I felt so helpless. It gave me such a feeling of failure and worthlessness that I could only go in and do what I could and then leave the room. The entire staff was affected. All of a sudden everyone walked around with a serious expression—almost a frown. I didn't want to come to work.

The disease-oriented philosophy considers that "life" is all that matters . . . to have a patient die is a sign of failure. When questioned concerning this approach to caring, some physicians may consider that raising such issues is an affront to their medical competence or integrity. After all, some physicians may feel that they are trained to treat, to cure at all costs, rather than practice a more humanitarian approach to the art of healing. Moreover, when the myth of "legal rightness" prevails, the patient and the family become victims of the tyranny of technology; technical considerations dominate decision making and push aside personal and family notions of right and wrong.

The second patient described obviously had suffered "brain death."[5] Despite this, his physicians maintained his vital functions and ignored the feelings and desires of the surviving family and nursing staff as they drifted in quiet desperation from day to day. Ironically, the physicians probably were unaware that this practice was inflicting harm. Without risking time or emotion, they simply examined the patient, wrote their orders, and walked out.

PERSON-ORIENTED CARE

In this philosophy, "quality of life" as seen by the patient (or his family when the patient is incompetent) is a primary concern. Patients and families need the opportunity and, if possible, the time to understand the condition, the treatment, and the limitations of outcomes. Then, if professionals are willing to share the responsibility and the agony of deciding care, one important aspect of a person-oriented philosophy becomes evident: the patient may be relieved of suffering from disease or pointless dehumanizing treatment. Simultaneously, the family may have the opportunity to adapt to their expected loss through anticipatory grieving. Just as close, early parent-infant contact may enhance the development of healthy relationships for a living child, so may similar contacts help the grieving relatives of a dying person at any age. The following story illustrates this point.

It was 4 A.M. when the attending staff gathered around the respirator which was attached to John and Mary's baby, Tommy. Tommy was blue; his heart rate slowed perceptively as he was watched. He had lived for 41 short days, and now it was time to die. His heart and lungs could be kept functioning indefinitely with the help of our machinery and drugs. But that would be treating ourselves—our feelings of helplessness and guilt over his irreversible damaged lungs. Once again we reviewed in detail the events of the past 41 days. As the attending physician, I suggested that it was time to remove the respirator and let him die peacefully.

First Mary, then John, put their hands in the incubator and rubbed Tommy's body with soft, soothing caresses. Then they both nodded in agreement. They were led to a nearby room, and I went back to Tommy. The wires attached from the patient to the cardiac monitor, as well as the temperature probe and the nasogastric tube were removed. The gauze packing was taken from his mouth and the endotracheal tube extracted from his airway. Carefully, his body was wrapped in a blanket and carried to his mother and father in the adjacent room.

Lisa, Tommy's nurse, and I left the parents alone with their baby. Oddly enough, I was not embarrassed to cry although I had thought that I would be. Later, Lisa and I sat quietly with John, Mary, and Tommy. As we sat and reminisced about Tommy's life, first one and then another of the night nurses wandered in, paused with tears in their eyes, and just touched one or the other of us. Several offered words of love. It was a touching scene.

John expressed his appreciation for the care they all had received. He said: "I've learned a lot during the last 41 days. Though Tommy weighed only 2 pounds at birth and has needed a respirator to help him breathe since he was born, all the nurses and doctors never stopped caring about him or us."

I interrupted briefly to listen to Tommy's chest for the sound of a heart beat. There was none. It was over.

No one seemed in a hurry to leave. Like iron drawn to a magnet, we just sat and looked at Tommy. "Tommy, we'll miss you," John said. "It has been a good six weeks." Strange, the past six weeks had been difficult for me . . . the worry, uncertainty, and guilt. But for John, it had been a good six weeks. I was touched by the feeling that flowed between us. Though we had spent long hours in caring for Tommy and his parents, they, in turn, had helped all of us as well.

In this example, physicians and nurses had maintained open and honest communication between themselves and with baby Tommy's parents from his birth. The physicians, nurses, and parents grew to appreciate the limitations of technology and together, after long and anguished hours of deliberations, arrived at the final decision to discontinue life support when all hope for survival was gone. Continued follow-up with these parents supports the belief that parents can participate as partners with their physician in difficult infant-care decisions, even when death results, and subsequently make a healthy adjustment to their loss.[6]

In a pluralistic society composed of persons of various backgrounds with differing values about terminal illness, dying, and death, some conflict is inevitable. On one hand, the patient or his family may resent the intrusion of others into their private lives. For those patients and families, a disease-orientation may meet their needs. On the other hand, patients and families usually welcome the opportunity to discuss their feelings and desires openly and honestly with a concerned caregiver. Handling this responsibility for caring requires hard work and a commitment from all parties concerned; it should include plans to care for the caretakers as well.

OBSTACLES TO PERSON-ORIENTED CARING

Just as the modern hospital may be the greatest enemy of meaningful death,[7] it may be the greatest enemy of meaningful living for patients, families, and personnel. There are at least five major factors which obstruct person-oriented caring.

One serious barrier to rendering care is the lack of teamwork among health care providers. In large measure, this is due to the classic, rigid, vertical structure of the system with the physician at the head of the team, the other caregivers under his administration, with the patient and family beneath them all.

A second deterrent, one faced by nurses in the hospital setting especially, is the scarcity of time. The hospital system rewards nurses for "getting work done" and keeping the organization running smoothly.

Third, the stereotype of the nurse as a technician in critical care areas hold that the nurse should be more concerned with the machinery surrounding the patient than with the patient's care. In the intensive-care atmosphere, patients or their families may be reluctant to express their fears of dying, or desires to die, and staff members may be too busy with monitoring the patient's physical condition to listen.

A fourth deterrent to caring is the feeling expressed at one time or another by caregivers that they lack training in caring for critically ill or dying patients and their families. When they have to meet the terminally ill face to face, classroom theory may prove woefully inadequate for the nurse, physician, social worker, minister, or hospital administrator.

Finally, communication is a major problem which relates to each of the first four factors. Caregivers frequently do not know what the patient or his family have been told by the physician. Yet, nonphysicians may be the very persons approached by the patient or family for clarification—perhaps because patients and families are more comfortable with those persons. In other instances, the physician may choose not to inform the patient of the diagnosis, a choice which may produce conflict among personnel.

According to Menninger, "It is not enough for physicians to provide the best technological care available; they also have a responsibility to treat the patient as a 'whole person.' "[8] Until physicians recognize the value of person-oriented care and take a leadership role in restoring the human touch, personalized caring will remain a latent dream in the heart of man.

An Afterthought

As I complete this article, my father lies stuporous before me in his hospital bed, dying of cancer. He is soaked with sweat, totally dependent on others to move him, feed him, bathe him and wipe him. This is the stark reality of man in need at the most basic level. There is no formalized caregiving team here, and there are no conferences to plan strategy for the terminally ill. It's a small community hospital like so many throughout the United States.

In this hospital, aides lift the patients, empty their excrement, bathe the patients, and change the beds. An aide shuffles by mumbling obscenities under his breath and doing his job grudgingly. I want to reach out and say to him: "Stop and listen to me . . . You have the most important job in this hospital. My father needs you; he depends on you; he is grateful to you." Somehow, I just can't say it. He doesn't even know that I exist, except as another meddling relative.

Imagine! The aide is more important to my father than all the nurses and doctors combined. *How little we know about caring!*

Acknowledgment: This paper was written to fulfill a course requirement in the Department of Philosophy, Kent State University. I am indebted to Raymond S. Duff, M.D., Department of Pediatrics, Yale University, and to Patricia James, Ph.D., Department of Philosophy, Kent State University, for sharing their ideas and for their continuing encouragement.

REFERENCES

1 Howard J: Humanization and dehumanization of health care, in Reich WT (ed): *The Encyclopedia of Bioethics,* New York, 1978, p 619.
2 Duff RS, Hollingshead AB: *Sickness and Society,* New York, Harper & Row, 1968.
3 Duff RS, Campbell AGM: On deciding the care of severely handicapped or dying persons: with particular reference to infants. *Pediatrics* **57**:487–493, 1976.
4 Caroline NL: Dying in academe, in Petetz D, et al (eds): *Death and Grief, Selected Readings for the Medical Student,* New York, Health Science Pub Corp, 1977, pp 17–20.
5 A definition of irreversible coma, Ad Hoc Committee of the Harvard Medical School to Examine the Definition of Brain Death. *JAMA* **205**:337–340, 1968.
6 Benfield DG, Leib SA, Vollman JH: Grief response of parents to neonatal death and parent participation in deciding care. *Pediatrics* **62**:171–177, 1978.
7 Carmody, J: A death, a radicalization. *Christian Century* **91**:639–640, 1974.
8 Menninger WW: 'Caring' as part of health care quality. *JAMA* **234**:836–837, 1975.

WHY CARE ABOUT CARING?

Nel Noddings

THE FUNDAMENTAL NATURE OF CARING

The main task in this chapter is a preliminary analysis of caring. I want to ask what it means to care and to lay down the lines along which analysis will proceed. . . . It seems obvious in an everyday sense why we should be interested in caring. Everywhere we hear the complaint "Nobody cares!" and our increasing immersion in bureaucratic procedures and regulations leads us to predict that the complaint will continue to be heard. As human beings we want to care and to be cared for. *Caring* is important in itself. It seems necessary, however, to motivate the sort of detailed analysis I propose; that is, it is reasonable in a philosophical context to ask: Why care about caring?

If we were starting out on a traditional investigation of what it means to be moral, we would almost certainly start with a discussion of moral judgment and moral reasoning. This approach has obvious advantages. It gives us something public and tangible to grapple with—the statements that describe our thinking on moral matters. But I shall argue that this is not the only—nor even the best— starting point. Starting the discussion of moral matters with principles, defini- tions, and demonstrations is rather like starting the solution of a mathematical problem formally. Sometimes we can and do proceed this way, but when the problematic situation is new, baffling, or especially complex, we cannot start

From Nel Noddings, *Caring: A Feminine Approach to Ethics and Moral Education*, pp. 7–29. © 1984 The Regents of the University of California. Used by permission of The University of California Press.

this way. We have to operate in an intuitive or receptive mode that is somewhat mysterious, internal, and nonsequential. After the solution has been found by intuitive methods, we may proceed with the construction of a formal demonstration or proof. As the mathematician Gauss put it: "I have got my result but I do not know yet how to get (prove) it."[1]

A difficulty in mathematics teaching is that we too rarely share our fundamental mathematical thinking with our students. We present everything ready-made as it were, as though it springs from our foreheads in formal perfection. The same sort of difficulty arises when we approach the teaching of morality or ethical behavior from a rational-cognitive approach. We fail to share with each other the feelings, the conflicts, the hopes and ideas that influence our eventual choices. We share only the justification for our acts and not what motivates and touches us.

I think we are doubly mistaken when we approach moral matters in this mathematical way. First, of course, we miss sharing the heuristic processes in our ethical thinking just as we miss that sharing when we approach mathematics itself formally. But this difficulty could be remedied pedagogically. We would not have to change our approach to ethics but only to the teaching of ethical behavior or ethical thinking. Second, however, when we approach moral matters through the study of moral reasoning, we are led quite naturally to suppose that ethics is necessarily a subject that must be cast in the language of principle and demonstration. This, I shall argue, is a mistake.

Many persons who live moral lives do not approach moral problems formally. Women, in particular, seem to approach moral problems by placing themselves as nearly as possible in concrete situations and assuming personal responsibility for the choices to be made. They define themselves in terms of *caring* and work their way through moral problems from the position of one-caring.[2] This position or attitude of caring activates a complex structure of memories, feelings, and capacities. Further, the process of moral decision making that is founded on caring requires a process of concretization rather than one of abstraction. An ethic built on caring is, I think, characteristically and essentially feminine—which is not to say, of course, that it cannot be shared by men, any more than we should care to say that traditional moral systems cannot be embraced by women. But an ethic of caring arises, I believe, out of our experience as women, just as the traditional logical approach to ethical problems arises more obviously from masculine experience.

One reason, then, for conducting the comprehensive and appreciative investigation of caring to which we shall now turn is to capture conceptually a feminine—or simply an alternative—approach to matters of morality.

WHAT DOES IT MEAN TO CARE?

Our dictionaries tell us that "care" is a state of mental suffering or of engrossment: to care is to be in a burdened mental state, one of anxiety, fear, or solicitude about something or someone. Alternatively, one cares for something or someone if one has a regard for or inclination toward that something or someone. If I have an inclination toward mathematics, I may willingly spend some time with it, and if I have a regard for you, what you think, feel, and desire will matter to me. And, again, to care may mean to be charged with the protection, welfare, or maintenance of something or someone.

These definitions represent different uses of "care" but, in the deepest human sense, we shall see that elements of each of them are involved in caring. In one sense, I may equate "cares" with "burdens"; I have cares in certain matters (professional, personal, or public) if I have burdens or worries, if I fret over current and projected states of affairs. In another sense, I *care* for someone if I feel a stir of desire or inclination toward him. In a related sense, I *care* for someone if I have regard for his views and interests. In the third sense, I have the care of an elderly relative if I am charged with the responsibility for his physical welfare. But, clearly, in the deep human sense that will occupy us, I cannot claim to care for my relative if my caretaking is perfunctory or grudging.

We see that it will be necessary to give much of our attention to the one-caring in our analysis. Even though we sometimes judge caring from the outside, as third-persons, it is easy to see that the essential elements of caring are located in the relation between the one-caring and the cared-for. In a lovely little book, *On Caring*, Milton Mayeroff describes caring largely through the view of one-caring. He begins by saying: "To care for another person, in the most significant sense, is to help him grow and actualize himself."[3]

I want to approach the problem a bit differently, because I think emphasis on the actualization of the other may lead us to pass too rapidly over the description of what goes on in the one-caring. Further, problems arise in the discussion of reciprocity, and we shall feel a need to examine the role of the cared-for much more closely also. But Mayeroff has given us a significant start by pointing to the importance of constancy, guilt, reciprocation, and the limits of caring. All of these we shall consider in some detail.

Let's start looking at caring from the outside to discover the limitations of that approach. In the ordinary course of events, we expect some action from one who claims to care, even though action is not all we expect. How are we to determine whether Mr. Smith cares for his elderly mother, who is confined to a nursing home? It is not enough, surely, that Mr. Smith should say, "I care." (But the possibility of his saying this will lead us onto another path of analysis shortly. We shall have to examine caring from the inside.) We, as observers, must look for some action, some manifestation in Smith's behavior, that will allow us to agree that he cares. To care, we feel, requires some action in behalf of the cared-for. Thus, if Smith never visits his mother, nor writes to her, nor telephones her, we would be likely to say that, although he is charged formallly with her care—he pays for her confinement—he does not really care. We point out that he seems to be lacking in regard, that he is not troubled enough to see for himself how his mother fares. There is no desire for her company, no inclination toward her. But notice that a criterion of action would not be easy to formulate from this case. Smith, after all, does perform some action in behalf of his mother: he pays for her physical maintenance. But we are looking for a qualitatively different sort of action.

Is direct, externally observable action necessary to caring? Can caring be present in the absence of action in behalf of the cared-for? Consider the problem of lovers who cannot marry because they are already committed to satisfactory and honorable marriages. The lover learns that his beloved is ill. All his instincts cry out for his presence at her bedside. Yet, if he fears for the trouble he may bring her, for the recriminations that may spring from his appearance, he may stay away from her. Surely, we would not say in such a case that the lover does not care. He is in a mental state of engrossment, even suffering; he feels the deepest regard and, charged by his love with the duty to protect, he denies his own need in order to spare her one form of pain. Thus, in caring, he chooses not to act directly and tenderly in response to the beloved's immediate physical pain. We see that, when we consider the action component of caring in depth, we shall have to look beyond observable action to acts of commitment, those acts that are seen only by the individual subject performing them.

In the case of the lover whose beloved has fallen ill, we might expect him to express himself when the crisis has passed. But even this might not happen. He might resolve never to contact her again, and his caring could then be known only to him as he renews his resolve again and again. We do not wish to deny that the lover cares, but clearly, something is missing in the relationship: caring is not completed in the cared-for. Or, consider the mother whose son, in young adulthood, leaves home in anger and rebellion. Should she act to bring about reconciliation? Perhaps. Are we sure that she does not care if she fails to act directly to bring him into loving contact with his family? She may, indeed, deliberately abstain from acting in the belief that her son must be allowed to work out his problem alone. Her regard for him may force her into anguished and carefully considered inaction. Like the lover, she may eventually express herself to her son—when the crisis has passed—but then again, she may not. After a period of, say, two years, the relationship may stabilize, and the mother's caring may resume its usual form. Shall we say, then, that she "cares again" and that for two years she "did not care"?

There are still further difficulties in trying to formulate an action criterion for caring. Suppose that I learn about a family in great need, and suppose that I decide to help them. I pay their back rent for them, buy food for them, and supply them with the necessities of life. I do all this cheerfully, willingly spending time with them. Can it be doubted that I care? This sort of case will raise problems also. Suppose both husband and wife in this family want to be independent, or at least have a latent longing in this direction. But my acts tend to suppress the urge toward independence. Am I helping or hindering?[4] Do I care or only seem to care? If it must be said that my relation to the needy family is not, properly, a caring relation, what has gone wrong?

Now, in this brief inspection of caring acts, we have already encountered problems. Others suggest themselves. What of indirect caring, for example? What shall we say about college students who engage in protests for the blacks of South Africa or the "boat people" of Indochina or the Jews of Russia? Under what conditions would we be willing to say that they care? Again, these may be questions that can be answered only by those claiming to care. We need to know, for example, what motivates the protest. Then, as we shall see, there is the recurring problem of "completion." How is the caring conveyed to the cared-for? What sort of meeting can there be between the one-caring and the cared-for?

We are not going to be able to answer all of these questions with certainty. Indeed, this essay is not aiming toward a systematic exposition of criteria for caring. Rather, I must show that such a systematic effort is, so far as the system is its goal, mistaken. We expend the effort as much to show what is not fruitful as what is. It is not my aim to be able to sort cases at the finish: A cares, B does not care, C cares but not about D, etc. If we can understand how complex and intricate, indeed how subjective, caring is, we shall perhaps be better equipped to meet the conflicts and pains it sometimes induces. Then, too, we may come to understand at least in part how it is that, in a country that spends billions on caretaking of various sorts, we hear everywhere the complaint, "Nobody cares."

In spite of the difficulties involved, we shall have to discuss behavioral indicators of caring in some depth, because we will be concerned about problems of entrusting care, of monitoring caretaking and assigning it. When we consider the possibility of institutional caring and what might be meant by the "caring school," we shall need to know what to look for. And so, even though the analysis will move us more and more toward first- and second-person views of caring, we shall examine caring acts and the "third-person" view also. In this initial analysis, we shall return to the third-person view after examining first- and second-person aspects.

So far, we have talked about the action component of caring, and we certainly have not arrived at a determinate set of criteria. Suppose, now, that we consider the engrossment we expect to find in the one-caring. When Mr. Smith, whose "caring" seems to us to be at best perfunctory, says, "I care," what can he mean? Now, clearly we can only guess, because Mr. Smith has to speak for himself on this. But he might mean: (1) I *do* care. I think of my mother often and worry about her. It is an awful burden. (2) I *do* care. I should see her more often, but I have so much to do—a houseful of kids, long working hours, a wife who needs my companionship. . . . (3) I *do* care. I pay the bills, don't I? I have sisters who could provide company. . . .

These suggested meanings do not exhaust Mr. Smith's possibilities, but they give us something to work with. In the first case, we might rightly conclude that Mr. Smith does not care for his mother as much as he does for himself as caretaker. He is burdened with cares, and the focus of his attention has shifted inward to himself and his worries. This, we shall see, is a risk of caring. There exists in all caring situations the risk that the one-caring will be overwhelmed by the responsibilities and duties of the task and that, as a result of being burdened, he or she will cease to care for the other and become instead the object of "caring." Now, here—and throughout our discussion on caring—we must try to avoid equivocation. There are, as we have noted, several common meanings of "to care," but no one of them yields the deep sense for which we are probing. When it is clear that "caring" refers to one of the restricted senses, or when we are not yet sure to what it refers, I shall enclose it in quotes. In the situation where Mr. Smith is *burdened with cares,* he is the object of "caring."

In the third case, also, we might justifiably conclude that Mr. Smith does not care. His interest is in equity. He wants to be credited with caring. By doing something, he hopes to find an acceptable substitute for genuine caring. We see similar behavior in the woman who professes to love animals and whisks every stray to the animal shelter. Most animals, once at the shelter, suffer death. Does one who cares choose swift and merciful death for the object of her care over precarious and perhaps painful life? Well, we might say, it depends. It depends on our caretaking capabilities, on traffic conditions where we live, on the physical condition of the animal. All this is exactly to the point. What we do depends not upon rules, or at least not wholly on rules—not upon a prior determination of what is fair or equitable—but upon a constellation of conditions that is viewed through both the eyes of the one-caring and the eyes of the cared-for. By and large, we do not say with any conviction that a person cares if that person acts routinely according to some fixed rule.

The second case is difficult. This Mr. Smith has a notion that caring involves a commitment of self, but he is finding it difficult to handle the commitments he has already made. He is in conflict over how he should spend himself. Undergoing conflict is another risk of caring, and we shall consider a variety of possible conflicts. Of special interest to us will be the question: When should I attempt to remove conflict, and when should I resolve simply to live with the conflict? Suppose, for example, that I care for both cats and birds. (I must use "care for" at this stage without attempting to justify its use completely.) Having particular cats of my own and *not* having particular birds of my own at the same time are indications of my concern for each. But there are wild birds in my garden, and they are in peril from the cats. I may give the matter considerable thought. I feed the cats well so that they will not hunt out of hunger. I hang small bells on their collars. I keep bird cages ready for victims I am able to rescue. I keep bird baths and feeders inaccessible to the cats. Beyond this, I live with the conflict. Others might have the cats declawed, but I will not do this. Now, the point here is not whether I care more for cats than birds, or whether Ms. Jones (who declaws her cats) cares more for birds than I do. The point lies in trying to discern the kinds of things I must think about when I am in a conflict of caring. When my caring is directed to living things, I must consider their natures, ways of life, needs, and desires. And, although I can never accomplish it entirely, I try to apprehend the reality of the other.

This is the fundamental aspect of caring from the inside. When I look at and think about how I am when I care, I realize that there is invariably this displacement of interest from my own reality to the reality of the other. (Our discussion now will be confined to caring for persons.) Kierkegaard has said that we apprehend another's reality as *possibility*.[5] To be touched, to have aroused in me something that will disturb my own ethical reality, I must see the other's reality as a possibility for my own. This is not to say that I cannot try to see the other's reality differently. Indeed, I can. I can look at it objectively by collecting factual data; I can look at it historically. If it is heroic, I can come to admire it. But this sort of looking does not touch my own ethical reality; it may even distract me from it. As Kierkegaard put it:

> Ethically speaking there is nothing so conducive to sound sleep as admiration of another person's ethical reality. And again ethically speaking, if there is anything that can stir and rouse a man, it is a possibility ideally requiring itself of a human being.[6]

But I am suggesting that we do not see only the direct possibilities for becoming better than we are when we struggle toward the reality of the other. We also have aroused in us the feeling, "I must do something." When we see the other's reality as a possibility for us, we must act to eliminate the intolerable, to reduce the pain, to fill the need, to actualize the dream. When I am in this sort of relationship with another, when the other's reality becomes a real possibility for me, I care. Whether the caring is sustained, whether it lasts long enough to be conveyed to the other, whether it becomes visible in the world, depends upon my sustaining the relationship or, at least, acting out of concern for my own ethicality as though it were sustained.

In this latter case, one in which something has slipped away from me or eluded me from the start but in which I strive to regain or to attain it, I experience a genuine caring for self. This caring for self, for the *ethical* self, can emerge only from a caring for others. But a sense of my physical self, a knowledge of what gives me pain and pleasure, precedes my caring for others. Otherwise, their realities as possibilities for my own reality would mean nothing to me. When we say of someone, "He cares only for himself," we mean that, in our deepest sense, he does not care at all. He has only a sense of that physical self— of what gives him pain and pleasure. Whatever he sees in others is pre-selected in relation to his own needs and desires. He does not see the reality of the other as a possibility for himself but only as an instance of what he has already determined as self or not-self. Thus, he is ethically both zero and finished. His only "becoming" is a physical becoming. It is clear, of course, that I must say more about what is meant by "ethical reality" and "ethical self," and I shall return to this question.

I need not, however, be a person who cares only for myself in order to behave occasionally as though I care only for myself. Sometimes I behave this way because I have not thought through things carefully enough and because the mode of the times pushes the thoughtless in its own direction. Suppose, for example, that I am a teacher who loves mathematics. I encounter a student who is doing poorly, and I decide to have a talk with him. He tells me that he hates mathematics. *Aha,* I think. *Here is the problem. I must help this poor boy to love mathematics, and then he will do better at it.* What am I doing when I proceed in this way? I am not trying to grasp the reality of the other as a possibility for myself. I have not even asked: *How would it feel to hate mathematics?* Instead, I project my own reality onto my student and say, *You will be just fine if only you learn to love mathematics.* And I have "data" to support me. There is evidence that intrinsic motivation is associated with higher achievement. (Did anyone ever doubt this?) So my student becomes an object of study and manipulation for me. Now, I have deliberately chosen an example that is not often associated with manipulation. Usually, we associate manipulation with trying to get our student to achieve some learning objective that we have devised and set for him. Bringing him to "love mathematics" is seen as a noble aim. And so it is, if it is held out to him as a possibility that he glimpses by observing me and others; but then I shall not be disappointed in him, or in myself, if he remains indifferent to mathematics. It is a possibility that may not be actualized. What matters to me, if I care, is that he find some reason, acceptable in his inner self, for learning the mathematics required of him or that he reject it boldly and honestly. How would it feel to hate mathematics? What reasons could I find for learning it? When I think this way, I refuse to cast about for rewards that might pull him along. He must find his rewards. I do not begin with dazzling performances designed to intrigue him or to change his attitude. I begin, as nearly as I can, with the view from his eyes: Mathematics is bleak, jumbled, scary, boring, boring, boring. . . . What in the world could induce me to engage in it? From that point on, we struggle together with it.

Apprehending the other's reality, feeling what he feels as nearly as possible, is the essential part of caring from the view of the one-caring. For if I take on the other's reality as possibility and begin to feel its reality, I feel, also, that I must act accordingly; that is, I am impelled to act as though in my own behalf, but in behalf of the other. Now, of course, this feeling that I must act may or may not be sustained. I must make a commitment to act. The commitment to act in behalf of the cared-for, a continued interest in his reality throughout the appropriate time span, and the continual renewal of commitment over this span of time are the essential elements of caring from the inner view. Mayeroff speaks of devotion and the promotion of growth in the cared-for. I wish to start with engrossment and motivational displacement. Both concepts will require elaboration.

PROBLEMS ARISING IN THE ANALYSIS OF ONE-CARING

As I think about how I feel when I care, about what my frame of mind is, I see that my caring is always characterized by a move away from self. Yet not all instances of caring are alike even from the view of one-caring. Conditions change, and the time spanned by caring varies. While I care for my children throughout our mutual lifetimes, I may care only momentarily for a stranger in need. The intensity varies. I care deeply for those in my inner circles and more lightly for those farther removed from my personal life. Even with those close to me, the intensity of caring varies; it may be calm and steady most of the time and desperately anxious in emergencies.

The acts performed out of caring vary with both situational conditions and type of relationship. It may bother me briefly, as a teacher, to learn that students in general are not doing well with the subject I teach, but I cannot really be said to care for each of the students having difficulty. And if I have not taken up a serious study of the difficulties themselves, I cannot be said to care about the problem qua problem. But if one of my own students is having difficulty, I may experience the engrossment and motivational displacement of caring. Does this caring spring out of the relationship I have formed with the student? Or, is it possible that I cared in some meaningful way before I even met the particular student?

The problems arising here involve time spans, intensity, and certain formal aspects of caring. Later, I shall explore the concept of chains of caring in which certain formal links to known cared-fors bind us to the possibility of caring. The construction of such formal chains places us in a state of readiness to care. Because my future students are related (formally, *as* students) to present, actual students for whom I do care, I am prepared to care for them also.

As we become aware of the problems involving time, intensity, and formal relationships, we may be led to reconsider the requirement of engrossment. We might instead describe caring of different sorts, on different levels and at varying degrees of intensity. Although I understand why several writers have chosen to speak of special kinds of caring appropriate to particular relationships, I shall claim that these efforts obscure the fundamental truth. At bottom, all caring involves engrossment. The engrossment need not be intense nor need it be pervasive in the life of the one-caring, but it must occur. This requirement does not force caring into the model of romantic love, as some critics fear,[7] for our engrossment may be latent for long periods. We may say of caring as Martin Buber says of love, "it endures, but only in the alternation of actuality and latency."[8] The difference that this approach makes is significant. Whatever roles I assume in life, I may be described in constant terms as one-caring. My first and unending obligation is to meet the other as one-caring. Formal constraints may be added to the fundamental requirement, but they do not replace or weaken it. When we discuss pedagogical caring, for example, we shall develop it from the analysis of caring itself and not from the formal requirements of teaching as a profession.[9]

Another problem arises when we consider situations in which we do not naturally care. Responding to my own child crying in the night may require a physical effort, but it does not usually require what might be called an ethical effort. I naturally want to relieve my child's distress. But receiving the other as he feels and trying to do so are qualitatively different modes. In the first, I am already "with" the other. My motivational energies are flowing toward him and, perhaps, toward his ends. In the second, I may dimly or dramatically perceive a reality that is a repugnant possibility for me. Dwelling in it may bring self-revulsion and disgust. Then I must withdraw. I do not "care" for this person. I may hate him, but I need not. If I do something in his behalf—defend his legal rights or confirm a statement he makes—it is because I care about my own ethical self. In caring for my ethical self, I grapple with the question: Must I try to care? When and for whom? A description of the ethical ideal and its construction will be essential in trying to answer these questions.

There are other limitations in caring. Not only are there those for whom I do not naturally care—situations in which engrossment brings revulsion and motivational displacement is unthinkable—but there are, also, many beyond the reach of my caring. I shall reject the notion of universal caring—that is, caring for everyone—on the grounds that it is impossible to actualize and leads us to substitute abstract problem solving and mere talk for genuine caring. Many of us think that it is not only possible to care for everyone but morally obligatory that we should do so. We can, in a sense that will need elaboration, "care about" everyone; that is, we can maintain an internal state of readiness to try to care for whoever crosses our path. But this is different from the caring-for to which we refer when we use the word "caring." If we are thoughtful persons, we know that the difference is great, and we may even deliberately restrict our contacts so that the caring-for of which we are capable does not deteriorate to mere verbal caring-about. I shall not try to maintain this linguistic distinction, because it seems somewhat unnatural, but we should keep in mind the real distinction we are pointing at: in one sense, "caring" refers to an actuality; in the other, it refers to a verbal commitment to the possibility of caring.

We may add both guilt and conflict to our growing list of problems in connection with the analysis of caring. Conflict arises when our engrossment is divided, and several cared-fors demand incompatible decisions from us. Another sort of conflict occurs when what the cared-for wants is not what we think would be best for him, and still another sort arises when we become overburdened and our caring turns into "cares and burdens." Any of these conflicts may induce guilt. Further, we may feel guilty when we fall short of doing what the cared-for wants us to do or when we bring about outcomes we ourselves did not intend to bring about. Conflict and guilt are inescapable risks of caring, and their consideration will suggest an exploration of courage.

The one-caring is, however, not alone in the caring relationship. Sometimes caring turns inward—as for Mr. Smith in his description of worries and burdens—because conditions are intolerable or because the cared-for is singularly difficult. Clearly, we need also to analyze the role of the cared-for.

THE CARED-FOR

We want to examine both the effects of caring on the cared-for and the special contributions that the cared-for makes to the caring relation. The first topic has received far more attention, and we shall start there also. We shall see that for (A, B) to be a caring relation, both A (the one-caring) and B (the cared-for) must contribute appropriately. Something from A must be received, completed, in B. Generally, we characterize this something as an attitude. B looks for something which tells him that A has regard for him, that he is not being treated perfunctorily.

Gabriel Marcel characterizes this attitude in terms of "disposability (*disponibilité*), the readiness to bestow and spend oneself and make oneself available, and its contrary, indisposability."[10] One who is disposable recognizes that she has a self to invest, to give. She does not identify herself with her objects and possessions. She is present to the cared-for. One who is indisposable, however, comes across even to one physically present as absent, as elsewhere. Marcel says: "When I am with someone who is indisposable, I am conscious of being with someone for whom I do not exist; I am thrown back on myself."[11]

The one-caring, in caring, is *present* in her acts of caring. Even in physical absence, acts at a distance bear the signs of presence: engrossment in the other, regard, desire for the other's well-being. Caring is largely reactive and responsive. Perhaps it is even better characterized as receptive. The one-caring is sufficiently engrossed in the other to listen to him and to take pleasure or pain in what he recounts. Whatever she does for the cared-for is embedded in a relationship that reveals itself as engrossment and in an attitude that warms and comforts the cared-for.

The caring attitude, this quality of disposability, pervades the situational time-space. So far as it is in my control, if we are conversing and if I care, I remain present to you throughout the conversation. Of couse, if I care and you do not, then I may put my presence at a distance, thus freeing you to embrace the absence you have chosen. This is the way of dignity in such situations. To be treated as though one does not exist is a threatening experience, and one has to gather up one's self, one's presence, and place it in a safer, more welcome environment. And, of course, it is the way of generosity.

The one cared-for sees the concern, delight, or interest in the eyes of the one-caring and feels her warmth in both verbal and body language. To the cared-for no act in his behalf is quite as important or influential as the attitude of the one-caring. A major act done grudgingly may be accepted graciously on the surface but resented deeply inwardly, whereas a small act performed generously may be accepted nonchalantly but appreciated inwardly. When the attitude of the one-caring bespeaks caring, the cared-for glows, grows stronger, and feels not so much that he has been given something as that something has been added to him. And this "something" may be hard to specify. Indeed, for the one-caring and the cared-for in a relationship of genuine caring, there is no felt need on either part to specify what sort of transformation has taken place.

The intangible something that is added to the cared-for (and often, simultaneously, to the one-caring) will be an important consideration for us when we discuss caring in social institutions and, especially, in schools. It may be that much of what is most valuable in the teaching-learning relationship cannot be specified and certainly not prespecified. The attitude characteristic of caring comes through in acquaintance. When the student associates with the teacher, feeling free to initiate conversation and to suggest areas of interest, he or she is better able to detect the characteristic attitude even in formal, goal-oriented situations such as lectures. Then a brief contact of eyes may say, "I am still the one interested in you. All of this is of variable importance and significance, but you still matter more." It is no use saying that the teacher who "really cares" wants her students to learn the basic skills which are necessary to a comfortable life; I am not denying that, but the notion is impoverished on both ends. On the one extreme, it is not enough to want one's students to master basic skills. I would not want to choose, but if I had to choose whether my child would be a reader or a loving human being, I would choose the latter with alacrity. On the other extreme, it is by itself too much, for it suggests that I as a caring teacher should be willing to do almost anything to bring my students to mastery of the basic skills. And I am not. Among the intangibles that I would have my students carry away is the feeling that the subject we have struggled with is both fascinating and boring, significant and silly, fraught with meaning and nonsense, challenging and tedious, and that whatever attitude we take toward it, it will not diminish our regard for each other. The student is infinitely more important than the subject.

So far in this discussion of the cared-for, I have emphasized the attitude of the one-caring and how its reception affects the cared-for. But we are interested also in the unique contribution of the cared-for to the relation. In chapter three, where we shall discuss the role of the cared-for in some detail, we shall encounter the problem of *reciprocity*. What exactly does the cared-for give to the relation, or does he simply receive? What responsibility does he have for the maintenance of the relation? Can he be blamed for ethical deterioration in the one-caring? How does he contribute to the construction of the ethical ideal in the one-caring?

AESTHETICAL CARING

I am going to use the expression "aesthetical caring" for caring about things and ideas, and I shall justify that use a bit later. Caring about things or ideas seems to be a qualitatively different form of caring. We do use "care about" and "care for" in relation to objects. We say, "Mr. Smith really cares about his lawn," and "Ms. Brown cares more for her kitchen than for her children." But we cannot mean by these expressions what we have been talking about in connection with caring for persons. We may be engrossed in our lawn or kitchen, but there is no "other" toward whom we move, no other subjective reality to grasp, and there is no second person to whom an attitude is conveyed. Such "caring" may be related to caring for persons other than ourselves and, of course, it is related to the ways in which we care for ourselves, but it may also distract us from caring about persons. We can become too busy "caring" for things to care about people.

We shall encounter challenging anomalies in this area of caring also. Most of us commonly take as pejorative, "He cares only about money"; but we have mixed feelings when we hear, "He cares only about mathematics," or "She cares only about music." In part, we react this way because we feel that a person who cares only about money is likely to hurt others in his pursuit of it, while one who cares only about mathematics is a harmless and, perhaps, admirable person who is denying himself the pleasures of life in his devotion to an esoteric object. But, again, our attitude may be partially conditioned by a traditional respect and regard for the intellectual and, especially, the aesthetic, here interpreted as a sort of passionate involvement with form and nonpersonal content. It will be a special problem for us to ask about the relation between the ethical and the aesthetic and how caring, which we shall take to be the very foundation of the ethical, may be enhanced, distorted, or even diminished by the aesthetic. From the writing of T. E. Lawrence on his Arabian adventures [12] to Kierkegaard's disinterested and skeptical "Mr. A,"[13] we see the loss of the ethical in a highly intellectualized aesthetic. To be always apart in human affairs, a critical and sensitive observer, to remain troubled but uncommitted, to be just so much affected or affected in just such a way, is to lose the ethical in the aesthetic.

And yet we feel, perhaps rightly, that the receptivity characteristic of aesthetic engagement is very like the receptivity of caring. Consciousness assumes a similar mode of being—one that attempts to grasp or to receive a reality rather than to impose it. Mozart spoke of hearing melodies in his head,[14] and the mathematician Gauss was "seized" by mathematics.[15] Similarly, one who cares for another is seized by the other's projects or plight and often "hears" without words having been spoken by the other. Further, the creative artist, in creating, is present to the work of art as it is forming: listening, watching, feeling, contributing. This exchange between artist and work, this sense of an apprehended or received reality that is nevertheless uniquely one's own, was attested to by Mozart when he asked: "Now, how does it happen that, while I am at work, my compositions assume the form or style which characterize Mozart and are not like anybody else's?"[16]

The sense of having something created through one and only incidentally *by* one is reported frequently by artists. In an interview celebrating his eighty-sixth birthday, Joan Miró tried to explain his creativity to questioning interviewers. He said such things as, "The paper has magnetism," "My hand is guided by a magnetic force," "It is like I am drunk."[17] Yet when we discuss creativity in schools our focus is almost invariably on the activity, the manipulation, the freedom. And, similarly, when we talk about caring, our emphasis is again on the action, on what might properly be called the caretaking. But the caring that gives meaning to the caretaking is too often dismissed as "sentiment." In part, our approaches to creativity and caring are induced by the dominating insistency on objective evaluation. How can we emphasize the receptivity that is at the core of both when we have no way of measuring it? Here we may ultimately decide that some things in life, and in education, must be undertaken and sustained by faith and not by objective evaluation.

Even though the receptivity characteristic of artistic creation resembles that of caring, we shall find important differences, and we are by no means convinced that artistic receptivity is correlated (in individual human beings) with the receptivity of caring. After all, we have known artistic monsters (Wagner comes to mind); men who have loved orchids and despised human life (Conan Doyle's fictional "Moriarity"); people such as some high in the Nazi command, who loved music and art and yet performed unbelievable cruelty on humans. And, of course, we are acquainted with those who care passionately for their families, tribes, or nations and tear the heads off enemies with gusto. We do not expect, then, to find a simple formula that will describe what our children should learn to care about in order to care meaningfully for persons. But we shall see, again, the great importance of the cared-for in contributing to caring relations. Perhaps some people find ideas and things more responsive than the humans they have tried to care for.

Finally, in our discussion of education, we shall be interested in aesthetical caring in its own right. Schools and teachers may, if they wish to do so, exercise some control over the nature and responsiveness of the potential "cared-fors" presented to students as subject matter, and there may be reasonable ways in which to give perceptive/creative modes an appropriate place alongside judgmental/evaluative modes.

CARING AND ACTING

Let's return briefly to the issue of action. Perhaps, with a better notion of what constitutes the first- and second-person aspects of caring, we can now say something more determinate about acts of caring. Our motivation in caring is directed toward the welfare, protection, or enhancement of the cared-for. When we care, we should, ideally, be able to present reasons for our action/inaction which would persuade a reasonable, disinterested observer that we have acted in behalf of the cared-for. This does not mean that all such observers have to agree that they would have behaved exactly as we did in a particular caring situation. They may, on the contrary, see preferred alternatives. They may experience the very conflicts that caused us anxiety and still suggest a different course of action; or they may proceed in a purely rational-objective way and suggest the same or a different course. But, frequently, and especially in the case of inaction, we are not willing to supply reasons to an actual observer; our ideal observer is, and remains, an abstraction. The reasons we would give, those we give to ourselves in honest subjective thinking, should be so well connected to the objective elements of the problem that our course of action clearly either stands a chance of succeeding in behalf of the cared-for, or can have been engaged in only with the hope of effecting something for the cared-for.

Caring involves stepping out of one's own personal frame of reference into the other's. When we care, we consider the other's point of view, his objective needs, and what he expects of us. Our attention, our mental engrossment is on the cared-for, not on ourselves. Our reasons for acting, then, have to do both with the other's wants and desires and with the objective elements of his problematic situation. If the stray cat is healthy and relatively safe, we do not whisk it off to the county shelter; instead, we provide food and water and encourage freedom. Why condemn it to death when it might enjoy a vagabond freedom? If our minds are on ourselves, however—if we have never really left our own a priori frame of reference—our reasons for acting point back at us and not outward to the cared-for. When we want to be thought of as caring, we often act routinely in a way that may easily secure that credit for us.

This gives us, as outsiders to the relation, a way, not infallible to be sure, to judge caretaking for signs of real caring. To care is to act not by fixed rule but by affection and regard. It seems likely, then, that the actions of one-caring will be varied rather than rule-bound; that is, her actions, while predictable in a global sense, will be unpredictable in detail. Variation is to be expected if the one claiming to care really cares, for her engrossment is in the variable and never fully understood other, in the particular other, in a particular set of circumstances. Rule-bound responses in the name of caring lead us to suspect that the claimant wants most to be credited with caring.

To act as one-caring, then, is to act with special regard for the particular person in a concrete situation. We act not to achieve for ourselves a commendation but to protect or enhance the welfare of the cared-for. Because we are inclined toward the cared-for, we want to act in a way that will please him. But we wish to please him for his sake and not for the promise of his grateful response to our generosity. Even this motivation—to act so that the happiness and pleasure of the cared-for will be enhanced—may not provide a sure external sign of caring. We are sometimes thrown into conflict over what the cared-for wants and what we think would be best for him. As caring parents, for example, we cannot always act in ways which bring immediate reactions of pleasure from our children, and to do so may bespeak a desire, again, to be credited with caring.

The one-caring desires the well-being of the cared-for and acts (or abstains from acting—makes an internal act of commitment) to promote that well-being. She is inclined to the other. An observer, however, cannot see the crucial motive and may misread the attitudinal signs. The observer, then, must judge caring, in part, by the following: First, the action (if there has been one) either brings about a favorable outcome for the cared-for or seems reasonably likely to do so; second, the one-caring displays a characteristic variability in her actions—she acts in a nonrule-bound fashion in behalf of the cared-for.

We shall have to spend some time and effort on the discussion of nonrule-bound, caring behavior. Clearly, I do not intend to advocate arbitrary and capricious behavior, but something more like the inconsistency advocated long ago by Ralph Waldo Emerson,[18] the sort of behavior that is conditioned not by a host of narrow and rigidly defined principles but by a broad and loosely defined ethic that molds itself in situations and has a proper regard for human affections, weaknesses, and anxieties. From such an ethic we do not receive prescriptions as to how we must behave under given conditions, but we are somewhat enlightened as to the kinds of questions we should raise (to ourselves and others) in various kinds of situations and the places we might look for appropriate answers. Such an ethic does not attempt to reduce the need for human judgment with a series of "Thou shalts" and "Thou shalt nots." Rather, it recognizes and calls forth human judgment across a wide range of fact and feeling, and it allows for situations and conditions in which judgment (in the impersonal, logical sense) may properly be put aside in favor of faith and commitment.

We establish funds, or institutions, or agencies in order to provide the caretaking we judge to be necessary. The original impulse is often the one associated with caring. It arises in individuals. But as groups of individuals discuss the perceived needs of another individual or group, the imperative changes from "I must do something" to "Something must be done." This change is accompanied by a shift from the nonrational and subjective to the rational and objective. What should be done? Who should do it? Why should the persons named do it? This sort of thinking is not in itself a mistake; it is needed. But it has buried within it the seed of major error. The danger is that caring, which is essentially nonrational in that it requires a constitutive engrossment and displacement of motivation, may gradually or abruptly be transformed into abstract problem solving. There is, then, a shift of focus from the cared-for to the "problem." Opportunities arise for self-interest, and persons entrusted with caring may lack the necessary engrossment in those to be cared-for. Rules are formulated and the characteristic variation in response to the needs of the cared-for may fade away. Those entrusted with caring may focus on satisfying the formulated requirements for caretaking and fail to be present in their interactions with the cared-for. Thus caring disappears and only its illusion remains.

It is clear, of course, that there is also danger in failing to think objectively and well in caring situations. We quite properly enter a rational-objective mode as we try to decide exactly what we will do in behalf of the cared-for. If I am ill informed, or if I make a mistake, or if I act impetuously, I may hurt rather than help the cared-for. But one may argue, here, that the failure is still at the level of engrossment and motivational displacement. Would I behave so carelessly in my own behalf?

It would seem, then, that one of the greatest dangers to caring may be premature switching to a rational-objective mode. It is not that objective thinking is of no use in problems where caring is required, but it is of limited and particular use, and we shall have to inquire deeply into what we shall call "turning points." If rational-objective thinking is to be put in the service of caring, we must at the right moments turn it away from the abstract toward which it tends and back to the concrete. At times we must suspend it in favor of subjective thinking and reflection, allowing time and space for *seeing* and *feeling*. The rational-objective mode must continually be re-established and redirected from a fresh base of commitment. Otherwise, we find ourselves deeply, perhaps inextricably, enmeshed in procedures that somehow serve only themselves; our thoughts are separated, completely detached, from the original objects of caring.

ETHICS AND CARING

It is generally agreed that ethics is the philosophical study of morality, but we also speak of "professional ethics" and a "a personal ethic." When we speak in the second way, we refer to something explicable—a set of rules, an ideal, a constellation of expressions—that guides and justifies our conduct. One can, obviously, behave ethically without engaging in ethics as a philosophical enterprise, and one can even put together an ethic of sorts—that is, a description of what it means to be moral—without seriously questioning what it means to be moral. Such an ethic, it seems to me, may or may not be a guide to moral behavior. It depends, in a fundamental way, on an assessment of the answer to the question: What does it mean to be moral? This question will be central to our investigation. I shall use "ethical" rather than "moral" in most of our discussions but, in doing so, I am assuming that to behave ethically is to behave under the guidance of an acceptable and justifiable account of what it means to be moral. To behave ethically is not to behave in conformity with just any description of morality, and I shall claim that ethical systems are not equivalent simply because they include rules concerning the same matters or categories.

In an argument for the possibility of an objective morality (against relativism), anthropologist Ralph Linton makes two major points that may serve to illuminate the path I am taking. In one argument, he seems to say that ethical relativism is false because it can be shown that all societies lay down rules of some sort for behavior in certain universal categories. All societies, for example, have rules governing sexual behavior. But Linton does not seem to recognize that the content of the rules, and not just their mere existence, is crucial to the discussion of ethicality. He says, for example ". . . practically all societies recognize adultery as unethical and punish the offenders. The same man who will lend his wife to a friend or brother will be roused to fury if she goes to another man without his permission."[19] But, surely, we would like to know what conception of morality makes adultery "wrong" and the lending of one's wife "right." Just as surely, an ethical system that renders such decisions cannot be equivalent to one that finds adultery acceptable and wife lending unacceptable.

In his second claim, Linton is joined by a substantial number of anthropologists. Stated simply, the claim is that morality is based on common human characteristics and needs and that, hence, an objective morality is possible. That morality is rooted somehow in common human needs, feelings, and cognitions is agreed. But it is not clear to me that we can move easily or swiftly from that agreement to a claim that objective morality is possible. We may be able to describe the moral impulse as it arises in response to particular needs and feelings, and we may be able to describe the relation of thinking and acting in relation to that impulse, but as we tackle these tasks, we may move farther away from a notion of objective morality and closer to the conviction that an irremovable subjective core, a longing for goodness, provides what universality and stability there is in what it means to be moral.

I want to build an ethic on caring, and I shall claim that there is a form of caring natural and accessible to all human beings. Certain feelings, attitudes, and memories will be claimed as universal. But the ethic itself will not embody a set of universalizable moral judgments. Indeed, moral judgment will not be its central concern. It is very common among philosophers to move from the question: What is morality? to the seemingly more manageable question: What is a moral judgment? Fred Feldman, for example, makes this move early on. He suggests:

> Perhaps we can shed some light on the meaning of the noun "morality" by considering the adjective "moral." Proceeding in this way will enable us to deal with a less abstract concept, and we may thereby be more successful. So instead of asking "What is morality?" let us pick one of the most interesting of these uses of the adjective "moral" and ask instead, "What is a moral judgment?"[20]

Now, I am not arguing that this move is completely mistaken or that nothing can be gained through a consideration of moral judgments, but such a move is not the only possibility. We might choose another interesting use of the adjective and ask, instead, about the moral impulse or moral attitude. The choice is important. The long-standing emphasis on the study of moral judgments has led to a serious imbalance in moral discussion. In particular, it is well known that many women—perhaps most women—do not approach moral problems as problems of principle, reasoning, and judgment. I shall discuss this problem at length in chapter four. If a substantial segment of humankind approaches moral problems through a consideration of the concrete elements of situations and a regard for themselves as caring, then perhaps an attempt should be made to enlighten the study of morality in this alternative mode. Further, such a study has significant implications, beyond ethics, for education. If moral education, in a double sense, is guided only by the study of moral principles and judgments, not only are women made to feel inferior to men in the moral realm but also education itself may suffer from impoverished and one-sided moral guidance.

So building an ethic on caring seems both reasonable and important. One may well ask, at this point, whether an ethic so constructed will be a form of "situation ethics." It is not, certainly, that form of act-utilitarianism commonly labeled "situation ethics."[21] Its emphasis is not on the consequences of our acts, although these are not, of course, irrelevant. But an ethic of caring locates morality primarily in the pre-act consciousness of the one-caring. Yet is is not a form of agapism. There is no command to love nor, indeed, any God to make the commandment. Further, I shall reject the notion of universal love, finding it unattainable in any but the most abstract sense and thus a source of distraction. While much of what will be developed in the ethic of caring may be found, also, in Christian ethics, there will be major and irreconcilable differences. Human love, human caring, will be quite enough on which to found an ethic.

We must look even more closely at that love and caring.

NOTES

1 Gauss's remark is quoted by Morris Kline, Why Johnny Can't Add (New York: Vintage Books, 1974), p. 58.

2 See Carol Gilligan, "In a Different Voice: Women's Conception of the Self and of Morality," *Harvard Educational Review* 47 (1977), 481–517. Also, "Woman's Place in Man's Life Cycle," *Harvard Educational Review* 49 (1979), 431–446. Also, *In a Different Voice* (Cambridge, Mass.: Harvard University Press), 1982.

3 Milton Mayeroff, *On Caring* (New York: Harper and Row, 1971), p. 1.

4 See David Brandon, *Zen in the Art of Helping* (New York: Dell Publishing Co., 1978), chap. 3.

5 Søren Kierkegaard, *Concluding Unscientific Postscript,* trans. David F. Swenson and Walter Lowrie (Princeton: Princeton University Press, 1941).

6 Ibid., p. 322.

7 See Mary Anne Raywid, "Up from Agape: Response to 'Caring' by Nel Noddings," *Journal of Curriculum Theorizing* (1981), 152–156.

8 Martin Buber, *I and Thou,* trans. Walter Kaufmann (New York: Charles Scribner's Sons, 1970), p. 69.

9 See Richard E. Hult, Jr., "On Pedagogical Caring," *Educational Theory* 29 (1979), 237–244.

10 See H. J. Blackham, *Six Existentialist Thinkers* (New York: Harper and Row, 1959), p. 80.

11 Ibid., p. 80.

12 T. E. Lawrence, *Seven Pillars of Wisdom* (New York: Garden City Publishing Co., 1938), pp. 549, 562–566.

13 Søren Kierkegaard, *Either/Or,* I, trans. David F. Swenson and Lillian M. Swenson (Princeton: Princeton University Press, 1959).

14 See the account in Jacques Hadamard, *The Psychology of Invention in the Mathematical Field* (New York: Dover Publications, Inc., 1954), pp. 16–17.

15 See E. T. Bell, *Men of Mathematics* (New York: Simon and Schuster, 1965), p. 254.

16 Quoted in Hadamard, *The Psychology of Invention in the Mathematical Field*, pp. 16–17.

17 On NBC's *Prime Time Sunday* (July 8, 1979).

18 Ralph Waldo Emerson, "Self-Reliance," in *Essays*, First Series (Boston and New York: Houghton Mifflin Company, 1903), pp. 45–90.

19 Ralph Linton, "An Anthropologist's Approach to Ethical Principles," in *Understanding Moral Philosophy*, ed. James Rachels (Encino, Calif.: Dickenson Publishing Company, Inc., 1976), p. 8.

20 Fred Feldman, *Introductory Ethics* (Englewood Cliffs, N.J.: Prentice-Hall, Inc., 1978), p. 2.

21 See, for example, Joseph Fletcher, *Situation Ethics* (Philadelphia: The Westminster Press, 1966).

WHAT IS MEDICAL ETHICS?

K. Danner Clouser

Medical ethics does not have its own unique methods and principles. Rather, medical ethics is the enterprise of understanding the specialized facts and relationships of the medical world, to apply more precisely the familiar moral rules of everyday life. Some general implications of this view for practitioners and medical ethicists are spelled out.

Reflecting on the *nature* of medical ethics can be helpful only in a limited way. It is not the colorful, zesty part of medical ethics. It does not determine what we should do and should not do. It does not intrigue us with those dramatic, mind-boggling, impossible dilemmas that confront the clinician almost daily. Reflecting on the *nature* of medical ethics is a step removed from all that. One doesn't ask, What ought we do and why?; instead one asks, What are we really doing when we are doing medical ethics? If discussing the nature of medical ethics is a practical help, it is so only remotely. That is, it may point us in the direction of the right ballpark, but it doesn't tell us how to play the game. On the other hand, there is *some* value in finding the right ballpark. In this case we want to know some general boundaries and directions. How is medical ethics different from other ethics? What kinds of questions does it deal with? What considerations are relevant? Are there specialists, and what do they do? This kind of question is very different from that asking, What ought I do in this

Reprinted by permission from the *Annals of Internal Medicine*, vol. 80, no. 5 (1974), p. 657–660. © 1974 The American College of Physicians.

situation?, and probably a lot less exciting. But still, finding the ballpark is not without value.

My plan is to blurt out in a sentence or two what I think to be the relationship between ethics and medical ethics and then to spend the rest of the time elaborating and explaining the basic point. In the end I will briefly discuss some implications of my view of medical ethics for the practitioner and for the medical ethicist.

I do not take myself to be saying anything imaginative or profound. I am simply suggesting an overview that could give some order and perspective to our scattered thoughts and confused immpressions of these phenomena we have come to label "medical ethics."

ETHICS AND MEDICAL ETHICS

Does medical ethics have its own special principles, or assumptions, or methods? Are there special obligations that only physicians have? What makes this realm so special that it has its own morality? What justifies or validates the ethics of medicine, and what is it that ethics is trying to accomplish in medicine?

My view of the matter can be stated very simply: medical morality is no different from normal, everyday morality. In medical ethics we are really working with the same moral rules that we acknowledge in other areas of life. It is just that in medical ethics these familiar moral rules are being applied to situations and relationships peculiar to the medical world. I shall go on to expand that simple notion.

Let's glance first at regular, everyday morality. Moral rules seem to be the core of ethics. That is, the moral rules to which we regularly appeal constitute the starting point in our thinking about ethics. They are the "givens," the phenomena present in our midst, in need of clarification and justification. The moral rules constitute morality; if they are not morality, nothing is. It is the job of the moral philosopher to articulate and describe the rules, to explicate them, and to search for their justification. "Do not kill" is certainly a moral rule; to deny it would be to pull the rug from under ethics. For if that rule doesn't count as an example of morality, what does? It is then up to the moral philosopher to discover why such a rule is so binding, what its characteristics are, what leads us to accept it, when exceptions are justified, and so on*. But these pursuits are not to the point. What is now at issue is how moral rules relate to medical morality. I believe these everyday moral rules apply to the situations and relations of the medical sphere. What makes them "medical ethics" is not something special about the rules or their justification, but something special about the situations and issues with which they are concerned. Medical ethics specializes in applying

---

*I am much indebted to years of discussion with Professor Bernard Gert for my view of philosophical ethics. I highly recommend his book, *The Moral Rules: A New Rational Foundation for Morality,* Harper and Row, 1970 (also in Harper Torchback, 1973).

the old familiar moral rules to one particular domain of activity, namely, the medical. It focuses on the minute details of the medical sector to see what would constitute acting in accord with a particular moral rule in that setting. It is as though it were the job or medical ethics to hold up a huge magnifying glass to the universe of medicine to see its workings more accurately, so that our standard moral rules might be applied more precisely.

But why in that case should we make so much fuss about "medical ethics"? Why are straight ordinary ethics not enough?

There are two answers to that question. One is that within the universe of things medical, the issues and dealings are so very sensitive, intimate, emotionally charged, and critical to lives. This calls for meticulous attention, fine distinctions, and careful surveillance. Hence the intense focus and highlighting of ethics in medicine—to the point of giving it its own name, "medical ethics."

The other main reason for special attention to this realm is its sheer complication. The facts, probabilities, distinctions, risks, and benefits are so involved that it is not easy to act in accord with the moral rules even if you want to. Hence, it becomes imperative to magnify this sector to work through its complicated, microscopic webs.

This latter point is the more important, and elaboration of it will help crystallize our central interest: the relation of ethics to medical ethics. For example, consider the moral rule, "do not kill." Although this rule is relatively easy to understand and to abide by in normal life, it is not at all easy in the biomedical world. Not only is it difficult to know what is life, but it is even difficult to know when one is killing. Is fetal life, life? Is comatose life life? Is isoelectric EEG life with artificial respiration, life? What if respiration is self-supported but the EEG is still flat? Is *that* life? And, as for killing, Is withholding therapy killing? Is it killing even if it is the more merciful death? Is withdrawing therapy in such cases, killing? Is giving massive doses of drugs that nullify the pain but shorten the life, killing? Is unplugging the heart bypass machine when it is discovered the heart cannot be repaired, killing?

Such problems illustrate my point, that medical ethics is esentially ordinary moral rules applied to a special subject matter. And it is the job of medical ethics to get clear about that subject matter.

Other quick examples may help clarify the point. Consider the ordinary moral rule, "Do not deceive." In the medical sphere, Are we deceiving when we don't tell the patient all the hypotheses we are entertaining about the symptoms? When we don't mention all the conceivable risks involved in a procedure? When we don't tell the patient all we know of his condition? When we order many extra tests just to be protected from malpractice suits or just to add some data to our clinical research?

Are we breaking a confidence when we discuss the case with another doctor, or when our secretary sees the patient's folder, or when medical-records personnel see the folder? Are we infringing on a patient's freedom when our social and value opinions are masked as medical judgments; for example, when we decide the options for the patient—ourselves doing all the weighing of risks, benefits, and the quality of life involved—and then give our conclusion as medical advice rather than as the personal value judgment it happens to be?

Another closely related point is the importance of knowing the *facts* of the biomedical world. So many moral decisions involve a weighing of risks against benefits or risk against risk. If we want to do that which causes the least suffering, the facts must be known. We must know what causes what, the probabilities of one result over another, the likelihood of this particular patient being at risk for one thing or another. Apart from these facts we cannot really know what action will cause less suffering, or less loss of freedom, or less deception. So, thorough knowledge of the facts in the medical world is critical to the moral deliberation that takes place there.

Unhappily, the "facts" themselves represent a kind of philosophical problem that needs careful attention. Values insinuate themselves so easily in, under, and through the "facts" of medicine that it sometimes takes a trained eye to see where the fact stops and the value starts. When medicine declares a man "healthy," more than sheer observations and lab reports are involved. Judging a man "healthy" presupposes norms about the state of medical technology, length of life expectations, and maybe even judgments as to quality of life. Similarly, we have become aware of the value judgments hidden in establishing the moment of death, even as we more obviously have in establishing the beginning of life. Both involve assumptions about what human functions, abilities, and qualities have value. Or again, labeling behavior "bizarre" or a child as "acting out" is more than a mere description of facts; it is the comparing of behavior with an implicit norm, involving value judgments. This problem does not call for the deletion of value-laden terms; it calls for vigilance. That is, if we are basing our moral decisions on the facts, then those facts should not be unwittingly distorted by built-in value biases. Such vigilance also becomes a task of medical ethics.

In short, the medical universe is rich in subtleties, nuances, and involved relationships. This makes our everyday moral rules especially difficult to apply and hence the need to prepare the factual and conceptual ground for the application of these moral rules: classifying, making distinctions, organizing the facts, sorting out causes and effects, teasing out implicit value-ladenness, formulating moral rules of thumb, and, of course, defending all these moves.

DO YOUR DUTY

So far I have argued that medical ethics is special because of subject matter and not because of special moral rules. But one of these standard moral rules, in being delineated with respect to medicine, would become uniquely "medical ethics." It it the moral rule, "Do your duty." This is a moral rule because it involves expectations; it involves what others have come to count on and have every reason to believe will be forthcoming. So to fail them is to harm them. This is particularly so in medicine where people's deepest hopes and fears pivot on what they take to be the doctor's obligation. That is, they really depend on the health professional doing his duty to them—or what they believe to be his duty.

This rule needs considerable elaboration. Unfortunately, we must limit it to three basic observations.

1. Much of what has generally been thought to be medical ethics has in reality been the delineation of this particular moral rule. That is, it has been the attempt to fill in what constitutes the duty of health professionals. Fathers have a duty as fathers, firemen as firemen, elected officials as elected officials—and doctors, as doctors. The duties thereby articulated are more *decided* on than derived from basic moral principles. They spell out what could reasonably be expected and what ought to be able to be counted on by others. No doubt this is how many human values that are not strictly ethical values come to be seen as obligations of the medical community. Dignity, compassion, privacy, and understanding are examples. These are important to most humans, and hence probably relevant to their health. So promoting these values may become an obligation of the medical world, under the auspices of this basic moral rule, "Do your duty," even though the promotion of these values would not be thought to be the obligation of people in general.

2. The second observation concerning "Do your duty" is that it is unlike other moral rules. The other moral rules generally tell us what *not* to do, and they are obligatory; it is expected of everyone to refrain from that which is proscribed. Very generally, they proscribe us from causing evil. Fulfillment of these rules is not particularly admirable or praiseworthy, it's just to be expected; these are basic, easily fulfilled obligations of all rational men. Notable for *not* being obligatory is that one go out of his way for someone else, to help them or to avert evil. It's great if he does; it's praiseworthy—but it's beyond the call of basic moral obligation.

Now, "do your duty," as applied to the medical profession, makes some of what is superogatory for others, *obligatory* for health professionals. That is, it become an obligation for health professionals to prevent suffering or death.

3. My final observation about this particular moral rule has to do with how the specifics of this "duty" are determined. They are not necessarily derived from ethical principles nor are they discovered in the nature of things; they must, in effect, be *decided*. What constitutes the duty of health professionals should ideally be reached by agreement between the professionals and their patients. Ideally, the details of this arrangement would be acceptable to any rational person who did not yet know whether he'd be doctor or patient. It might well be that what was considered duty would differ from one community to another. In fact, this may well be why medical ethics seems to differ from one time and place to another, although this is by no means evidence that basic moral rules differ. In any case, what is of prime importance in the "do your duty" rule is that expectations be fair and be clearly understood by all. The crux of the moral issue is that the patient knows what to count on, for to fail him in these expectations is to cause suffering.

SUMMARY

Before considering some of the implications of all this, it may be helpful to get a perspective on my claim about the nature of medical ethics. It is that medical ethics does not have different methods of different principles. Rather, medicine is a specialized body of knowledge and practices to which the ordinary moral rules are applicable. Medical ethics is the enterprise of understanding these specialized and complicated facts with an eye to seeing how the familiar moral rules relate thereto. Additionally, medicine spins its own particular web under the directive of the standard moral rule, "do your duty." Much of what has gone by the name medical ethics has in fact been the spelling out of what constitutes duty. I am arguing that this elaborate spelling out really falls under one standard moral rule, and calls more for agreement and decision than for moral reasoning.

What I am *not* talking about is how our ordinary moral rules come to be or how they come to be discovered. I am not talking about what they are precisely or how we would justify them. Rather, in response to the question, "What is the nature of medical ethics?," I am simply saying that it is really just like ordinary ethics except for certain elaborations in deference to the special facts and relationships of medicine. But these elaborations are, nevertheless, filigree *on* and *within* the house of ethics. The whole point of morality would seem to be the same for both: to allow each of us to realize as much of our own aims and desires as is compatible with everyone else's realizing their own aims and desires and partially to accomplish this with a set of rules that all rational persons would feel compelled (for one reason or another) to urge on each other.

IMPLICATIONS

It may help to discuss explicitly some implications of my view.

1. It is appropriate for doctors to make moral decisions. It is not necessary for them to await word from the medical ethicist. The health professional knows (roughly) the moral rules we all acknowledge, and he knows the specialized facts and relationships to which they are being applied. He therefore is in as good a position as many, and a better position than most, to make a moral judgment. He should proceed with confidence—at least with no less confidence than we all manage to muster in our everyday moral judgments. This is not to say there are not many times when the situation is very complicated and a "specialist" would be a valuable consultant. But it is to counteract the current trend of trying to keep the practitioner from ever making a moral judgment, with the argument that he is stepping outside the domain of competence.

But, as in the rest of medicine, it becomes crucial to know when to consult a specialist. Guidelines are difficult to formulate. Simply saying, "When in doubt, consult a specialist," may be helpful, but it is clearly not enough. I tremble to think how often individuals have been put at risk by an experimenter who confidently believed that "the public interest" or "the good of society" amply justified his action! I know of no formal safeguard against this. It calls for medical people to become familiar with some of the basics of ethical theory just as we would demand that medical ethicists become familiar with some of the facts of medicine. A constant and focused interchange is necessary.

2. The particular tasks of medical ethics are more focused. Its job is neither to discover some new principles on which to build an ethical system nor to evolve some new line of medically appropriate ethical reasoning. Neither is it to articulate the moral rules, nor explicate their nature, nor formulate their justification. That is all more appropriately the domain of philosophical ethics.

But it is the task of medical ethics to prepare the ground for the "application" of the moral rules. As we have seen, this involves knowing the facts of this special realm, making helpful distinctions, and clarifying and creating fruitful concepts so that ethics can rigorously and perceptively be done in this realm.

Having distinguished these two foci—philosophical ethics and medical ethics—one can see that they need each other. Those who daily confront the problems and who know medical facts, probabilities, causes, and effects are indispensable. And to know where to go and what to do with all this, we need those who know ethics—its rules, distinctions, justifications, exceptions, and lines of reasoning.

Needless to say, influence filters both ways: the detailed data force some changes in the theoretical structures, and the theoretical frameworks lead to a new understanding of the data. That is, pressed by actual moral dilemmas and recalcitrant facts, philosophical ethics might well be forced to certain conceptual changes; likewise, medical ethics, enlightened by some theoretical clarification or distinction, might be led to find new data or a new construing of old data.

3. Finally, there are some implications in all this for our expectations. As in ordinary ethics, we should not expect a decision procedure in medical ethics. That is, we should not expect an automatic, deductive procedure for arriving at "the" ethical answer. We must rid ourselves of the confidence that there is a right answer in the back of the book; there is no sure way to arrive at a solution; there is no assurance there is a solution. On the other hand, there may well be a dozen different but equally moral solutions.

Also, as in everyday ethics, we must not expect medical ethics as a discipline to motivate us to be moral or to reprimand us when we aren't. And its role is neither to promote life styles nor to campaign for particular life values. Rather, it should show us how we can implement the familiar moral rules in this new and changing medical context—rules that for the most part tell us what not to do and that have a rational basis, in that we would unhesitatingly urge all others to follow them with respect to ourselves. Again, just like normal, everyday ethics.

APPENDIX

SELECTED PROFESSIONAL CODES OF ETHICS

AMERICAN NURSES' ASSOCIATION CODE FOR NURSES

Preamble

The *Code for Nurses* is based on belief about the nature of individuals, nursing, health, and society. Recipients and providers of nursing services are viewed as individuals and groups who possess basic rights and responsibilities, and whose values and circumstances command respect at all times. Nursing encompasses the promotion and restoration of health, the prevention of illness, and the alleviation of suffering. The statements of the *Code* and their interpretation provide guidance for conduct and relationships in carrying out nursing responsibilities consistent with the ethical obligations of the profession and quality in nursing care.

Code for Nurses

1 The nurse provides services with respect for human dignity and the uniqueness of the client unrestricted by considerations of social or economic status, personal attributes, or the nature of health problems.

2 The nurse safeguards the client's right to privacy by judiciously protecting information of a confidential nature.

Adopted by the American Nurses' Association in 1976 and reprinted by permission.

3 The nurse acts to safeguard the client and the public when health care and safety are affected by the incompetent, unethical, or illegal practice of any person.

4 The nurse assumes responsibility and accountability for individual nursing judgments and actions.

5 The nurse maintains competence in nursing.

6 The nurse exercises informed judgment and uses individual competence and qualifications as criteria in seeking consultation, accepting responsibilities, and delegating nursing activities to others.

7 The nurse participates in activities that contribute to the ongoing development of the profession's body of knowledge.

8 The nurse participates in the profession's efforts to implement and improve standards of nursing.

9 The nurse participates in the profession's efforts to establish and maintain conditions of employment conducive to high quality nursing care.

10 The nurse participates in the profession's effort to protect the public from misinformation and misrepresentation and to maintain the integrity of nursing.

11 The nurse collaborates with members of the health professions and other citizens in promoting community and national efforts to meet the health needs of the public.

INTERNATIONAL COUNCIL OF NURSES CODE FOR NURSES: ETHICAL CONCEPTS APPLIED TO NURSING

The fundamental responsibility of the nurse is fourfold: to promote health, to prevent illness, to restore health and to alleviate suffering.

The need for nursing is universal. Inherent in nursing is respect for life, dignity and rights of man. It is unrestricted by considerations of nationality, race, creed, color, age, sex, politics or social status.

Nurses render health services to the individual, the family and the community and coordinate their services with those of related groups.

Nurses and People

The nurse carries personal responsibility for nursing practice and for maintaining competence by continual learning.

The nurse maintains the highest standards of nursing care possible within the reality of a specific situation.

Adopted by the International Council of Nurses, May 1973. Reprinted by permission.

The nurse uses judgement in relation to individual competence when accepting and delegating responsibilities.

The nurse when acting in a professional capacity should at all times maintain standards of personal conduct which reflect credit upon the profession.

Nurses and Society

The nurse shares with other citizens the responsibility for initiating and supporting action to meet the health and social needs of the public.

Nurses and Co-Workers

The nurse sustains a cooperative relationship with co-workers in nursing and other fields.

The nurse takes appropriate action to safeguard the individual when his care is endangered by a co-worker or any other person.

Nurses and the Profession

The nurse plays the major role in determining and implementing desirable standards of nursing practice and nursing education.

The nurse is active in developing a core of professional knowledge.

The nurse, acting through the professional organization, participates in establishing and maintaining equitable social and economic working conditions in nursing.

THE HIPPOCRATIC OATH

I swear by Apollo Physician and Asclepius and Hygieia and Panaceia and all the gods and goddesses, making them my witnesses, that I will fulfil according to my ability and judgment this oath and this covenant:

To hold him who has taught me this art as equal to my parents and to live my life in partnership with him, and if he is in need of money to give him a share of mine, and to regard his offspring as equal to my brothers in male lineage and to teach them this art—if they desire to learn it—without fee and covenant; to give a share of precepts and oral instruction and all the other learning to my sons and to the sons of him who has instructed me and to pupils who have signed the covenant and have taken an oath according to the medical law, but to no one else.

I will apply dietetic measures for the benefit of the sick according to my ability and judgment; I will keep them from harm and injustice.

I will neither give a deadly drug to anybody if asked for it, nor will I make a suggestion to this effect. Similarly I will not give to a woman an abortive remedy. In purity and holiness I will guard my life and my art.

I will not use the knife, not even on sufferers from stone, but will withdraw in favor of such men as are engaged in this work.

Whatever houses I may visit, I will come for the benefit of the sick, remaining free of all intentional injustice, of all mischief and in particular of sexual relations with both female and male persons, be they free or slaves.

What I may see or hear in the course of the treatment or even outside of the treatment in regard to the life of men, which on no account one must spread abroad, I will keep to myself holding such things shameful to be spoken about.

If I fulfill this oath and do not violate it, may it be granted to me to enjoy life and art, being honored with fame among all men for all time to come; if I transgress it and swear falsely, may the opposite of all this be my lot.

PRINCIPLES OF MEDICAL ETHICS OF THE AMERICAN MEDICAL ASSOCIATION

Preamble

These principles are intended to aid physicians individually and collectively in maintaining a high level of ethical conduct. They are not laws but standards by which a physician may determine the propriety of his conduct in his relationship with patients, with colleagues, with members of allied professions, and with the public.

Section 1

The principal objective of the medical profession is to render service to humanity with full respect for the dignity of man. Physicians should merit the confidence of patients entrusted to their care, rendering to each a full measure of service and devotion.

Section 2

Physicians should strive continually to improve medical knowledge and skill, and should make available to their patients and colleagues the benefits of their professional attainments.

Section 3

A physician should practice a method of healing founded on a scientific basis; and he should not voluntarily associate professionally with anyone who violates this principle.

Section 4

The medical profession should safeguard the public and itself against physicians deficient in moral character or professional competence. Physicians should observe all laws, uphold the dignity and honor of the profession and accept its self-imposed disciplines. They should expose, without hesitation, illegal or unethical conduct of fellow members of the profession.

Section 5

A physician may choose whom he will serve. In an emergency, however, he should render service to the best of his ability. Having undertaken the care of a patient, he may not neglect him; and unless he has been discharged he may discontinue his services only after giving adequate notice. He should not solicit patients.

Section 6

A physician should not dispose of his services under terms or conditions which tend to interfere with or impair the free and complete exercise of his medical judgment and skill or tend to cause a deterioration of the quality of medical care.

Section 7

In the practice of medicine a physician should limit the source of his professional income to medical services actually rendered by him, or under his supervision, to his patients. His fee should be commensurate with the services rendered and the patient's ability to pay. He should neither pay nor receive a commission for referral of patients. Drugs, remedies or appliances may be dispensed or supplied by the physician provided it is in the best interests of the patient.

Section 8

A physician should seek consultation upon request; in doubtful or difficult cases, or whatever it appears that the quality of medical service may be enhanced thereby.

Section 9

A physician may not reveal the confidences entrusted to him in the course of medical attendance, or the deficiencies he may observe in the character of patients, unless he is required to do so by law or unless it becomes necessary in order to protect the welfare of the individual or of the community.

Section 10

The honored ideals of the medical profession imply that the responsibilities of the physician extend not only to the individual, but also to society where these responsibilities deserve his interest and participation in activities which have the purpose of improving both the health and the well-being of the individual and the community.

AMERICAN MEDICAL RECORD ASSOCIATION: CODE OF ETHICS

Preamble

The medical record professional abides by a set of ethical principles developed to safeguard the public and to contribute within the scope of the profession to quality and efficiency in health care. This code of ethic, adopted by members of the American Medical Record Association, defines the standards of behavior which promote ethical conduct.

1 The Medical Record Professional demonstrates behavior that reflects integrity, supports objectivity, and fosters trust in professional activities.

2 The Medical Record Professional respects the dignity of each human being.

3 The Medical Record Professional strives to improve personal competence and quality of services.

4 The Medical Record Professional represents truthfully and accurately professional credentials, education, and experience.

5 The Medical Record Professional refuses to participate in illegal or unethical acts and also refuses to conceal the illegal, incompetent, or unethical acts of others.

6 The Medical Record Professional protects the confidentiality of primary and secondary health records as mandated by law, professional standards, and the employer's policies.

Adopted by the American Medical Record Association, October 1985. Reprinted by permission.

7 The Medical Record Professional promotes to others the tenets of confidentiality.

8 The Medical Record Professional adheres to pertinent laws and regulations while advocating changes which serve the best interest of the public.

9 The Medical Record Professional encourages appropriate use of health record information and advocates policies and systems that advance the management of health records and health information.

10 The Medical Record Professional recognizes and supports the association's mission.

CONSTITUTION OF THE WORLD HEALTH ORGANIZATION

The States Parties to this Constitution declare, in conformity with the Charter of the United Nations, that the following principles are basic to the happiness, harmonious relations and security of all peoples:

Health is a state of complete physical, mental and social well-being and not merely the absence of disease or infirmity.

The enjoyment of the highest attainable standard of health is one of the fundamental rights of every human being without distinction of race, religion, political belief, economic or social condition.

The health of all peoples is fundamental to the attainment of peace and security and is dependent upon the fullest co-operation of individuals and States.

The achievement of any State in the promotion and protection of health is of value to all.

Unequal development in different countries in the promotion of health and control of disease, especially communicable disease, is a common danger.

Healthy development of the child is of basic importance; the ability to live harmoniously in a changing total environment is essential to such development.

The extension to all peoples of the benefits of medical, psychological and related knowledge is essential to the fullest attainment of health.

Informed opinion and active co-operation on the part of the public are of the utmost importance in the improvement of the health of the people.

Governments have a responsibility for the health of their peoples which can be fulfilled only by the provision of adequate health and social measures.

Accepting these principles, and for the purpose of co-operation among themselves and with others to promote and protect the health of all peoples, the Contracting Parties agree to the present Constitution and hereby establish the World Health Organization as a specialized agency within the terms of Article 57 of the Charter of the United Nations.

AMERICAN HOSPITAL ASSOCIATION: A PATIENT'S BILL OF RIGHTS

The American Hospital Association presents a Patient's Bill of Rights with the expectation that observance of these rights will contribute to more effective patient care and greater satisfaction for the patient, his physician, and the hospital organization. Further, the Association presents these rights in the expectation that they will be supported by the hospital on behalf of its patients, as an integral part of the healing process. It is recognized that a personal relationship between the physician and the patient is essential for the provision of proper medical care. The traditional physician-patient relationship takes on a new dimension when care is rendered within an organizational structure. Legal precedent has established that the institution itself also has a responsibility to the patient. It is in recognition of these factors that these rights are affirmed.

1 The patient has the right to considerate and respectful care.

2 The patient has the right to obtain from his physician complete current information concerning his diagnosis, treatment, and prognosis in terms the patient can be reasonably expected to understand. When it is not medically advisable to give such information to the patient, the information should be made available to an appropriate person in his behalf. He has the right to know, by name, the physician responsible for coordinating his care.

3 The patient has the right to receive from his physician information necessary to give informed consent prior to the start of any procedure and/or treatment. Except in emergencies, such information for informed consent should include but not necessarily be limited to the specific procedure and/or treatment, the medically significant risks involved, and the probable duration of incapacitation. Where medically significant alternatives for care or treatment exist, or when the patient requests information concerning medical alternatives, the patient has the right to such information. The patient also has the right to know the name of the person responsible for the procedures and/or treatment.

4 The patient has the right to refuse treatment to the extent permitted by law and to be informed of the medical consequences of his action.

5 The patient has the right to every consideration of his privacy concerning his own medical care program. Case discussion, consultation, examination, and treatment are confidential and should be conducted discreetly. Those not directly involved in his care must have the permission of the patient to be present.

6 The patient has the right to expect that all communications and records pertaining to his care should be treated as confidential.

7 The patient has the right to expect that within its capacity a hospital must make reasonable response to the request of a patient for services. The hospital must provide evaluation, service, and/or referral as indicated by the urgency of the case. When medically permissible, a patient may be transferred to another facility only after he has received complete information and explanation concerning the needs for and alternatives to such a transfer. The institution to which the patient is to be transferred must first have accepted the patient for transfer.

8 The patient has the right to obtain information as to any relationship of his hospital to other health care and educational institutions insofar as his care is concerned. The patient has the right to obtain information as to the existence of any professional relationships among individuals, by name, who are treating him.

9 The patient has the right to be advised if the hospital proposes to engage in or perform human experimentation affecting his care or treatment. The patient has the right to refuse to participate in such research projects.

10 The patient has the right to expect reasonable continuity of care. He has the right to know in advance what appointment times and physicians are available and where. The patient has the right to expect that the hospital will provide a mechanism whereby he is informed by his physician or a delegate of the physician of the patient's continuing health care requirements following discharge.

11 The patient has the right to examine and receive an explanation of his bill regardless of source of payment.

12 The patient has the right to know what hospital rules and regulations apply to his conduct as a patient.

No catalog of rights can guarantee for the patient the kind of treatment he has a right to expect. A hospital has many functions to perform, including the prevention and treatment of disease, the education of both health professionals and patients, and the conduct of clinical research. All these activities must be conducted with an overriding concern for the patient, and, above all, the recognition of his dignity as a human being. Success in achieving this recognition assures success in the defense of the rights of the patient.

THE NUREMBURG CODE

The great weight of the evidence before us is to the effect that certain types of medical experiments on human beings, when kept within reasonably well-defined bounds, conform to the ethics of the medical profession generally. The protagonists of the practice of human experimentation justify their views on the basis that such experiments yield results for the good of society that are unprocurable by other methods or means of study. All agree, however, that certain basic principles must be observed in order to satisfy moral, ethical and legal concepts:

Reprinted from *Trials of War Criminals before The Nuremberg Military Tribunals under Control Council Law No. 10, vol. 2* U.S. Government Printing Office, Washington D.C., 1949, p. 181–182.

1 The voluntary consent of the human subject is absolutely essential.

This means that the person involved should have legal capacity to give consent; should be so situated as to be able to exercise free power of choice, without the intervention of any element of force, fraud, deceit, duress, over-reaching, or other ulterior form of constraint or coercion; and should have sufficient knowledge and comprehension of the elements of the subject matter involved as to enable him to make an understanding and enlightened decision. This latter element requires that before the acceptance of an affirmative decision by the experimental subject there should be made known to him the nature, duration, and purpose of the experiment; the method and means by which it is to be conducted; all inconveniences and hazards reasonably to be expected; and the effects upon his health or person which may possibly come from his participation in the experiment.

The duty and responsibility for ascertaining the quality of the consent rests upon each individual who initiates, directs or engages in the experiment. It is a personal duty and responsibility which may not be delegated to another with impunity.

2 The experiment should be such as to yield fruitful results for the good of society, unprocurable by other methods or means of study, and not random and unnecessary in nature.

3 The experiment should be so designed and based on the results of animal experimentation and a knowledge of the natural history of the disease or other problem under study that the anticipated results will justify the performance of the experiment.

4 The experiment should be so conducted as to avoid all unnecessary physical and mental suffering and injury.

5 No experiment should be conducted where there is an a priori reason to believe that death or disabling injury will occur; except, perhaps, in those experiments where the experimental physicians also serve as subjects.

6 The degree of risk to be taken should never exceed that determined by the humanitarian importance of the problem to be solved by the experiment.

7 Proper preparations should be made and adequate facilities provided to protect the experimental subject against even remote possibilities of injury, disability, or death.

8 The experiment should be conducted only by scientifically qualified persons. The highest degree of skill and care should be required through all stages of the experiment of those who conduct or engage in the experiment.

9 During the course of the experiment the human subject should be at liberty to bring the experiment to an end if he has reached the physical or mental state where continuation of the experiment seems to him to be impossible.

10 During the course of the experiment the scientist in charge must be prepared to terminate the experiment at any stage, if he has probable cause to believe, in the exercise of the good faith, superior skill and careful judgment required of him that a continuation of the experiment is likely to result in injury, disability, or death to the experimental subject.

THE WORLD MEDICAL ASSOCIATION: DECLARATION OF HELSINKI

Introduction

It is the mission of the medical doctor to safeguard the health of the people. His or her knowledge and conscience are dedicated to the fulfillment of this mission.

The Declaration of Geneva of the World Medical Association binds the doctor with the words, "The health of my patient will be my first consideration," and the International Code of Medical Ethics declares that, "Any act or advice which could weaken physical or mental resistance of a human being may be used only in his interest."

The purpose of biomedical research involving human subjects must be to improve diagnostic, therapeutic and prophylactic procedures and the understanding of the aetiology and pathogenesis of disease.

In current medical practice most diagnostic, therapeutic or prophylactic procedures involve hazards. This applies a fortiori to biomedical research.

Medical progress is based on research which ultimately must rest in part on experimentation involving human subjects.

In the field of biomedical research a fundamental distinction must be recognized between medical research in which the aim is essentially diagnostic or therapeutic for a patient, and medical research, the essential object of which is purely scientific and without direct diagnostic or therapeutic value to the person subjected to the research.

Special caution must be exercised in the conduct of research which may affect the environment, and the welfare of animals used for research must be respected.

Because it is essential that the results of laboratory experiments be applied to human beings to further scientific knowledge and to help suffering humanity, The World Medical Association has prepared the following recommendations as a guide to every doctor in biomedical research involving human subjects. They should be kept under review in the future. It must be stressed that the standards as drafted are only a guide to physicians all over the world. Doctors are not relieved from criminal, civil and ethical responsibilities under the laws of their own countries.

I. Basic Principles

1 Biomedical research involving human subjects must conform to generally accepted scientific principles and should be based on adequately performed laboratory and animal experimentation and on a thorough knowledge of the scientific literature.

2 The design and performance of each experimental procedure involving human subjects should be clearly formulated in an experimental protocol which should be transmitted to a specially appointed independent committee for consideration, comment and guidance.

3 Biomedical research involving human subjects should be conducted only by scientifically qualified persons and under the supervision of a clinically competent medical person. The responsibility for the human subject must always rest with a medically qualified person and never rest on the subject of the research, even though the subject has given his or her consent.

4 Biomedical research involving human subjects cannot legitimately be carried out unless the importance of the objective is in proportion to the inherent risk to the subject.

5 Every biomedical research project involving human subjects should be preceded by careful assessment of predictable risks in comparison with foreseeable benefits to the subject or to others. Concern for the interests of the subject must always prevail over the interests of science and society.

6 The right of the research subject to safeguard his or her integrity must always be respected. Every precaution should be taken to respect the privacy of the subject and to minimize the impact of the study on the subject's physical and mental integrity and on the personality of the subject.

7 Doctors should abstain from engaging in research projects involving human subjects unless they are satisfied that the hazards involved are believed to be predictable. Doctors should cease any investigation if the hazards are found to outweigh the potential benefits.

8 In publication of the results of his or her research, the doctor is obliged to preserve the accuracy of the results. Reports of experimentation not in accordance with the principles laid down in this Declaration should not be accepted for publication.

9 In any research on human beings, each potential subject must be adequately informed of the aims, methods, anticipated benefits and potential hazards of the study and the discomfort it may entail. He or she should be informed that he or she is at liberty to abstain from participation in the study and that he or she is free to withdraw his or her consent to participation at any time. The doctor should then obtain the subject's freely-given informed consent, preferably in writing.

10 When obtaining informed consent for the research project the doctor should be particularly cautious if the subject is in a dependent relationship to him or her or may consent under duress. In that case the informed consent should be obtained by a doctor who is not engaged in the investigation and who is completely independent of this official relationship.

11 In case of legal incompetence, informed consent should be obtained from the legal guardian in accordance with national legislation. Where physical or mental incapacity makes it impossible to obtain informed consent, or when the subject is a minor, permission from the responsible relative replaces that of the subject in accordance with national legislation.

12 The research protocol should always contain a statement of the ethical considerations involved and should indicate that the principles enunciated in the present Declaration are complied with.

II. Medical Research Combined with Professional Care (Clinical Research)

1 In the treatment of the sick person, the doctor must be free to use a new diagnostic and therapeutic measure, if in his or her judgment it offers hope of saving life, reestablishing health or alleviating suffering.

2 The potential benefits, hazards and discomfort of a new method should be weighed against the advantages of the best current diagnostic and therapeutic methods.

3 In any medical study, every patient—including those of a control group, if any—should be assured of the best proven diagnostic and therapeutic method.

4 The refusal of the patient to participate in a study must never interfere with the doctor-patient relationship.

5 If the doctor considers it essential not to obtain informed consent, the specific reasons for this proposal should be stated in the experimental protocol for transmission to the independent committee (1,2).

6 The doctor can combine medical research with professional care, the objective being the acquisition of new medical knowledge, only to the extent that medical research is justified by its potential diagnostic or therapeutic value for the patient.

III. Non-therapeutic Biomedical Research Involving Human Subjects (Non-clinical Biomedical Research)

1 In the purely scientific application of medical research carried out on a human being, it is the duty of the doctor to remain the protector of the life and health of that person on whom biomedical research is being carried out.

2 The subjects should be volunteers—either healthy persons or patients for whom the experimental design is not related to the patient's illness.

3 The investigator or the investigating team should discontinue the research if in his/her or their judgment it may, if continued, be harmful to the individual.

4 In research on man, the interest of science and society should never take precedence over considerations related to the wellbeing of the subject.

DEPARTMENT OF HEALTH, EDUCATION, AND WELFARE: REGULATIONS ON THE PROTECTION OF HUMAN SUBJECTS

§46.101 Applicability

(a) The regulations in this part are applicable to all Department of Health, Education, and Welfare grants and contracts supporting research, development, and related activities in which human subjects are involved.

(b) The Secretary may, from time to time, determine in advance whether specific programs, methods, or procedures to which this part is applicable place subjects at risk, as defined in §46.103(b). Such determinations will be published as notices in the FEDERAL REGISTER and will be included in an appendix to this part.

§46.102 Policy

(a) Safeguarding the rights and welfare of subjects at risk in activities supported under grants and contracts from DHEW is primarily the responsibility of the institution which receives or is accountable to DHEW for the funds awarded for the support of the activity. In order to provide for the adequate discharge of this institutional responsibility, it is the policy of DHEW that no activity involving human subjects to be supported by DHEW grants or contracts shall be undertaken unless an Institutional Review Board has reviewed and approved such activity, and the institution has submitted to DHEW a certification of such review and approval, in accordance with the requirements of this part.

(b) This review shall determine whether these subjects will be placed at risk, and, if risk is involved, whether:

1 The risks to the subject are so outweighed by the sum of the benefit to the subject and the importance of the knowledge to be gained as to warrant a decision to allow the subject to accept these risks;

2 The rights and welfare of any such subjects will be adequately protected; and

3 Legally effective informed consent will be obtained by adequate and appropriate methods in accordance with the provisions of this part.

(c) Unless the activity is covered by subpart B of this part, if it involves as subjects women who could become pregnant, the Board shall also determine as part of its review that adequate and appropriate steps will be taken to avoid involvement of women who are in fact pregnant (as evidenced by any of the presumptive signs of pregnancy, such as missed menses, or by a medically acceptable pregnancy test), when such activity would involve risk to a fetus.

(d) Where the Board finds risk is involved under paragraph (b) of this section, it shall review the conduct of the activity at timely intervals.

(e) No grant or contract involving human subjects at risk shall be made to an individual unless he is affiliated with or sponsored by an institution which can and does assume responsibility for the subjects involved.

§46.103 Definitions

(a) "Institution" means any public or private institution or agency (including Federal, State, and local government agencies).

(b) "Subject at risk" means any individual who may be exposed to the possibility of injury, including physical, psychological, or social injury, as a consequence of participation as a subject in any research, development, or related activity which departs from the application of those established and accepted methods necessary to meet his needs, or which increases the ordinary risks of daily life, including the recognized risks inherent in a chosen occupation or field of service.

(c) "Informed consent" means the knowing consent of an individual or his legally authorized representative, so situated as to be able to exercise free power of choice without undue inducement or any element of force, fraud, deceit, duress, or other form of constraint or coercion. The basic elements of information necessary to such consent include:

1 A fair explanation of the procedures to be followed, and their purposes, including identification of any procedures which are experimental;

2 A description of any attendant discomforts and risks reasonably to be expected;

3 A description of any benefits reasonably to be expected;

4 A disclosure of any appropriate alternative procedures that might be advantageous for the subject;

5 An offer to answer any inquiries concerning the procedures; and

6 An instruction that the person is free to withdraw his consent and to discontinue participation in the project or activity at any time without prejudice to the subject . . .

INDEX